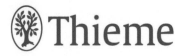

Neuromuscular Spine Deformity

Amer F. Samdani, MD
Chief of Surgery
Shriners Hospitals for Children-Philadelphia
Philadelphia, Pennsylvania

Peter O. Newton, MD
Professor, Department of Orthopedic Surgery
UC San Diego School of Medicine
Chief, Division of Orthopedics & Scoliosis
Rady Children's Hospital-San Diego
San Diego, California

Paul D. Sponseller, MD
Sponseller Professor and Head of Pediatric Orthopaedic Surgery
Johns Hopkins Medical Institutions
Baltimore, Maryland

Harry L. Shufflebarger, MD
Director
Division of Spinal Surgery
Nicklaus Children's Hospital
Miami, Florida

Randal R. Betz, MD
Pediatric Scoliosis and Spine Surgeon
Institute for Spine & Scoliosis
Lawrenceville, New Jersey

264 illustrations

Thieme
New York • Stuttgart • Delhi • Rio de Janeiro

Executive Editor: William Lamsback
Managing Editor: Sarah Landis
Editorial Assistant: Nikole Connors
Director, Editorial Services: Mary Jo Casey
Production Editor: Sean Woznicki
International Production Director: Andreas Schabert
Editorial Director: Sue Hodgson
International Marketing Director: Fiona Henderson
International Sales Director: Louisa Turrell
Director of Institutional Sales: Adam Bernacki
Senior Vice President and Chief Operating Officer: Sarah Vanderbilt
President: Brian D. Scanlan

Library of Congress Cataloging-in-Publication Data

Names: Samdani, Amer F., editor. | Newton, Peter O., editor. |
    Sponseller, Paul D., editor. | Shufflebarger, Harry L., editor. | Betz,
    Randal R., editor.
Title: Neuromuscular spine deformity / [edited by] Amer F.
    Samdani, Peter O. Newton, Paul D. Sponseller,
    Harry L. Shufflebarger, Randal R. Betz.
Description: New York : Thieme, [2018] | Includes bibliographical
    references.
Identifiers: LCCN 2017058030| ISBN 9781626232600 (print) |
    ISBN 9781626232617 (eISBN)
Subjects: | MESH: Spinal Curvatures–surgery | Neuromuscular
    Diseases–complications | Orthopedic Procedures–methods |
    Perioperative Care | Child
Classification: LCC RD771.S3 | NLM WE 735 | DDC 617.5/6059–dc23
    LC record available at https://lccn.loc.gov/2017058030

Thieme Publishers New York
333 Seventh Avenue, New York, NY 10001 USA
+1 800 782 3488, customerservice@thieme.com

Thieme Publishers Stuttgart
Rüdigerstrasse 14, 70469 Stuttgart, Germany
+49 [0]711 8931 421, customerservice@thieme.de

Thieme Publishers Delhi
A-12, Second Floor, Sector-2, Noida-201301
Uttar Pradesh, India
+91 120 45 566 00, customerservice@thieme.in

Thieme Publishers Rio de Janeiro, Thieme Publicações Ltda.
Edifício Rodolpho de Paoli, 25º andar
Av. Nilo Peçanha, 50 – Sala 2508
Rio de Janeiro 20020-906C Brasil
+55 21 3172-2297 / +55 21 3172-1896

Cover design: Thieme Publishing Group
Typesetting by DiTech Process Solutions

Printed in the United States by King Printing   5 4 3 2 1

ISBN 978-1-62623-260-0

Also available as an e-book:
eISBN 978-1-62623-261-7

Important note: Medicine is an ever-changing science undergoing continual development. Research and clinical experience are continually expanding our knowledge, in particular our knowledge of proper treatment and drug therapy. Insofar as this book mentions any dosage or application, readers may rest assured that the authors, editors, and publishers have made every effort to ensure that such references are in accordance with **the state of knowledge at the time of production of the book.**

Nevertheless, this does not involve, imply, or express any guarantee or responsibility on the part of the publishers in respect to any dosage instructions and forms of applications stated in the book. **Every user is requested to examine carefully** the manufacturers' leaflets accompanying each drug and to check, if necessary in consultation with a physician or specialist, whether the dosage schedules mentioned therein or the contraindications stated by the manufacturers differ from the statements made in the present book. Such examination is particularly important with drugs that are either rarely used or have been newly released on the market. Every dosage schedule or every form of application used is entirely at the user's own risk and responsibility. The authors and publishers request every user to report to the publishers any discrepancies or inaccuracies noticed. If errors in this work are found after publication, errata will be posted at www.thieme.com on the product description page.

Some of the product names, patents, and registered designs referred to in this book are in fact registered trademarks or proprietary names even though specific reference to this fact is not always made in the text. Therefore, the appearance of a name without designation as proprietary is not to be construed as a representation by the publisher that it is in the public domain.

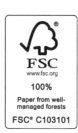

FSC
www.fsc.org
100%
Paper from well-managed forests
FSC® C103101

This book would not have been possible without the support of my wife and best friend, Besma, and many thanks to our children, Umar, Hiba, Zara, and Aman, for their understanding of their dad's work schedule.

—Amer F. Samdani, MD

In hopes of changing their lives for the better, we dedicate this book to the patients with neuromuscular scoliosis, their families and the future generations of patients stricken by spinal deformity.

—Peter O. Newton, MD

I would like to dedicate the work to my family, Amy, Matt, and Nina Sponseller, and to my wonderful colleagues in the Harms Study Group.

—Paul D. Sponseller, MD

To patients with neuromuscular spinal deformity: those of the past from whom what we have learned constitutes the material of this book; and those of the future who will benefit from this book and from whom we will continue to learn.

—Harry L. Shufflebarger MD

To the children who live with neuromuscular conditions and for their strength of spirit, which is such an inspiration to their physicians and surgeons.

—Randal R. Betz, MD

Contents

Foreword ix

Preface x

Acknowledgments xii

Contributors xiii

I. Surgical and Medical Considerations

1. **Preoperative Evaluation and Optimization** 2
    Michael P. Kelly and Scott J. Luhmann

2. **Nonoperative Management** 7
    Stefan Parent

3. **Surgical Indications in Neuromuscular Scoliosis** 11
    Cheryl R. Lawing, Michael P. Kelly, and Paul D. Sponseller

4. **Intraoperative Issues: Anesthesia, Neuromonitoring, Estimated Blood Loss** 20
    Paul D. Kiely, Akhil A. Tawari, Jahangir K. Asghar, and Harry L. Shufflebarger

5. **Unique Challenges with Scoliosis and Dislocated Hips** 25
    Firoz Miyanji and Randal R. Betz

6. **Predicting Complications: When to Operate or Not** 30
    Mark F. Abel and Anuj Singla

II. Diagnosis Specific

7. **Scoliosis in Cerebral Palsy** 40
    Paul D. Sponseller and Stuart L. Mitchell

8. **Surgical Treatment of Spinal Deformity in Myelomeningocele** 49
    Peter G. Gabos

9. **The Patient with Spinal Cord Injury: Surgical Considerations** 59
    Joshua M. Pahys, Amer F. Samdani, and Randal R. Betz

10. **The Spine in Duchenne Muscular Dystrophy** 66
     Benjamin Alman

11. **Spinal Muscular Atrophy** 71
     Benjamin D. Roye and Michael G. Vitale

12. **Other Neuromuscular Conditions: Rett Syndrome, Charcot–Marie–Tooth Disease, and Friedreich's Ataxia** 78
     Keith R. Bachman and Vidyadhar V. Upasani

Contents

13. **Neurosurgical Causes of Scoliosis** 88
Marie Roguski, Steven W. Hwang, and Amer F. Samdani

14. **Sagittal Plane Spinal Deformity in Patients with Neuromuscular Disease** 95
Kirk W. Dabney

15. **Spinal Deformity Associated with Neurodegenerative Disease in Adults** 104
Dana L. Cruz, Shaleen Vira, Virginie Lafage, Themistocles Protopsaltis, and Thomas J. Errico

III. **Surgical Techniques**

16. **Sacropelvic Fixation Techniques** 114
Suken A. Shah

17. **Comparison of Unit Rods with Modular Constructs in Cerebral Palsy** 122
Mark Shasti and Paul D. Sponseller

18. **Halo-Gravity Traction: An Adjunctive Treatment for Severe Spinal Deformity** 126
Joshua M. Pahys and Amer F. Samdani

19. **Osteotomies: Ponte and Vertebral Column Resection** 132
Scott C. Wagner, Ronald A. Lehman Jr., and Lawrence G. Lenke

20. **Growing Spine Options for Neuromuscular Scoliosis** 136
Joshua S. Murphy and Burt Yaszay

21. **Anterior Approaches to the Spine for Neuromuscular Spinal Deformity** 143
Peter O. Newton

IV. **Postoperative Management and Complications**

22. **Incidence of Major Complications in Surgery for Neuromuscular Spine Deformity** 150
Andrew H. Milby and Patrick J. Cahill

23. **Management of Early and Late Infection** 155
Mark Shasti, Paul D. Sponseller, and Stefan Parent

24. **Postoperative Intensive Care Unit Management** 161
Sandeep Khanna and Kathleen Gorenc

25. **Reoperations: Instrumentation Failure, Junctional Kyphosis, and Cervical Extension** 167
Vidyadhar V. Upasani, Corey B. Fuller, and Munish Gupta

26. **Health-Related Quality of Life in Neuromuscular Scoliosis** 173
James H. Stephen, Eve Hoffman, Unni G. Narayanan, Paul D. Sponseller, and Amer F. Samdani

27. **Baclofen Pump: Preoperative, Intraoperative, and Postoperative Management** 179
Brian P. Scannell and Burt Yaszay

Index 184

Foreword

Managing neuromuscular spinal deformities is an awesome responsibility. These patients present with the most challenging pathologies of the deformed spine. For too long we've had to depend on the limited resource recommendations of those who've treated these children as our source of surgical strategies. Limited individual surgeon experience driven resources include a lot of less than satisfactory results with the patients paying a tremendous price to educate the surgical teams. Finally with this book we have under one cover a tome on management of neuromuscular spinal deformities not only in children but also in adults. It's a multi-authored book that draws on the strength of two concepts not previously espoused together: disease-specific intervention strategies and multidisciplinary teaming. These experienced authors have enjoyed a tremendous time-line rapport communicating directly with each other over the years regarding the entire range of spinal deformities and have now decided to publish this book. It has been developed as a result of their research on prospective and retrospective clinical trials and publications, providing evidence-based measures of success.

The Harms Study Group has been quite active mostly in research of the adolescent spine, concentrating on correcting and stabilizing idiopathic deformities. The team approach to managing the perioperative complexities of neuromuscular spinal deformities had not been thoroughly validated. This group's investigation in managing neuromuscular spinal deformities has coincided with increased molecular genetic delineation of specific neurodevelopmental disorders. This collateral research specifically into atrophies and dystrophies in patients with neuropathic disorders has improved life expectancy and quality of life enough to justify the risk of spine surgery. The teams alluded to in this text are virtual and include Neuroscience (neurorehabilitation and spinal cord monitoring), Spine (orthopaedic surgeon or neurosurgeon as the prime mover in this endeavor), Surgery (Urology, VATS access, Plastics), Anesthesia, Critical Care, Rehabilitation (Orthotic, Physical/Occupational Therapy), GI, Radiology, Infectious Disease, and Family Support (skilled nursing, research coordinators and case managers). These virtual teams developed seamlessly from the Harms Study Group "Prospective Database Registry Study of Scoliosis in Children with Cerebral Palsy" and patient education handbook "Navigating Your Journey: Guide for You and Your Family." The virtual team is omnipresent, and various elements weave in and out of the fabric when necessary to manage these patients.

Also found in this book are various strategies to assess patient health factors, modification of mobility aids, and nonoperative management. Attention is given to disease-specific presurgical planning, consenting (including indications-contraindications), hematologic, and gastroenteric/nutritional assessments. They carefully identify specific pulmonary issues, urinary imaging, and consenting issues regarding when to consider avoiding surgery. Every section contains detailed approaches and discussions of risks, benefits, expectations with family regarding the post-surgical course, and critical care of static and progressive congenital and syndromic disorders including spinal deformity associated with neurodegenerative disease in adults.

The book further identifies practical tips of OR table positioning, specific benefits of traction, preoperative and intraoperative issues, anterior releases (anterior thoracolumbar, TLIF, video-assisted thoracoscopy and VCR), as well as anatomic specific implants for EOS conditions (VEPTR, growth modulating, lumbopelvic stabilizing, etc.), identifying advantages and disadvantages of each.

Having this comprehensive information in one source is powerful. Some surgical techniques rarely seen in Pediatric Spine texts such as TLIF are beneficial in avoiding the morbidity of anterior releases. Also discussed is Health Related Quality of Life, a very necessary component of this team endeavor as we enter an uncertain and potentially challenging time in healthcare compensation.

Finally, the scientific curiosity of the Harms Study Group has resulted in publication of an abundance of peer reviewed, innovative articles on spinal biomechanics, techniques, and instrumentation resulting in best practices. Its members continue to advance in leadership positions of our academic and scientific societies. This sentinel book documents the need to align with all disciplines involved in managing correction of these oftentimes severe and complex neuromuscular conditions in order to achieve best outcomes. I've been fortunate to participate in and observe the development of this group of master surgeons and feel especially proud of their work. This book will become a reference in the library of spine surgeons who have the awesome responsibility of managing patents with neuromuscular spinal deformities.

Alvin H. Crawford, MD, FACS, Hon Caus. GR.
Past President, Scoliosis Research Society
Founding Director, Crawford Spine Center
Professor Emeritus, Pediatrics and Spine
University of Cincinnati College of Medicine

Preface

Neuromuscular scoliosis is a very common condition, but it presents the pediatric spine surgeon with many treatment challenges. The patient population is diverse, and the deformities can be complex. Most surgeons have developed their surgical treatment plans and intraoperative techniques through experience. While many different treatments work in a given surgeon's hands, there is currently no one resource to which a younger, inexperienced surgeon or an experienced surgeon presented with a challenging deformity can go to gain knowledge from the vast experience of experts in the field.

The purpose of this book is to present some of the experiences of master surgeons, including key aspects of their surgical technique, ways to avoid problems, and advice on dealing with complications. In addition, the authors will provide evidence-based knowledge from both the literature and from the studies performed by the Harms Study Group. The authors assume that the reader has a basic knowledge of neuromuscular disease and some experience treating paralytic spine deformities using basic instrumentation.

Section I: Surgical and Medical Considerations deals with nonoperative management and indications for surgery. Preoperative planning and intraoperative issues including anesthesia and neuromonitoring are addressed in this section. The management of subluxed or dislocated hips, which may be very familiar to the pediatric orthopaedist but not to a spine-fellowship trained surgeon, are discussed. The presence of subluxed or dislocated hips in the patient with neuromuscular scoliosis presents particular challenges. The majority of neuromuscular disorders that include subluxed or dislocated hips usually fall into one of three diagnoses, which include 1) spinal cord injury; 2) myelomeningocele; and 3) cerebral palsy. However, the highest prevalence of dislocation is probably caused by sepsis, and it is essential that any relatively acute, radiographically identified dislocated hip have an aspiration and adequate work-up to rule out sepsis. Generally, for the noninfected case, the spine deformity is treated first followed by the hip because of the high incidence of deep vein thrombosis if the hip surgery were to be performed first. Perioperative medical management, both for prevention of deep vein thrombosis and heterotopic ossification about the hip following surgery, presents additional challenges for the spine surgeon. The final chapter in this section concerns predicting complications and trying to assess the risk vs. benefit in recommending surgery to the parents of a child with severe deformity.

Section II: Disease Specific highlights the key components of the surgeons' techniques in treating neuromuscular scoliosis arising from different diagnoses. One can no longer use the same surgical strategy and execution of surgery for all patients with scoliosis of neuromuscular origins. The age at intervention maybe very different, requiring a growing spine (for example, Chapter 11: Spinal Muscular Atrophy). Sagittal profile can be very different in these patients and must be considered. Spinal deformity secondary to cerebral palsy presents unique issues especially with regards to a hyperlordotic (Chapter 7) or hyperkyphotic spine (Chapter 14). The authors of these two chapters will present some of their correction techniques and discuss how they capitalize on some of the technical advances such as reduction pedicle screws for hyperlordosis. One recommendation for a thoracic kyphosis would be to start placing the rods proximally first instead of in the pelvis.

In Chapter 8 ("Surgical Treatment of Spinal Deformity in Myelomeningocele"), Dr. Gabos will discuss three major things that have changed his practice and resulted in significant improvements for patients with myelodysplasia and spine deformity: 1) He includes posterior lumbar interbody fusions (PLIFs) where there are no lamina; 2) he uses S2 screws (S2AI screw fixation) to provide a low profile but solid fixation to the pelvis; and 3) he enlists the help of plastic surgeons to complete the closure to help reduce the high infection rate.

In Chapter 9 ("The Patient with Spinal Cord Injury: Surgical Considerations"), Drs. Pahys, Samdani and Betz will describe treatment of patients with spinal cord injury and matters to consider during preoperative planning. For example, many of these patients use compensatory spinal motion to assist with raising their hand to their mouth/face for feeding/grooming. Placing them in a standard, prefixed sagittal profile (unit rod) may eradicate this compensatory motion and render these patients completely dependent, whereas they were independent with feeding/grooming prior to the spinal fusion. These patients may need a different sagittal profile emulating their normal sitting posture in a wheelchair which requires a reduced lumbar lordosis and enhanced thoracolumbar kyphosis. The authors will also describe how to assess the sagittal profile preoperatively and execute it intraoperatively.

As noted in *Section III: Surgical Techniques*, a key component of correction of neuromuscular scoliosis is that the instrumentation in the majority of cases extends down into the sacrum and the ileum. In Chapter 16 ("Sacropelvic Fixation Techniques"), Dr. Shah will present multiple options for fixation including the new sacral ala iliac screw approach to reduce profile issues. Some surgeons are now using halofemoral traction as described in Chapter 18 to correct some of the pelvic obliquity before a surgical incision is made. The surgeon should keep in mind that the use of halofemoral traction may be counterproductive in cases of hyperlordosis because the hips must be kept flexed to correct the hyperlordosis, and pulling with femoral traction is also counterproductive.

Finally, *Section IV: Postoperative Management and Complications* covers postoperative management and the complications that can occur in patients with neuromuscular scoliosis. The most common and more devastating for the patient is wound infection, and Drs. Milby and Cahill discuss suggestions for prevention and treatment based on evidence from the literature. This section also includes some prospectively collected health-related quality of life outcomes in children with cerebral palsy and scoliosis surgery (Chapter 26) generated over the last 5 years by the Harms Study Group.

The authors are very appreciative of the opportunity to collectively incorporate our experience into this book. We also thank Carolyn Hendrix and Sarah Landis for their editorial assistance with this project.

Amer F. Samdani, MD
Randal R. Betz, MD

Acknowledgments

A project of this magnitude cannot be completed without the tireless work of numerous people, including our esteemed editors, section editors, and chapter authors. In addition, the editors would like to thank Sarah Landis and Nikole Connors at Thieme Medical Publishers for their unwavering support and belief in us as we worked on this project. We also wish to thank Michelle Marks, Executive/ Research Director of the Setting Scoliosis Straight Foundation, and her staff for managing all of the research data and projects associated with the Harms Study Group. Finally, we would like to thank Carolyn Hendrix, Academic Assistant at Shriners Hospitals-Philadelphia, for her indispensable organizational and editorial skills.

Contributors

Mark F. Abel, MD
Charles Frankel Professor of Orthopaedic Surgery
Division Head Pediatric Orthopaedics
Department of Orthopaedics
University of Virginia Health System
Charlottesville, Virginia

Benjamin Alman, MD
James R. Urbaniak, MD, Professor of Orthopaedic Surgery
Chair, Department of Orthopaedic Surgery
Duke University School of Medicine
Durham, North Carolina

Jahangir K. Asghar, MD
Orthopaedic Spine Surgeon
Miami, Florida

Keith R. Bachmann, MD
Assistant Professor of Orthopaedic Surgery
Department of Orthopaedic Surgery
University of Virginia Health System
Charlottesville, Virginia

Randal R. Betz, MD
Pediatric Scoliosis and Spine Surgeon
Institute for Spine & Scoliosis
Lawrenceville, New Jersey

Patrick J. Cahill, MD
Associate Professor
The Perelman School of Medicine at The University of
  Pennsylvania
Division of Orthopaedic Surgery
The Children's Hospital of Philadelphia
Philadelphia, Pennsylvania

Dana L. Cruz, MD
Resident Physician
Temple Orthopaedics & Sports Medicine
Philadelphia, Pennsylvania

Kirk W. Dabney, MD, MHCD
Department of Orthopedics
Co-Director, Cerebral Palsy Program
Nemours Children's Health System
Wilmington, Delaware

Thomas J. Errico, MD
Chief, Division of Spine Surgery
NYU Langone Medical Center
New York, New York

Corey B. Fuller, MD
Orthopaedic Spine Surgeon
Department of Orthopaedic Surgery
Loma Linda University Medical Center
Loma Linda, California

Peter G. Gabos, MD
Assistant Professor
Department of Orthopaedic Surgery
Thomas Jefferson University Hospital/Jefferson Medical
  College
Philadelphia, PA
Co-Director
Spine and Scoliosis Center
Nemours/Alfred I. duPont Hospital for Children
Wilmington, Delaware

Kathleen Gorenc, CPNP-AC
Pediatric Intensive Care Unit
Rady Children's Hospital
San Diego, California

Munish Gupta, MD
Mildred B. Simon Distinguished Professor of Orthopaedic
  Surgery
Professor of Neurological Surgery
Chief of Pediatric and Adult Spinal Surgery
Co-director of Pediatric and Adult Spinal Deformity Service
Washington University
St. Louis, Missouri

Eve Hoffman, MD
Resident Physician
Department of Orthopaedics
University of Maryland Medical Center
Baltimore, Maryland

Steven W. Hwang, MD
Neurosurgeon
Shriners Hospitals for Children-Philadelphia
Philadelphia, Pennsylvania

Michael P. Kelly, MD, MSc
Assistant Professor
Department of Orthopaedic Surgery
Washington University
St. Louis, Missouri

Sandeep Khanna, MD
Clinical Director
Division of Pediatric Critical Care Medicine
Clinical Assistant Professor
Department of Anesthesia
University of California San Diego
San Diego, California

Paul D. Kiely, MCh, FRCS
Center for Spinal Disorders
Nicklaus Children's Hospital
Miami, Florida

Virginie Lafage, PhD
Director, Spine Research
Hospital for Special Surgery
New York, New York

Cheryl R. Lawing, MD
Pediatric Orthopaedic Surgery
Shriners Hospitals for Children-Tampa
Tampa, Florida

Ronald A. Lehman Jr., MD
Professor of Orthopaedic Surgery, Tenure
Chief, Degenerative, MIS and Robotic Spine Surgery
Director, Athletes Spine Center
Director, Spine Research
Co-Director, Adult and Pediatric Spine Fellowship
Advanced Pediatric and Adult Deformity Service
The Spine Hospital
New York-Presbyterian/The Allen Hospital
New York, New York

Lawrence G. Lenke, MD
Professor of Orthopedic Surgery
Columbia University Medical Center
Surgeon-in-Chief
The Spine Hospital at New York-Presbyterian/Allen
Chief, Spine Division
Co-Director, Adult and Pediatric Comprehensive Spine
   Fellowship
New York, New York

Scott J. Luhmann, MD
Professor, Pediatric Orthopaedic Surgery
Washington University
Head of Surgery, Pediatric Orthopaedics
Shriners Hospitals for Children-St. Louis
St. Louis, Missouri

Andrew H. Milby, MD
Assistant Professor
Department of Orthopaedic Surgery
University of Pennsylvania
Philadelphia, Pennsylvania

Stuart L. Mitchell, MD
Resident Physician
Department of Orthopaedic Surgery
Johns Hopkins University
Baltimore, Maryland

Firoz Miyanji, MD, FRCSC
Clinical Associate Professor
UBC Faculty of Medicine, Department of Orthopedics, Pediatric Orthopedics, and Spine Surgery British Columbia
   Children's Hospital,
Vancouver, British Columbia, Canada

Joshua S. Murphy, MD
Orthopaedic Surgeon
Children's Orthopaedics of Atlanta
Atlanta, Georgia

Unni G. Narayanan, MBBS, MSc, FRCS(C)
Associate Professor, Department of Surgery
Division of Orthopaedic Surgery
Senior Associate Scientist
Child Health Evaluative Sciences Program
Director, Paediatric Orthopaedic Fellowship Program
The Hospital for Sick Children
University of Toronto
Adjunct Senior Scientist
Bloorview Research Institute
Holland Bloorview Kids Rehabilitation Hospital
Toronto, Ontario, Canada

Peter O. Newton, MD
Professor, Department of Orthopedic Surgery
UC San Diego School of Medicine
Chief, Division of Orthopedics & Scoliosis
Rady Children's Hospital- San Diego
San Diego, California

Joshua M. Pahys, MD
Orthopaedic Surgeon
Shriners Hospitals for Children-Philadelphia
Philadelphia, Pennsylvania

Stefan Parent, MD, PhD
Associate Professor
Department of Surgery
Faculty of Medicine
University of Montreal
Chief, Paediatric Orthopaedic Surgery
CHU Ste-Justine
Montreal, Quebec, Canada

Themistocles Protopsaltis, MD
Associate Professor of Orthopaedic Surgery and
    Neurosurgery
Department of Orthopaedic Surgery
NYU Langone Medical Center
New York, New York

Marie Roguski, MD, MPH
Chief Resident
Department of Neurosurgery
Tufts Medical Center
Boston, Massachusetts

Benjamin D. Roye, MD, MPH
Assistant Professor
Department of Orthopaedic Surgery
Columbia University Medical Center
Attending Physician
New York-Presbyterian Hospital
New York, New York

Amer F. Samdani, MD
Chief of Surgery
Shriners Hospitals for Children-Philadelphia
Philadelphia, Pennsylvania

Brian P. Scannell, MD
Associate Professor of Orthopaedic Surgery
Levine Children's Hospital
Carolinas Healthcare System
Charlotte, North Carolina

Suken A. Shah, MD
Division Chief, Spine and Scoliosis Center
Clinical Fellowship Director
Department of Orthopaedic Surgery
Nemours/Alfred I. duPont Hospital for Children
Wilmington, Delaware
Associate Professor of Orthopaedic Surgery and Pediatrics
Sidney Kimmel Medical College of Thomas Jefferson
    University
Philadelphia, Pennsylvania

Mark Shasti, MD
Resident Physician
Department of Orthopaedic Surgery
University of Maryland Medical Center
Baltimore, Maryland

Harry L. Shufflebarger, MD
Director
Division of Spinal Surgery
Nicklaus Children's Hospital
Miami, Florida

Anuj Singla, MD
Instructor, Spine Surgery
Department of Orthopaedics
University of Virginia Health System
Charlottesville, Virginia

Paul D. Sponseller, MD, MBA
Sponseller Professor and Head, Pediatric Orthopaedic
    Surgery
Johns Hopkins Medical Institutions
Baltimore, Maryland

James H. Stephen, MD
Resident Physician
Department of Neurosurgery
Hospital of the University of Pennsylvania
Philadelphia, Pennsylvania

Akhil Tawari, MD
Orthopaedic Spine Fellow
Nicklaus Children's Hospital
Miami, Florida

Vidyadhar V. Upasani, MD
Orthopaedic Surgeon
Rady Children's Hospital- San Diego
San Diego, California

Shaleen Vira, MD
Resident Physician
Department of Orthopaedic Surgery
NYU Langone Medical Center
New York, New York

Michael G. Vitale, MD, MPH
Ana Lucia Professor of Pediatric Orthopedic Surgery
Chief, Pediatric Spine and Scoliosis Surgery
Co-Director, Division of Pediatric Orthopedics
Chief Quality Officer, Department of Orthopedic Surgery
Columbia University Medical Center
New York, New York

Scott C. Wagner, MD
Orthopaedic Surgeon
Walter Reed National Military Medical Center
Bethesda, Maryland

Burt Yaszay, MD
Pediatric Orthopaedic Surgeon
Rady Children's Hospital-San Diego
Associate Clinical Professor
University of California, San Diego
San Diego, California

Part I

Surgical and Medical Considerations

1 Preoperative Evaluation and
   Optimization   2

2 Nonoperative Management   7

3 Surgical Indications in Neuromuscular
   Scoliosis   11

4 Intraoperative Issues: Anesthesia,
   Neuromonitoring, Estimated Blood Loss   20

5 Unique Challenges with Scoliosis and
   Dislocated Hips   25

6 Predicting Complications: When to
   Operate or Not   30

1 Preoperative Evaluation and Optimization

Michael P. Kelly and Scott J. Luhmann

Abstract

Pediatric neuromuscular spinal deformity surgeries are complex due to the multisystem involvement of the diseases commonly encountered. Complication rates may exceed 25%, in a stark contrast to adolescent idiopathic scoliosis. A multidisciplinary approach is mandatory to minimize the risk of complication. Furthermore, the perioperative team should be well versed in the care of these complex patients. Malnutrition is not uncommon and nutrition should be optimized before surgery, as these are generally elective and not performed on an emergent basis. Some comorbidities are "fixed" and not modifiable, such as cardiomyopathy or seizure disorders. Thus, knowledge of perioperative management of these comorbid conditions is required to avoid potentially common pitfalls. The physical examination helps define patient needs and assists with surgical planning, including patient positioning, which may not be overlooked. The radiographic evaluation helps indicate surgery and define the fusion levels through an examination of curve rigidity. Magnetic resonance imaging is sometimes needed to ensure there is no intraspinal pathology. Computed tomography scanning helps identify landmarks for fixation and reveals areas of dorsal bone deficiency, such as spina bifida or prior surgeries. Finally, anticipation of postoperative needs must occur at the preoperative visit so that families and caretakers are prepared at the time of discharge.

Keywords: cardiomyopathy, indications, neuromuscular scoliosis, perioperative care, preoperative plan, pulmonary, radiographic evaluation

1.1 Introduction

Pediatric neuromuscular spinal deformity patients are among the most challenging faced due to the number of comorbid conditions that often exist, potentially affecting the intraoperative and postoperative course and outcomes.[1] Complication rates approach 25%, and these patients are more prone to perioperative complications, especially infection, than adolescent idiopathic scoliosis patients.[2,3,4,5] Careful preoperative evaluation and optimization will help minimize complications related to neuromuscular spinal surgery. Additionally, input from other specialists can be important contributions to risk stratification, surgical planning and decision making, and, ultimately, informed consent.

Neuromuscular scoliosis is a heterogeneous disease with a wide array of causes, each requiring different preoperative evaluations. Neuromuscular disease can present anywhere along the spectrum from high muscular tone (spastic) to low muscular tone (flaccid). In addition, there are varying levels of cognition. Cerebral palsy (CP) is a heterogeneous diagnosis itself, again requiring an understanding of the underlying disease state to allow for appropriate preoperative optimization. In the authors' experience, a formulaic approach to the preoperative evaluation for all neuromuscular patients, with a standard checklist applied to all patients regardless of diagnosis, is

helpful. A thorough standardized checklist will help minimize missed data, which may, in turn, improve outcomes in this complicated population.

Several groups treating adult spinal deformity have shown that preoperative, multidisciplinary conferences and standardized care protocols are able to reduce complications and improve outcomes.[6,7,8] At the foundation of these care pathways are evidence-based reviews of the literature. A multidisciplinary team consisting of neurological and orthopaedic spine surgeons, anesthesiologists, intensivists, internists, and internists, use the review to develop preoperative, intraoperative, and postoperative care protocols.[6,7] The institution of a preoperative multidisciplinary conference has been shown to reduce postoperative complications and 30-day readmissions.[6] Zeeni et al have shown that an intraoperative care protocol reduced operative time and the need for allogenic blood transfusion.[8] The "team" approach to care was emphasized, with protocol violations rarely reported (2.6%). While no published evidence exists, yet, for this approach in neuromuscular spinal deformity, it stands to reason that this is an approach that centers should consider. At a minimum, "virtual" conferences can be held via electronic mail, where the concerns of all may be addressed and the patients optimized for these complex surgeries.

1.2 History and Review of Systems

All preoperative evaluations begin with a comprehensive medical history and review of systems. Polypharmacy is common in neuromuscular scoliosis, and all medications, with dosages, must be recorded. Of particular importance are cardiac medications, such as B-blockers and calcium channel blockers. In addition to providing the impetus for a cardiology consultation, these medications should be discussed with the anesthesia team to ensure proper perioperative administration. Cessation of some antihypertensives is associated with rebound hypertension, which can be dangerous and cause delays with surgery. In some cases of muscular dystrophy, cardiac arrhythmias may be present and prophylactic anticoagulation may be required. Appropriate risk stratification of anticoagulation cessation versus a bridge to shorter acting agents, such as enoxaparin, will require multidisciplinary input. Postoperative anticoagulation plans should be made before surgery.

1.2.1 Cardiopulmonary System

The cardiopulmonary system review must be exhaustive. Respiratory disease, and thus pulmonary complications, is common in neuromuscular spinal.[4] A comprehensive history will include details regarding any prior history of sleep apnea and prior sleep studies. The surgeon must also know whether the patient has a history of pneumonia, asthma, prior aspiration events, and any history of prolonged intubation. Consultation of a pulmonologist is recommended for all children confined to a wheelchair with a vital capacity less than 80% of expected.[9] The benefit in engaging a pulmonologist goes beyond the preoperative workup of optimization. Additionally, the pulmonologist can familiarize themselves with the patients, their history, baseline conditions, and preoperative workup. This permits more rapid and appropriate postoperative pulmonary care. When possible, pulmonary function tests (PFTs), via spirometry, should be obtained. In some cases, these are not possible due to patient cognition or participation. Other methods of PFT include whole-body plethysmography, gas dilution, and diffusion capacity. These methods are more complicated than spirometry and their benefit in neuromuscular spinal has not been shown. At a minimum, when spirometry is not possible, oxyhemoglobin saturation should be assessed with pulse oximetry. The benefit of PFTs is that they allow for more accurate informed discussion with patients and caregivers, while also helping plan postoperative care. The need for prolonged ventilation, prolonged intensive care unit time, and, in some cases, tracheostomy should be anticipated prior to surgery.[10] While interventions to improve PFTs before surgery are unlikely to be successful, knowledge of current lung function is necessary to provide informed consent to the patient and caretakers, as there is an immediate decrement in lung function after scoliosis surgery.[11] Low PFTs (forced vital capacity < 30%) are not an absolute contraindication to surgery.[12,13] However, neuromuscular spinal patients with low PFTs may be more likely to sustain perioperative complications, such as pneumonia, prolonged ventilator times, and postoperative tracheostomy.[10,14] Noninvasive intermittent positive-pressure ventilation is useful in the postoperative period, after extubation, and may help avoid postoperative tracheostomy.[15,16]

The "difficult airway" should be identified before the operating room and induction of anesthesia. This includes patients with severe cervicothoracic deformities and small facies/airways. In these cases, preoperative evaluation should include the otolaryngology (ear, nose, and throat [ENT]) service for possible postoperative tracheostomy needs. Patients deemed to have "difficult airways" are marked as such in their chart and in their hospital rooms, with signs, notifying caretakers of this status and providing the emergency number to alert a code team, ENT, and a trauma attending in the case of airway compromise.

As noted, cardiovascular abnormalities are common in some muscular dystrophies but are entirely uncommon in other forms of neuromuscular spinal, such as CP and myelomeningocele.[17] Muscular dystrophies, such as Duchenne muscular dystrophy and Becker's muscular dystrophy are commonly associated with a cardiomyopathy. It is important to recognize this, as the cardiomyopathy may go unnoticed and can be a cause of mortality in these patients. Furthermore, the phenotype expressed by patients with muscular dystrophies varies and the cardiomyopathy may be worse than the exhibited skeletal muscle involvement. Beyond assisting with perioperative planning, early identification of the cardiomyopathy offers a chance for intervention with protective therapies. Historically, electrocardiogram (ECG) and echocardiography have been used to assess cardiac status. More recently, however, cardiac magnetic resonance imaging (MRI) has been shown effective in identifying cardiomyopathy before ECG or echocardiogram changes are present.[17]

Duchenne and Becker's Muscular Dystrophies

Identification of cardiomyopathy in these patients may be delayed due to the profound skeletal myopathy exhibited. In Duchenne muscular dystrophy (DMD), cardiomyopathy often begins at age 3 to 7 years, prior to a definitive spinal fusion surgery. All patients with DMD who survive to the third decade of life suffer from cardiomyopathy. Decreased cardiac output and arrhythmias are complications most commonly associated with DMD and Becker's muscular dystrophy (BMD). Recommended screening for cardiomyopathy currently consists of biannual ECG and echocardiograms in boys until age 10, then yearly thereafter; in girls, ECG and echocardiograms are recommended every 5 years after the age of 16. Evidence of cardiomyopathy has been found in girls without DMD and BMD, but with relatives suffering from these diseases, and a cardiac evaluation must be performed in these patients as well. Current evidence supports the use of angiotensin-converting enzyme (ACE) inhibitors or, in those patients intolerant of ACE inhibitors, angiotensin receptor blockers (ARB).

Congenital Muscular Dystrophy/Myotonic Dystrophy

This is a heterogeneous group of muscular diseases with varying degrees of associated cardiomyopathy. Myotonic dystrophy I (Steinert's disease) can be profoundly affected and is associated with sudden cardiac death. Atrial and ventricular arrhythmias occur. Screening consists of annual ECG and echocardiography, with biannual Holter monitor testing. Management can include pacemaker/defibrillator placement. Placement of pacemaker pads during surgery may be advisable.

1.3 Neurology

For patients with a history of seizures, knowing the history of seizure activity is necessary. This includes prior seizure episodes, most recent seizure, and current antiseizure medications, with most recent serum levels of the medication. In addition to optimizing seizure control, a neurologist can provide specific medication management strategies for bridging patients off of valproic acid, which may increase blood product requirements, during surgery.[18] In many cases, neuromuscular disease affects bowel and bladder function, and these habits are queried at the preoperative evaluation. Patients with neurogenic bladder, such as those with myelomeningocele, commonly have urine/bladders colonized with bacteria and may have indwelling catheters. Incontinent patients receive an occlusive dressing postoperatively, and postoperative dressing changes are with the same dressing to ensure an impervious seal over the wound and minimize the risk of contamination with stool and urine. If containment of urine is problematic, then an indwelling urinary catheter may be advisable until the surgical wound is epithelialized. If the patient has a history of hydrocephalus treated with a shunt, it must be determined by the neurosurgeon that it is functioning properly prior to spine surgery; this usually requires a computed tomography (CT) of the head. Acute intraoperative death has been reported from acute hydrocephalus expansion during spinal surgery secondary to a nonfunctioning shunt.[19]

In some cases, patients will have had prior spine surgeries such as baclofen pump placement or rhizotomy. If a pump has been placed, the entry site of the pump tubing into the spinal canal must be known to assist made with the surgical approach.

Furthermore, the course of the catheter must be known to minimize the risk of damaging the catheter during the approach. Finally, the contents of the pump must be known in addition to when it was last filled. Intrathecal baclofen achieves much higher effective doses than are possible by oral administration, and death from baclofen withdrawal has been reported with a damaged pump not identified. Some surgeons request that patients wean the baclofen pumps to "off" prior to surgery, though this is not possible in all cases. The symptoms of baclofen withdrawal include increased spasticity, fever, and hypertension.[20] Identification of baclofen withdrawal is mandatory to avoid death, and members of the perioperative care team must know the symptoms of baclofen withdrawal. Preoperatively it is important to have a surgeon who implants, and cares for, baclofen pumps in case there are problems or questions postoperatively. If there is suspicion of baclofen withdrawal postoperatively, it is important to identify early. A test dose of oral or intrathecal baclofen (one shot) can aid in the assessment. While recording the surgical history, it is useful to ask about prior perioperative complications that may have occurred, including malignant hyperthermia.[21] Duchenne muscular dystrophy and Becker's dystrophy have been associated with malignant hyperthermia-"like" conditions, including rhabdomyolysis and hyperkalemia due to succinylcholine administration, and this medication should be avoided in these patients.

A review of endocrine systems will include any history of diabetes mellitus or corticosteroid use, the latter being common and effective in DMD patients.[22] Chronic corticosteroid use and, more commonly, malnutrition put this patient population at risk for osteopenia or osteoporosis. We do not routinely check bone mineral density (BMD) via dual-energy X-ray absorptiometry, though CT scans have been used to estimate bone density by measuring Hounsfield units (HU) in the vertebral body.[23] Pharmacologic interventions for osteopenia/osteoporosis include anti-catabolic medications (e.g. bisphosphonates) and anabolic medications (e.g. teriparatide). Bisphosphonates have been shown effective in increasing BMD in pediatric patients with osteoporosis.[24] The mechanism of action of bisphosphonates may impede early bone healing and fusion mass maturation and, as such, these are avoided in the early postoperative period.[25] Teriparatide has not been studied in neuromuscular spinal fusions, although we commonly employ this in our adult patients as there is evidence to support a benefit in fusion mass formation.[26]

1.4 Hematologic

The most common hematologic abnormality seen in these patients is anemia of chronic disease, due to the many systemic insults associated with severe neuromuscular disease. This emphasizes the need for attention to preoperative nutritional intake, including iron supplementation as appropriate.[27] Pharmacologic interventions for preoperative anemia include administration of recombinant erythropoietin (EPO). While EPO is able to raise hemoglobin levels, there was no appreciable benefit to this in a series of neuromuscular spinal patients, and transfusion rates were similar to untreated patients. Vitale et al concluded that while effective, EPO is not a cost-effective intervention.[28] Preoperative planning for neuromuscular spinal surgery should include the use of an antifibrinolytic, such as tranexamic acid, as this has been shown effective in reducing blood loss in pediatric scoliosis surgeries.[29]

1.5 Physical Examination

The physical examination begins by assessing the cognitive status of the patient. The Gross Motor Function Classification System (GMFCS) is used in CP to describe the level of systemic involvement of disease.[30] Patients with more severe involvement are more likely to develop a progressive scoliosis.[31] Understanding the severity of disease burden is important for disease prognostication and to allow for informed consent from caretakers.

Head control and sitting position should be assessed. In many deformities, there is a pelvic obliquity associated with the scoliosis. The pelvic obliquity can cause decubitus ulcers and difficulty with positioning, particularly within a wheelchair when used. In cases of flaccid neuromuscular disease, kyphosis is often present and may cause difficulty with maintaining horizontal gaze. As the goal of surgery is a stabilized spine with a head centered over the pelvis, the surgeon must understand the upright position of the head relative to the pelvis.

A standard motor and sensory exam should follow, if the patient can cooperate. In some cases, rigid spasticity causes flexion contractures of the upper and/or lower extremities, making intraoperative patient positioning very difficult. Infrequently, muscle and tendon releases about the knee or hip may be necessary. The surgeon will have to manage these while positioning in the operating room, and this should be planned prior to arriving in the operating room. Reflexes should be checked, again as possible, including abdominal reflexes and investigation for pathologic reflexes such as sustained clonus, asymmetric clonus, and the plantar (Babinski) reflex. While these pathologic reflexes may be a result of the neuromuscular disease, some consideration to intraspinal pathology should be given in cases where the finding is not expected (e.g., a muscular dystrophy). The skin should be examined, again looking for stigmata of intraspinal pathology such as a deep dimple or hairy patch. The lumbar spine should be carefully examined in cases of myelomeningocele and correlated with the MRI or CT scan. The posterior approach to the lumbar spine in myelomeningocele cases can be complicated, and one must plan the exposure to reach the spine without causing an iatrogenic dural opening. In some cases, a paraspinal (Wiltse-like) approach is used when the spine becomes bifid, leaving the skin over the underlying dura. Not infrequently, children present having undergone prior intradural surgery. This may complicate intraoperative neuromonitoring data and a Stagnara wake-up test must be rehearsed, if possible, prior to surgery.

The soft tissues and scar should be examined to ensure that sufficient tissue remains to allow for wound closure. This is true also for revision procedures, particularly those complicated by deep wound infection. In cases where there is insufficient tissue for wound coverage, we will often obtain a consultation from the plastic surgery service for assistance with wound closure. In some extreme cases, we will place tissue expanders for several months before spine surgery to increase the amount of locally available tissue.

1.6 Imaging

The radiographic workup begins with upright (weightbearing) full-length posterior to anterior (PA) and lateral (LAT) spine radiographs. If available, and the patient is ambulatory, standing whole-body radiographs should be obtained. Supine radiographs, anterior to posterior (AP) and LAT, are obtained next. These are useful in evaluating the flexibility of the spinal deformity, as some passive correction with gravity removed is often obtained. Traction films, with assistants pulling gentle traction on the skull and both lower extremities, are also helpful to evaluate flexibility.[32] These are particularly useful in cases with pelvic obliquity. In many cases, we will plan for a distal femoral traction pin on the side of the higher ilium to assist with leveling the pelvis. Side-bending radiographs are also used to evaluate flexibility in compliant patients. A push-prone radiograph, applying three-point bending forces to the deformity, offers more insight into the flexibility of the deformity.

Weight-bearing, full-length radiographs can be obtained with specialized EOS radiography machines or by stitching films. For ambulatory patients, the standing film is essential to understand the contribution of leg-length inequality and pelvic obliquity to the overall coronal plane alignment. Similarly, full-length lateral radiographs allow for a comprehensive assessment of the pelvic parameters and the contours of the spine. For those patients unable to stand, a radiolucent chair has been described and weight-bearing radiographs will help surgeons understand the overall sitting balance.[33] Suspension radiographs have been shown to be reliable for assessment of curve flexibility in adolescent idiopathic scoliosis.[34] These suspension radiographs may be useful for evaluating neuromuscular deformity, in particular the degree of pelvic obliquity correction that may be obtained with intraoperative traction and posterior instrumentation.

To assess skeletal maturity, a separate AP image of the pelvis may be necessary to accurately evaluate the iliac apophyses.[35] Patients with significant kyphosis can additionally be assessed with a supine lateral hyperextension view while positioned on a dorsal bolster. This can help with determining the stiffness of the deformity and the need for additional osteotomies.

Higher level imaging such as CT or MRI is not routinely obtained. In any case with an abnormal neurological examination, we will obtain a full-spine MRI. The MRI should be scrutinized with the assistance of a musculoskeletal radiologist for syrinx, Arnold Chiari malformation, tethered cord, fatty filum, or other intraspinal pathologies. In the case of an intraspinal finding, we will obtain a neurosurgical consultation to evaluate for the necessity of intervention prior to the spinal deformity surgery. MRI is necessary in cases of myelomeningocele, as this will assist with safe exposure. Preoperative CT scans are useful in cases with dysplastic spinal elements, such as myelomeningocele and other congenital malformations. Fluoroscopy or a multitude of plain radiographs can offer more detail regarding pedicle size and vertebral body morphology, though our preference is a CT scan. A review of imaging will assist with surgical planning, including implant needs, as some cases may require a combination of hooks, screws, and clamps.

1.7 Postoperative Planning

Finally, one must plan for the postoperative recovery period. This begins with anticipated discharge disposition and needs at the time of discharge. Arranging for rehabilitation facilities, wheelchair modifications, or other unique postoperative needs in advance of surgery will prevent delays in discharge. A complete discussion of postoperative limitations and expectations must be discussed with the patient and family/caretakers. It is not uncommon that patients and families are surprised at the duration of the recovery period. Warning in advance will limit disappointment and frustration. A discussion of the risks of surgery in neuromuscular scoliosis, with attention to the frequency of complications, both minor and major, is absolutely necessary given their relative frequency. Again, this will help with a smooth recovery process as expectations will be set in advance and all involved will understand the difficult course. The engagement of medical subspecialists preoperatively, such as cardiology and pulmonary specialists, can assist in setting expectations and evaluating the risks/benefits of a reconstructive spine surgery

1.8 Conclusion

Neuromuscular spinal deformity surgery is among the most challenging pathologies in spine surgery. Often, the deformities are severe, requiring technical excellence when performing the procedure. The patients are equally complex, however, and a complete preoperative evaluation and plan is necessary to achieve the best outcome possible. Complications are common in the surgeries and all efforts must be made to optimize the patient for surgery. Medical comorbidities, particularly malnutrition, must be addressed as possible. In cases where the comorbidity is not modifiable, one must be prepared for any particular associated pitfalls related to it.

References

[1] Basques BA, Chung SH, Lukasiewicz AM, et al. Predicting short-term morbidity in patients undergoing posterior spinal fusion for neuromuscular scoliosis. Spine. 2015; 40(24):1910–1917

[2] Murphy NA, Firth S, Jorgensen T, Young PC. Spinal surgery in children with idiopathic and neuromuscular scoliosis. What's the difference? J Pediatr Orthop. 2006; 26(2):216–220

[3] Mackenzie WG, Matsumoto H, Williams BA, et al. Surgical site infection following spinal instrumentation for scoliosis: a multicenter analysis of rates, risk factors, and pathogens. J Bone Joint Surg Am. 2013; 95(9):800–806, S1–S2

[4] Sharma S, Wu C, Andersen T, Wang Y, Hansen ES, Bünger CE. Prevalence of complications in neuromuscular scoliosis surgery: a literature meta-analysis from the past 15 years. Eur Spine J. 2013; 22(6):1230–1249

[5] Duckworth AD, Mitchell MJ, Tsirikos AI. Incidence and risk factors for postoperative complications after scoliosis surgery in patients with Duchenne muscular dystrophy : a comparison with other neuromuscular conditions. Bone Joint J. 2014; 96-B(7):943–949

[6] Buchlak QD, Yanamadala V, Leveque JC, Sethi R. Complication avoidance with pre-operative screening: insights from the Seattle spine team. Curr Rev Musculoskelet Med. 2016; 9(3):316–326

[7] Halpin RJ, Sugrue PA, Gould RW, et al. Standardizing care for high-risk patients in spine surgery: the Northwestern high-risk spine protocol. Spine. 2010; 35(25):2232–2238

[8] Zeeni C, Carabini LM, Gould RW, et al. The implementation and efficacy of the Northwestern High Risk Spine Protocol. World Neurosurg. 2014; 82(6):e815–e823

[9] Finder JD, Birnkrant D, Carl J, et al. American Thoracic Society. Respiratory care of the patient with Duchenne muscular dystrophy: ATS consensus statement. Am J Respir Crit Care Med. 2004; 170(4):456–465

[10] Yuan N, Skaggs DL, Dorey F, Keens TG. Preoperative predictors of prolonged postoperative mechanical ventilation in children following scoliosis repair. Pediatr Pulmonol. 2005; 40(5):414–419

[11] Yuan N, Fraire JA, Margetis MM, Skaggs DL, Tolo VT, Keens TG. The effect of scoliosis surgery on lung function in the immediate postoperative period. Spine. 2005; 30(19):2182–2185

[12] Chong HS, Moon ES, Park JO, et al. Value of preoperative pulmonary function test in flaccid neuromuscular scoliosis surgery. Spine. 2011; 36(21):E1391–E1394

[13] Gill I, Eagle M, Mehta JS, Gibson MJ, Bushby K, Bullock R. Correction of neuromuscular scoliosis in patients with preexisting respiratory failure. Spine. 2006; 31(21):2478–2483

[14] Kang GR, Suh SW, Lee IO. Preoperative predictors of postoperative pulmonary complications in neuromuscular scoliosis. J Orthop Sci. 2011; 16(2):139–147

[15] Bach JR, Sabharwal S. High pulmonary risk scoliosis surgery: role of noninvasive ventilation and related techniques. J Spinal Disord Tech. 2005; 18(6):527–530

[16] Khirani S, Bersanini C, Aubertin G, Bachy M, Vialle R, Fauroux B. Non-invasive positive pressure ventilation to facilitate the post-operative respiratory outcome of spine surgery in neuromuscular children. Eur Spine J. 2014; 23 Suppl 4:S406–S411

[17] Verhaert D, Richards K, Rafael-Fortney JA, Raman SV. Cardiac involvement in patients with muscular dystrophies: magnetic resonance imaging phenotype and genotypic considerations. Circ Cardiovasc Imaging. 2011; 4(1):67–76

[18] Winter SL, Kriel RL, Novacheck TF, Luxenberg MG, Leutgeb VJ, Erickson PA. Perioperative blood loss: the effect of valproate. Pediatr Neurol. 1996; 15(1):19–22

[19] Winston K, Hall J, Johnson D, Micheli L. Acute elevation of intracranial pressure following transection of non-functional spinal cord. Clin Orthop Relat Res. 1977(128):41–44

[20] Coffey RJ, Edgar TS, Francisco GE, et al. Abrupt withdrawal from intrathecal baclofen: recognition and management of a potentially life-threatening syndrome. Arch Phys Med Rehabil. 2002; 83(6):735–741

[21] Gurnaney H, Brown A, Litman RS. Malignant hyperthermia and muscular dystrophies. Anesth Analg. 2009; 109(4):1043–1048

[22] Lebel DE, Corston JA, McAdam LC, Biggar WD, Alman BA. Glucocorticoid treatment for the prevention of scoliosis in children with Duchenne muscular dystrophy: long-term follow-up. J Bone Joint Surg Am. 2013; 95(12):1057–1061

[23] Schreiber JJ, Anderson PA, Rosas HG, Buchholz AL, Au AG. Hounsfield units for assessing bone mineral density and strength: a tool for osteoporosis management. J Bone Joint Surg Am. 2011; 93(11):1057–1063

[24] Ward L, Tricco AC, Phuong P, et al. Bisphosphonate therapy for children and adolescents with secondary osteoporosis. Cochrane Database Syst Rev. 2007 (4):CD005324

[25] Hirsch BP, Unnanuntana A, Cunningham ME, Lane JM. The effect of therapies for osteoporosis on spine fusion: a systematic review. Spine J. 2013; 13(2):190–199

[26] Lehman RA, Jr, Dmitriev AE, Cardoso MJ, et al. Effect of teriparatide [rhPTH (1,34)] and calcitonin on intertransverse process fusion in a rabbit model. Spine. 2010; 35(2):146–152

[27] Hals J, Ek J, Svalastog AG, Nilsen H. Studies on nutrition in severely neurologically disabled children in an institution. Acta Paediatr. 1996; 85(12):1469–1475

[28] Vitale MG, Privitera DM, Matsumoto H, et al. Efficacy of preoperative erythropoietin administration in pediatric neuromuscular scoliosis patients. Spine. 2007; 32(24):2662–2667

[29] Verma K, Errico T, Diefenbach C, et al. The relative efficacy of antifibrinolytics in adolescent idiopathic scoliosis: a prospective randomized trial. J Bone Joint Surg Am. 2014; 96(10):e80

[30] Gorter JW, Ketelaar M, Rosenbaum P, Helders PJ, Palisano R. Use of the GMFCS in infants with CP: the need for reclassification at age 2 years or older. Dev Med Child Neurol. 2009; 51(1):46–52

[31] Persson-Bunke M, Hägglund G, Lauge-Pedersen H, Wagner P, Westbom L. Scoliosis in a total population of children with cerebral palsy. Spine. 2012; 37(12):E708–E713

[32] Vaughan JJ, Winter RB, Lonstein JE. Comparison of the use of supine bending and traction radiographs in the selection of the fusion area in adolescent idiopathic scoliosis. Spine. 1996; 21(21):2469–2473

[33] Bouloussa H, Dubory A, Seiler C, Morel B, Bachy M, Vialle R. A radiolucent chair for sitting-posture radiographs in non-ambulatory children: use in biplanar digital slot-scanning. Pediatr Radiol. 2015; 45(12):1864–1869

[34] Lamarre ME, Parent S, Labelle H, et al. Assessment of spinal flexibility in adolescent idiopathic scoliosis: suspension versus side-bending radiography. Spine. 2009; 34(6):591–597

[35] Gupta MC, Wijesekera S, Sossan A, et al. Reliability of radiographic parameters in neuromuscular scoliosis. Spine. 2007; 32(6):691–695

2 Nonoperative Management

Stefan Parent

Abstract

Scoliosis is a common deformity in neuromuscular disorders. This spinal deformity usually presents at an early age, rapidly progresses during growth, and continues to progress even after skeletal maturity. In this chapter, nonoperative management of pediatric neuromuscular spine deformities and treatment protocols for these specific pathologies are discussed in detail, along with the most recent scientific evidence. Nonoperative management of pediatric neuromuscular spine deformities has several limitations. A clear understanding of the natural history of the condition, including life expectancy and functional outcomes, can help formulate goals of treatment. Bracing may help limit progression and/or postpone surgery in some forms of neuromuscular spinal deformity but is not thought to be effective, especially for spastic curves. Patients with more severe involvement are at higher risk of developing a spinal deformity and are also at higher risk of progression.

Keywords: baclofen pumps, Botox, bracing, cerebral palsy, Charcot–Marie–Tooth disease, corticosteroids, Duchenne muscular dystrophy, Friedreich's ataxia, neuromuscular scoliosis, spinal muscular atrophy, Rett syndrome, wheelchair modifications

2.1 Introduction and Background

Spinal deformities are commonly associated with neuromuscular disorders. When using the standard definition of scoliosis (a curve greater than 10 degrees in the coronal plane using the Cobb method), the prevalence of scoliotic deformities is much higher than in the general population, ranging from 15 to 80% in some series. Comparatively, adolescent idiopathic scoliosis prevalence is only 2 to 3% in the general population. This difference is thought to be related to the muscular imbalance found in neuromuscular disorders and is further supported by the fact that more severely affected individuals have not only a higher prevalence, but also more severe scoliotic deformities. The wide range of reported incidence is probably due to the variations in the populations used in the different studies. Patient impairment, neurological dysfunction, and the nature of the neurological condition affecting the patient will significantly affect the prevalence of scoliosis. In a review of children attending an outpatient clinic, Balmer and MacEwen[1] reported a prevalence of 21% of patients with a scoliosis greater than 10 degrees. In contrast, studies reporting on the prevalence of scoliosis in institutionalized patients with cerebral palsy (CP; thus probably more involved) have reported much higher prevalence for spinal deformities. Thometz and Simon[2] reported that 61% of institutionalized patients had a scoliosis of more than 10 degrees and Saito et al[3] reported a similar prevalence of 68%. Prevalence of scoliosis also seems to be associated with neurological involvement with more severe involvement presenting a higher prevalence of scoliosis. Koop et al reported that patients with quadriplegia had a prevalence of scoliosis greater than 40 degrees in 30% of the patients, while those with diplegia had a prevalence of 10 and 2% for those with hemiplegia.[4]

2.1.1 Long-Term Risk of Progression

As for idiopathic scoliosis, the long-term risk of progression increases with curve severity. Thometz and Simon found that the risk of progression in adult patients with CP was 0.8% per year when the deformity was less than 50 degrees, whereas the rate of progression was 1.4 degrees when the curve was greater than 50 degrees.[2] In another study of adult patients by Saito et al, 85% of patients with curves over 40 degrees at age 15 years progressed over 60 degrees, whereas only 13% of patients with curves less than 40 degrees progressed over 60 degrees into adulthood.[3]

2.2 Managing Patient and Family Expectations

Patients with neuromuscular conditions have a wide range of presentations from minimal involvement in certain forms of hemiplegia to full-body involvement in severe quadriplegic CP. This wide array of clinical presentations underscores the personalized nature of the treatment to be offered to patients and families. It is essential to openly communicate with the caregiver and, when possible with the patient, to establish clear expectations and limitations of different treatment options. The benefits of nonoperative treatment versus surgical treatment must be discussed and the risk of long-term progression must be clearly explained. The goals of nonoperative treatment should also be clearly stated and realistic expectations should be set.

2.3 Bracing

Although bracing has been shown to be effective for adolescent idiopathic scoliosis, the same does not apply to neuromuscular spinal deformities. Nonetheless, many clinicians use bracing as a means to improve sitting balance and to limit progression in younger patients. Pulmonary function does not seem to be negatively affected by bracing and it may even decrease the work of breathing by improved positioning.[5] In a review of 90 patients, Olafsson et al found that curve progression was prevented in only 23 patients with neuromuscular disorders treated with bracing.[6] The main cause for progression in 41 of the 60 patients was brace discontinuation, whereas 19 patients progressed despite adequate brace wear. The authors concluded that success of bracing was more likely to occur in ambulatory patients with muscle hypotonia and short lumbar/thoracolumbar curves less than 40 degrees and nonambulating patients with spastic short lumbar curves. Rate of progression was found to be influenced only by age and initial correction in the orthosis in a study by Terjesen et al.[7] In another study concentrating on the results of bracing in patients with CP, Renshaw et al reported success (progression of < 5 degrees) in only 22% of their 46 patients. Curve magnitude was 47 degrees at the time of bracing, and the degree of correction in the brace was small (13 degrees).[8]

Bracing in the setting of spinal cord injury (SCI) has been shown to delay surgery if initiated early. Mehta et al[9] found that if bracing was initiated when the curve was less than 10 degrees, not only did the proportion of patients requiring surgery decrease, but also the surgery was often delayed by 8.5 years compared to 4.2 years for nonbraced patients. Similar trends were observed in patients with curves less than 20 degrees.

2.4 Wheelchair Modifications

More severely involved children are often confined to their wheelchair. As these patients are often difficult to brace effectively, molded wheelchair inserts became more widely used in an attempt to improve sitting balance (▶ Fig. 2.1). These molded inserts can be used in combination with or without a brace. Although it is unclear whether these inserts have any impact on curve progression or preventing surgery, they are particularly useful in everyday activities as they help maintain a

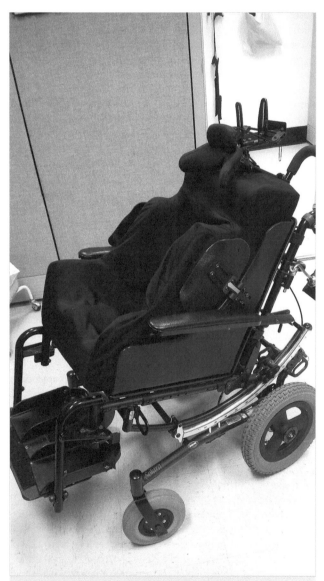

Fig. 2.1 Molded wheelchair insert to improve posture.

stable sitting balance. These inserts can also help during clinical and radiological evaluation with the patient sitting in the chair to confirm improved position and decreased curve magnitude. It remains unclear, however, whether these molded inserts have any role in preventing or slowing curve progression.

2.5 Baclofen Pumps

Although not truly a nonoperative option, baclofen pumps can play an important role in the preoperative or perioperative phase of patients with CP. Intrathecal baclofen (ITB) pumps are approved for the treatment of moderate to severe spasticity related to several disorders including CP.[10] The efficacy of ITB is well documented in children with CP.[11] Several studies have shown improvement in care of patients with CP from both the caretaker standpoint[12] and improved ease of care.[13]

2.6 Botox Injections

In at least one small series,[14] *Botulinum* toxin injection has been used with some success as an adjuvant measure to retard curve progression. Nuzzo et al found that among the 12 patients for which the toxin was used as a counterparalysis measure, none progressed significantly in the short-term study follow-up.

2.7 Diagnosis-Specific Considerations

2.7.1 Cerebral Palsy

Patients with CP represent a significant proportion of patients with neuromuscular scoliosis. These patients often exhibit significant spasticity and tend to have significant progression of their deformity, especially for patients with significant spastic quadriplegia. The spasticity seen in these patients may respond to baclofen treatment, but significant progression has been reported with the use of baclofen pumps.[15] Other reports have not shown a significant difference in scoliosis progression.[16]

2.7.2 Duchenne Muscular Dystrophy

Since the advent of corticoids treatment for Duchenne muscular dystrophy,[17] the rate of surgical intervention has drastically decreased.[18,19] This is thought to be due to the fact that the disease process is delayed and that patients do not develop spinal deformities prior to their growth spurt. Corticosteroids are thought to provide an initial increase in muscle strength and to reduce the loss of strength over time in boys with Duchenne muscular dystrophy. When spinal deformity occurs, early intervention to prevent later cardiopulmonary compromise is warranted. Bracing for these patients has not been shown to be effective in preventing deformity but could delay surgery.[20] As spinal deformities tend to occur later in the disease process as patients become nonambulatory, it is important to carefully monitor the spine at this stage for any developing deformities. Before the advent of corticosteroids, most authors recommended early spinal fusion as pulmonary function tended to decrease with age. A forced vital capacity of less than 35% may require prolonged intubation and possibly permanent tracheotomy.[21]

2.7.3 Spinal Muscular Atrophy

Spinal muscular atrophy represents a group of disorders involving the anterior horn cells. Patients with spinal muscular atrophy have significant involvement of their trunk muscles and have a limited respiratory function. The nonoperative management of these patients is often driven by their respiratory status. Aggressive respiratory therapy can help limit the impact of the scoliotic deformity and chest-limited expansion, but conservative treatment is often unsuccessful in preventing scoliosis progression and its effect on respiratory function.

2.7.4 Rett Syndrome

Rett syndrome is a neurodevelopmental disorder that is caused by a mutation in the *MECP2* gene[22,23] that affects approximately 1 in 9,000 female live births. Factors that have been found to influence the progression of scoliosis include ambulatory status and genotype. Several publications have found relationships between genotype and clinical severity and several comorbidities. Evidence- and consensus-based guidelines were created for the management of Rett syndrome.[24] These guidelines state that if bracing is tolerated, it should be used in skeletally immature patients to delay surgery and when active seating and trunk activation cannot be achieved. However, there is no consensus that bracing is beneficial in reducing the progression of scoliosis in Rett syndrome.[24]

2.7.5 Charcot–Marie–Tooth Disease

Charcot–Marie–Tooth disease is an inherited sensory neuropathy that affects 1 in 5,000 individuals.[25] It is an autosomal-dominant disease with variable penetrance and there are several types, each based on its genetic etiology.[26] In a cohort of 45 patients with Charcot–Marie–Tooth disease also presenting with scoliosis, Karol et al[27] reviewed their clinical experience. All patients who were followed up for more than 1 year progressed (24/24 patients), and brace treatment was successful in only 3 of 16 patients.[27] The deformity is often associated with increased kyphosis and one-third of the curves were left thoracic.

2.7.6 Friedreich's Ataxia

Friedreich's ataxia is a recessively inherited spinocerebellar degenerative disease. It is the most common form of hereditary ataxia affecting about 1 in 50,000 people in the United States. The mutated gene is *FRDA* located on Chromosome 9. In a series of 78 patients, Labelle et al evaluated the risk of progression and natural history of this condition.[28] They concluded that several curves behaved like adolescent idiopathic curves and that many curves were not progressive or only slowly progressive and that there was no relationship to muscle weakness. They propose surgically treating patients with curves more than 60 degrees because of the high rate of progression and suggest observing patients with curves under 40 degrees. They advocate surgical treatment or observation for curves between 40 and 60 degrees depending on the age of the patient at onset of the deformity and/or evidence of progression. As this was a study evaluating the natural history of scoliosis in Friedreich's ataxia, outcomes of bracing were specifically not evaluated. Onset of the disease at an early age and the presence of scoliosis prior to puberty were major factors in progression.[28]

2.7.7 Spinal Cord Injury

The overall occurrence of SCI in children is rare with an overall incidence of 1.99 spinal cord injuries per 100,000 children in the United States, and most of these children are older than 15 years. Although SCI in children is relatively rare, it can have devastating consequences for the family and the patient.[29,30,31,32] Younger patients are more likely to develop a significant spinal deformity especially if they are injured before the adolescent growth spurt.[33,34,35] There is weak evidence that bracing initiated before 20 degrees may in fact delay surgical correction and that bracing before 10 degrees may prevent scoliosis progression.[9] Based on this evidence and the relatively innocuous nature of bracing, it is suggested to aggressively treat these curves prior to the growth spurt.[32] Although bracing is often viewed as a low-risk treatment, care must be taken in patients having loss of sensation as they run the risk of pressure sores if not properly fitted.

References

[1] Balmer GA, MacEwen GD. The incidence and treatment of scoliosis in cerebral palsy. J Bone Joint Surg Br. 1970; 52(1):134–137

[2] Thometz JG, Simon SR. Progression of scoliosis after skeletal maturity in institutionalized adults who have cerebral palsy. J Bone Joint Surg Am. 1988; 70 (9):1290–1296

[3] Saito N, Ebara S, Ohotsuka K, Kumeta H, Takaoka K. Natural history of scoliosis in spastic cerebral palsy. Lancet. 1998; 351(9117):1687–1692

[4] Koop SE, Lonstein JE, Winter RB, Denis F. The natural history of spine deformity in cerebral palsy. Scoliosis Research Society Annual Meeting, Minneapolis, MN, September 24–27, 1991

[5] Leopando MT, Moussavi Z, Holbrow J, Chernick V, Pasterkamp H, Rempel G. Effect of a Soft Boston Orthosis on pulmonary mechanics in severe cerebral palsy. Pediatr Pulmonol. 1999; 28(1):53–58

[6] Olafsson Y, Saraste H, Al-Dabbagh Z. Brace treatment in neuromuscular spine deformity. J Pediatr Orthop. 1999; 19(3):376–379

[7] Terjesen T, Lange JE, Steen H. Treatment of scoliosis with spinal bracing in quadriplegic cerebral palsy. Dev Med Child Neurol. 2000; 42(7):448–454

[8] Renshaw TS, Green NE, Griffin PP, Root L. Cerebral palsy: orthopaedic management. Instr Course Lect. 1996; 45:475–490

[9] Mehta S, Betz RR, Mulcahey MJ, McDonald C, Vogel LC, Anderson C. Effect of bracing on paralytic scoliosis secondary to spinal cord injury. J Spinal Cord Med. 2004; 27 Suppl 1:S88–S92

[10] Lynn AK, Turner M, Chambers HG. Surgical management of spasticity in persons with cerebral palsy. PM R. 2009; 1(9):834–838

[11] Albright AL, Cervi A, Singletary J. Intrathecal baclofen for spasticity in cerebral palsy. JAMA. 1991; 265(11):1418–1422

[12] Gooch JL, Oberg WA, Grams B, Ward LA, Walker ML. Care provider assessment of intrathecal baclofen in children. Dev Med Child Neurol. 2004; 46 (8):548–552

[13] Armstrong RW, Steinbok P, Cochrane DD, Kube SD, Fife SE, Farrell K. Intrathecally administered baclofen for treatment of children with spasticity of cerebral origin. J Neurosurg. 1997; 87(3):409–414

[14] Nuzzo RM, Walsh S, Boucherit T, Massood S. Counterparalysis for treatment of paralytic scoliosis with botulinum toxin type A. Am J Orthop. 1997; 26 (3):201–207

[15] Ginsburg GM, Lauder AJ. Progression of scoliosis in patients with spastic quadriplegia after the insertion of an intrathecal baclofen pump. Spine. 2007; 32(24):2745–2750

[16] Senaran H, Shah SA, Presedo A, Dabney KW, Glutting JW, Miller F. The risk of progression of scoliosis in cerebral palsy patients after intrathecal baclofen therapy. Spine. 2007; 32(21):2348–2354

[17] Griggs RC, Moxley RT, III, Mendell JR, et al. Duchenne dystrophy: randomized, controlled trial of prednisone (18 months) and azathioprine (12 months). Neurology. 1993; 43(3, Pt 1):520–527

[18] Alman BA. Duchenne muscular dystrophy and steroids: pharmacologic treatment in the absence of effective gene therapy. J Pediatr Orthop. 2005; 25 (4):554–556

[19] Alman BA, Raza SN, Biggar WD. Steroid treatment and the development of scoliosis in males with Duchenne muscular dystrophy. J Bone Joint Surg Am. 2004; 86-A(3):519–524

[20] Seeger BR, Sutherland AD, Clark MS. Orthotic management of scoliosis in Duchenne muscular dystrophy. Arch Phys Med Rehabil. 1984; 65(2):83–86

[21] Miller F, Moseley CF, Koreska J. Spinal fusion in Duchenne muscular dystrophy. Dev Med Child Neurol. 1992; 34(9):775–786

[22] Gabel HW, Kinde B, Stroud H, et al. Disruption of DNA-methylation-dependent long gene repression in Rett syndrome. Nature. 2015; 522(7554):89–93

[23] Amir RE, Zoghbi HY. Rett syndrome: methyl-CpG-binding protein 2 mutations and phenotype-genotype correlations. Am J Med Genet. 2000; 97 (2):147–152

[24] Downs J, Bergman A, Carter P, et al. Guidelines for management of scoliosis in Rett syndrome patients based on expert consensus and clinical evidence. Spine. 2009; 34(17):E607–E617

[25] Holmberg BH. Charcot-Marie-Tooth disease in northern Sweden: an epidemiological and clinical study. Acta Neurol Scand. 1993; 87(5):416–422

[26] Ouvrier R. Correlation between the histopathologic, genotypic, and phenotypic features of hereditary peripheral neuropathies in childhood. J Child Neurol. 1996; 11(2):133–146

[27] Karol LA, Elerson E. Scoliosis in patients with Charcot-Marie-Tooth disease. J Bone Joint Surg Am. 2007; 89(7):1504–1510

[28] Labelle H, Tohmé S, Duhaime M, Allard P. Natural history of scoliosis in Friedreich's ataxia. J Bone Joint Surg Am. 1986; 68(4):564–572

[29] Reilly CW. Pediatric spine trauma. J Bone Joint Surg Am. 2007; 89 Suppl 1:98–107

[30] Platzer P, Jaindl M, Thalhammer G, et al. Cervical spine injuries in pediatric patients. J Trauma. 2007; 62(2):389–396, discussion 394–396

[31] Dogan S, Safavi-Abbasi S, Theodore N, Horn E, Rekate HL, Sonntag VK. Pediatric subaxial cervical spine injuries: origins, management, and outcome in 51 patients. Neurosurg Focus. 2006; 20(2):E1

[32] Parent S, Dimar J, Dekutoski M, Roy-Beaudry M. Unique features of pediatric spinal cord injury. Spine. 2010; 35(21) Suppl:S202–S208

[33] Dearolf WW, III, Betz RR, Vogel LC, Levin J, Clancy M, Steel HH. Scoliosis in pediatric spinal cord-injured patients. J Pediatr Orthop. 1990; 10(2):214–218

[34] Lancourt JE, Dickson JH, Carter RE. Paralytic spinal deformity following traumatic spinal-cord injury in children and adolescents. J Bone Joint Surg Am. 1981; 63(1):47–53

[35] Mayfield JK, Erkkila JC, Winter RB. Spine deformity subsequent to acquired childhood spinal cord injury. J Bone Joint Surg Am. 1981; 63(9):1401–1411

3 Surgical Indications in Neuromuscular Scoliosis

Cheryl R. Lawing, Michael P. Kelly, and Paul D. Sponseller

Abstract

Neuromuscular spinal deformity surgery carries significant risks of perioperative complication. A thorough knowledge of the common comorbid conditions and common complications will allow for the safest surgery possible, with patients, families, and caregivers prepared for the postoperative course. These spinal deformities are, in general, refractory to bracing and require observation with a shared decision-making approach to indicate surgery. Most neuromuscular deformities tend to progress once greater than 40 degrees. Similarly, fixing deformities measuring greater than 90 degrees often carries greater risk of complications, and it is likely prudent to initiate surgery before a severe curve has developed. Growing spine techniques, such as growing rods and trolleys, are useful in early-onset cases of neuromuscular scoliosis. Duchenne muscular dystrophy is a unique deformity, where treatment with corticosteroids has reduced the number of progressive spinal deformities and subsequent surgeries. Many neuromuscular diagnoses now carry longer life expectancies. As such, attention to care of the spinal deformity is needed to mitigate the long-term risks of a severe deformity such as a decline in pulmonary function or skin care difficulties. Until more advanced genetic and pharmacologic treatments are available, instrumented spinal fusions will be the standard for the care of neuromuscular spinal deformities.

Keywords: cerebral palsy, Duchenne, indications, neuromuscular scoliosis, spinal cord injury, spinal muscular atrophy, syndromic scoliosis

3.1 Patient Health Factors

Before any decision is made to take a patient to the operating room for neuromuscular scoliosis, the surgeon must ensure that the patient is healthy enough to tolerate surgery and that the potential risks associated with neuromuscular spinal surgeries are outweighed by the potential benefits.[1,2,3,4] Given the multitude of pathologies that constitute neuromuscular spinal, the surgeon and team must be aware of the many systems outside of the musculoskeletal system that are affected in each case. While Chapter 1 is devoted to the preoperative evaluation of the patient, it is prudent to reiterate certain points here.

3.1.1 Pulmonary

In many cases of neuromuscular spinal, the pulmonary system is affected by both the neuromuscular disease and the presence of the spinal deformity. This is true whether the diagnosis is totally involved cerebral palsy with a 100-degree coronal deformity or a Duchenne muscular dystrophy (DMD) patient with a 20-degree deformity and progressive muscle weakness.[5] While pulmonary function testing (PFT) is not always possible in this diverse patient population due to cognitive comorbidity, spirometry should be obtained when possible. Other methods to test pulmonary function include diffusion capacity and gas dilution methods. Poor PFTs may preclude surgery in the most extreme cases. Otherwise, knowledge of PFTs preoperatively allows for an informed decision-making process with the patient and caretakers. Those patients with poor PFTs are at a higher risk for perioperative complications such as prolonged intubation, ventilator-acquired pneumonia, and need for tracheostomy. Thus, all involved in the care of the patient should be prepared for these events.[5]

3.1.2 Cardiovascular

Patients undergoing surgery for neuromuscular spinal are at an estimated threefold higher risk of intraoperative cardiopulmonary arrest, when compared with other causes of pediatric scoliosis.[6] While this complication remains rare, knowledge of those at risk will improve response to any event, as well as allow for careful discussion with patients and caretakers. Particular attention must be paid to those diagnosed with muscular dystrophies, including DMD, Becker's muscular dystrophy, and some cases of congenital muscular dystrophy. These diseases are associated with early-onset cardiomyopathy, and preoperative evaluation must include electrocardiogram (ECG) and echocardiogram.[7] Congenital muscular dystrophy is also associated with arrhythmias, and pacemaker pad placement at the time of surgery is advisable. Appropriate pharmacologic management of cardiovascular disease is necessary as well, which includes angiotensin-converting enzyme inhibitors in DMD.

3.1.3 Gastroenterology/Nutrition

Malnutrition is not uncommon among patients with neuromuscular disease. This may put them at increased risk for perioperative complications including infection, wound healing difficulties, and pseudarthrosis.[8] It may be helpful to check preoperative serum albumin, prealbumin, and transferrin. These serve as some measure of nutritional status and may alert the surgeon to the severely malnourished patient, though the physical appearance will likely lead to this diagnosis before any laboratory value. For those patients that are malnourished, placement of an enteral feeding tube with several months of augmented caloric intake may help optimize them.[9] Some authors have promoted the use of parenteral feeding in the perioperative period, though the benefits of this are unclear and this intervention comes at high costs and some risk to the patient.[10] Consultation with gastroenterology and a nutrition service may help improve the nutritional status of the patient. Bowel habits must be assessed preoperatively to prepare for postoperative care, as prevention of wound contamination is essential. Immobility may also lead to obesity in this patient population.[11] A high body mass index (BMI) has been associated with larger deformities, which is concerning in an already "at-risk" population.[12,13] Furthermore, obesity has been associated with an increased risk of perioperative complications in adolescent idiopathic scoliosis and adult spinal deformity surgery.[14,15] It stands to reason that obesity conveys similar risks in neuromuscular scoliosis, given the already high rate of perioperative complication.

3.1.4 Genitourinary

Genitourinary abnormalities such as uncontrolled voiding and bacterial colonization of the bladder are not uncommon, particularly in patients with myelomeningocele. While not serving as contraindications to spine surgery, bladder habits should be evaluated preoperatively. Again, knowledge of preoperative habits and risk factors will optimize postoperative care through anticipation of complications and appropriate counseling of the patient and caregivers. Patients with myelomeningocele and their caregivers may find catheterization difficult and require Mitrofanoff procedures or other rerouting procedures to allow for safe and clean catheterization. A discussion of the potential needs should occur at a preoperative visit. In some cases, the patient or family may prefer to have the rerouting procedure performed before the spine fusion. Patients with frequent urinary tract infections should consider such a procedure before the spine surgery to reduce the risk of bacteremic seeding of the spine.

3.1.5 Ambulatory Status

The ambulatory status of the patient should be evaluated preoperatively as this will influence the choice of lowest instrumented vertebrae as well as call attention to the position of the pelvis with walking. Fusion to the sacrum and ilium likely alters gait mechanics. This is an important point for those patients using platform crutches to bear the majority of weight through the upper extremities. These patients require trunk flexibility to accommodate the paralytic lower extremities, and fusion to the sacrum and pelvis may affect gait to an unacceptable degree.[16] For this reason in ambulatory patients we will try to stop at L4 or higher and avoid fixing to the sacrum and ilium. For nonambulatory patients, the degree of pelvic obliquity and sitting imbalance should be assessed, as these two factors will influence the decision to fuse to the sacrum and ilium.

3.2 Disease-Specific Indications

3.2.1 Cerebral Palsy

The development of scoliosis in patients with cerebral palsy varies with the severity of neurologic involvement, though the deformities are often progressive if present before skeletal maturity (▶ Fig. 3.1 **a-d**, ▶ Fig. 3.2). Spastic cerebral palsy is often characterized by early onset and progression that persists through skeletal maturity.[17] Patients with quadriplegic involvement and those who are bedridden have the worst prognosis.[18] Deformities that measure 40 degrees or more may progress into large curves during adulthood, and one may consider surgery at this point in skeletally mature individuals.[19,20] Scoliosis in the setting of a baclofen pump may progress at a rate faster than the normal natural history, and intervention may be considered when a curve has progressed to 40 degrees or higher.[21] These findings have not been ubiquitous, however, and the dichotomy of findings emphasizes the importance of the informed decision-making process.[22,23,24]

The risk of surgery increases significantly once a curve reaches 90 degrees and therefore intervention is recommended if a curve reaches this point at a young age. Bracing is ineffective; therefore, in order to prevent crankshaft phenomenon and allow adequate development of trunk height, growing constructs may be needed if a curve exceeds 90 degrees before the skeletal age of about 9 to 10 years. Fusion for those patients near 10 years of age with curves of this magnitude (>90 degrees) may be the most appropriate option.[25]

Growing rods in patients with cerebral palsy have been shown not only to provide control of the deformity, but also to have a high infection rates, up to 30%.[26] Iliac fixation has shown superiority over sacral screws for distal fixation (67% correction vs. 40% for pelvic obliquity and 47% correction for scoliosis vs. 29%) when pelvic obliquity is present. Dual rods also afford better correction and are recommended.[26,27] More frequent

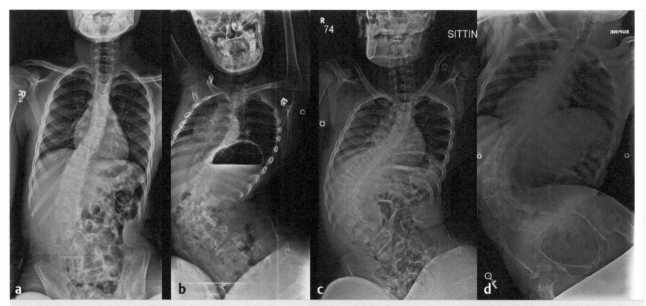

Fig. 3.1 (a-d) Progression of neuromuscular scoliosis over 6 years in a patient with tetraplegic cerebral palsy. Note the pelvic obliquity and hyperlordotic lumbar spine in **(d)**.

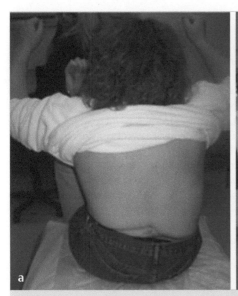
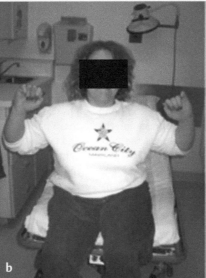
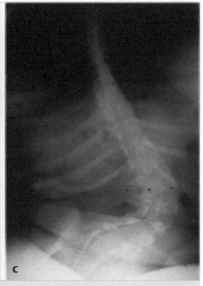

Fig. 3.2 (a-c) Large neuromuscular spinal deformity in a patient with myelomeningocele. The absence of severe pelvic obliquity allowed for maintained sitting balance, and surgery was avoided.

implant-related complication rates have been reported with growing constructs compared to fusion, and thus it is obviously ideal to delay insertion of growing rods for as long as possible.[28] The vertical expandable prosthetic titanium rib (VEPTR) may be useful in cases of early onset neuromuscular scoliosis.[29] A rib-to-pelvic construct avoids disruption of the spine and may maximize growth potential. Magnetically controlled growing rods require limited spinal fusion and allow for lengthening without a return to the operating room. They have shown promise in cases of early-onset scoliosis, including neuromuscular deformity.[30,31]

Consideration for surgical approach is of key importance. Posterior approaches offer excellent correction, similar to combined anterior and posterior, with shorter intensive care unit (ICU) stays and less morbidity.[32,33] However, for severe and rigid curves, or those with significant lordosis, an anterior approach may be beneficial by shortening the spine and decreasing the muscle tension needed.[34] Baclofen pumps are often present, though these do not affect complication rates or outcomes.[35] The importance of preoperative optimization, as discussed earlier, cannot be over emphasized in these complicated patients.

3.2.2 Duchenne Muscular Dystrophy

DMD is an X-linked recessive mutation in the gene coding for dystrophin. Historically, the progressive muscle weakness associated with DMD has led to scoliosis notorious for steady progression, necessitating surgical intervention. Scoliosis usually occurs once the child is no longer ambulatory and takes the form of a long C-shaped paralytic curve involving the thoracic and lumbar spine. Surgical indications in DMD have changed dramatically with the regular use of steroids. Glucocorticoids have been shown to prolong walking for 2.5 years, in addition to slowing the decline in lung function.[36] Fifteen-year follow-up of patients with DMD found that scoliosis developed in 20% of patients receiving the glucocorticoid deflazacort, a derivative of prednisone, versus 92% of patients not receiving steroids.

Seventy-eight percent of the glucocorticoid group in this study were able to avoid surgery, whereas only 8.3% of patients in the nonsteroid group did not need surgery. Corticosteroid treatment is not without risk, however, and cataract formation was common (70%) in those treated with deflazacort.[37] While further work to determine appropriate dosing regimens needs to be done, it is clear that corticosteroids positively affect spinal deformity progression and reduce the need for spinal fusions.

Historically, treatment of scoliosis was recommended prior to the decline of cardiopulmonary function, once the curve reached 20 degrees.[38] This was due, in part, to the combination of progressive weakness of muscles of respiration with the restrictive disease associated with a collapsing deformity as well as the ineffectiveness of bracing in controlling the deformity. However, with glucocorticoid treatment, fusion can now be avoided or delayed until curves are larger, around 50 degrees, or when sitting balance is becoming affected.[39,40] Of note, anterior approaches are contraindicated, given the potential to further compromise pulmonary function. If nonoperative management is chosen, then serial PFTs should be obtained and followed for evidence of progressive decline. Spinal fusion may help prevent decline in pulmonary function and consideration to surgery should be made in such a case.[41] Furthermore, a plateau of the vital capacity at 1,900 mL has been associated with rapid progression of the spinal deformity, particularly in those patients younger than 14 years.[42]

There is general consensus that spinal fusion should be performed before forced vital capacity (FVC) is less than 30 to 35% predicted, though FVC lower than this is not a strict contraindication to surgery and successful surgeries have been reported.[43,44] Marsh et al compared a group of patients with FVC < 30% (average 24%) to patients with FVC > 30% and found that there were similar times for postoperative ventilator support and hospitalization between the groups, when one patient in the less than 30% group requiring tracheostomy was excluded. Overall complication rates were 30% in each group, further suggesting that spinal surgery can be performed on patients with FVC < 30%.[44] Additionally, Kennedy et al found that there was high patient satisfaction in patients with FVC < 30% (mean 21.6%), with no major complications and all patients extubated immediately postoperatively.[45] However, there is also documentation of prolonged ventilator time and respiratory complications in patients with FVC < 30% and therefore the risks and benefits of surgery must seriously be considered in this patient population. It is important to realize that the decline in FVC will continue postoperatively, as a consequence of the ongoing disease process, and this is important to discuss with the family preoperatively.[45,46]

Cardiomyopathy is indicative of more advanced disease and needs to be factored into surgical considerations. ECG commonly shows abnormalities and echocardiogram should be performed to evaluate left ventricle function. The most common pathologies encountered include inferobasal wall motion abnormalities, which is then followed by left ventricular dilatation.[47] Echocardiogram should be performed preoperatively and a multidisciplinary team assessment performed.[48] Left ventricular dysfunction on echocardiogram, unlike ECG changes, is predictive of perioperative mortality.[49] A normal preoperative cardiac evaluation does not exclude all risks, however, as a fatal cardiac event has been reported in a child with a normal preoperative evaluation (FVC 87%, echocardiogram normal).[50] Important to consider and discuss with the anesthesia team is that patients with DMD can have rhabdomyolysis with anesthesia that can cause hyperkalemia and cardiac arrest, in a reaction similar to malignant hyperthermia.[47]

3.2.3 Myelomeningocele

In cases of myelomeningocele, curves of less than 20 degrees are unlikely to progress, though clinical motor level, ambulatory status, and last intact laminar arch all affect risk for progression and should be factored into treatment.[51,52] In a review of 46 patients, Muller et al[52] outlined the tendency for progression based on Cobb angles and found that curves less than 20 degrees progressed only 1.2 degrees per year, curves between 20 and 39 degrees progressed 3.8 degrees per year, and curves greater than 40 degrees progressed 12.5 degrees per year. While some surgeons feel that when the curve worsens to 50 degrees and sitting balance becomes affected, surgery is indicated, others feel that surgery should be recommended only if there is clear impairment of skin or sitting balance, as there is a high complication rate in patients with myelomeningocele.[53] Spinal fusion has been shown to have an uncertain impact on health-related quality of life, with some studies showing no relation between coronal deformity and self-perception or physical function. Thus, the decision to intervene surgically in these patients must include very careful consideration of risks and benefits[54] (▶ Fig. 3.3).

In the ambulatory patient, special consideration of levels are indicated, as fusion to the pelvis can potentially interfere with ambulation.[55] Fusion short of the pelvis can be performed if the apex of the curve is above T12 and there is minimal lumbar rotation. Surgical procedures may need to be coordinated with neurosurgical procedures to address tethered cord and shunt function.

3.2.4 Spinal Muscular Atrophy

Spinal muscular atrophy (SMA) involves a spectrum of disease. Patients with type I SMA, diagnosed between 3 and 6 months, are usually unable to roll or sit and have a life expectancy of only 2 years. Patients with type II SMA are diagnosed up to 18 months and are usually able to sit. The involvement of the disease varies, as does the life expectancy, and some patients may live into young adulthood. Patients with type III and IV SMA are able to walk and with good care may live normal life spans. Progressive scoliosis is a common problem in patients with SMA types I–III, occurring in about 60 to 95% of patients, and natural history shows progressive decline in respiratory function in these patients as they develop rib collapse that causes a triangular-shaped thorax[56] (▶ Fig. 3.3). Bracing has been shown to be ineffective in these patients, and the resulting chest wall constriction can have serious pulmonary complications.[57] Growing rods are able to increase trunk height (average of 1.2 ± 0.6 cm/year) and the space available for the lung ratio (8.6 ± 0.15 preoperatively to 0.94 ± 0.21 postoperatively). However, these improvements were less than the increase seen in a control cohort consisting of patients with infantile idiopathic scoliosis (IIS)/ juvenile idiopathic scoliosis (JIS; trunk height increase of 2.3 ± 3.3 cm/year and space available for the lung

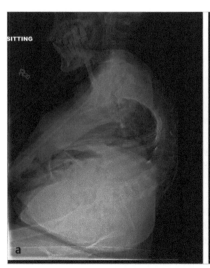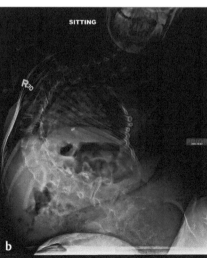

Fig. 3.3 (a,b) A patient with spinal muscular atrophy and a characteristic "C"-shaped deformity with scoliosis and a sweeping kyphosis. Given the magnitude of the deformity, she was treated with halo-gravity traction for 2 weeks prior to the posterior spinal fusion.

ratio of 0.93 ± 0.12 to 1.01 ± 0.08). Most importantly, there was continued rib collapse in patients with SMA despite growing rods, whereas there was not in the idiopathic comparison group. This is thought to be due to the progressive dysfunction of the intercostal muscles.[58]

Timing of definitive fusion is debated in this patient population, who develop scoliosis at an early age. Given the extremely poor prognosis for patients with SMA type I, no intervention for the early-onset scoliosis is usually performed. Studies are currently underway investigating intrathecal nusinersen, which may have promise in extending life for SMA type I patients.[59] Should this drug, or other gene therapy, prove beneficial, then intervention for scoliosis with SMA type I may be required. Zebala et al have shown that fusion can be performed in patients with the other types of SMA while skeletally immature with open triradiate cartilage.[60] Fujak et al recommended fusion in patients aged 10 to 12 years and older, justified by less annual loss of correction with fusion (1.0 degree/year) compared to telescoping rods (2.7 degrees/year), based on the estimation that 80 to 84% of expected maximum height has been achieved by this age for boys (84–91% for girls).[61] Mesfin et al have recommended that curves greater 70 degrees in children aged 9 years and under should be treated with growing rod constructs, while children aged 10 years and older benefit from posterior spinal fusion (PSF).[56] With modern pedicle screw instrumentation, anterior spinal fusion (ASF) is usually not indicated.

3.2.5 Spinal Cord Injury

Neuromuscular scoliosis is common following traumatic spinal cord injury (SCI). There is increased risk of progression the younger the age of the patient is at the time of injury and with skeletal immaturity.[62,63] neuromuscular spinal is far more likely to develop if the injury occurs prior to the growth spurt, rather than after it (97 vs. 52%).[64] Resultant scoliosis is thought to be due to spasticity and paralysis, rather than residual fracture deformity.[65] SCI without radiographic abnormality (SCIWORA) is a particular SCI more common in younger patients that accounts for up to 20% of all pediatric SCI.[66] SCIWORA occurs in the cervical spine more often than the thoracic spine, often leading to more affected trunk musculature and support than a thoracic-level SCI.

Brace treatment can be effective if started early but is thought to only slow progression once the curve reaches 20 degrees, as documented in a cohort study of 123 patients with SCI.[67] Only coronal deformities less than 10 degrees seemed to benefit from bracing, though this is likely to be due to the nature of the deformity itself and not the brace. Mehta et al found that curve progression, with subsequent surgery, was common for deformities greater than 20 degrees. Bracing is not without risk in SCI patients, as there may be an increased risk of pressure ulcers if insensate. Compliance with brace wear may be difficult as well, as bracing significantly interferes with the ability of children to use their arms normally.[68]

Dearolf et al[64] found that the risk of surgery for spinal deformity resulting from SCI was 67% if the injury occurred prior to maturity. In a study of 217 children with SCI, Mulcahey et al[63] reported that children injured at younger than 12 years were 3.7 times more likely to require a spinal fusion as compared to those injured after 12 years of age.

The degree of SCI (complete vs. incomplete) was not associated with risk of progression; only age at the time of injury was associated with curve progression and surgery.

Surgery for neuromuscular spinal associated with SCI should follow protocols similar to those of neuromuscular diseases. As skeletally immature patients with SCI are at the highest risk, we will consider growth modulation in these patients for certain progressive curves. Definitive fusions can be considered for those patients who have limited growth potential remaining and have coronal curves greater than 45 degrees or pelvic obliquity that makes sitting balance difficult. Extension of the fusion to the sacrum and ilium may be indicated in cases of pelvic obliquity. The treating physician should have a high level of concern for progression in skeletally immature patients and keep close surveillance. Once the curve has progressed significantly, surgical correction of the deformity becomes necessary according to standard neuromuscular techniques.[69]

3.2.6 Arthrogryposis

The incidence of scoliosis in arthrogryposis varies from 2.5 to 69% in various studies.[70,71,72] In a review of 46 patients with arthrogryposis, bracing was found to be successful in ambulatory patients with curves less than 30 degrees, but curves greater than 30 degrees in nonambulators tended to progress and usually needed surgery.[72] Other studies have shown that bracing is not effective and that curve progression is common.[71,73]

Scoliosis often develops at an early age in these patients, in which case growth-preserving treatment needs to be considered.[71,74] The VEPTR has been shown to be successful in allowing for continued thoracic cavity growth for early-onset scoliosis in association with arthrogryposis, though proximal junctional kyphosis greater than 20 degrees (average 45 degrees) occurred in 6 of their 10 patients. In this same study, they were able to obtain 89% of expected thoracic volume.

There are a variety of curve patterns, but long thoracolumbar patterns appear to be the most common in the literature with a high incidence of pelvic obliquity.[75] In Drummond and Mackenzie's series, congenital vertebral anomalies were found in 50% of cases, but this has not been found in other studies.[71,75,76] Hip pathology can be associated with these curves and hyperlordosis of the lumbar spine is often present.[71] Hip range of motion needs to be considered, as fusing to the pelvis in a patient with less than 90 degrees of hip motion can create difficulty with ambulation.[16,72] However, Herron et al found progression below L4 in three of six patients not fused to the pelvis.[71] As an additional consideration, O'Brien et al described the potential for excellent correction of rigid paralytic pelvic obliquity in patients with preoperative halo-femoral traction followed by combined anterior and posterior releases and fusion.[77] It is important to keep in mind and discuss with the family preoperatively that curves associated with arthrogryposis tend to be stiff and complete correction is very difficult to obtain.[73,76]

3.2.7 Syndromic Neuromuscular Scoliosis

Rett Syndrome

The prevalence of scoliosis in children with Rett syndrome is close to 90%, with increasing risk in more involved children.[78] Most children with Rett syndrome survive into adulthood, thus making treatment of scoliosis important to this population. Long-term survival is good, with 78% survival at 20 years, 72% at 25 years, and 60% at 37 years in an Australian registry.[79] A recent study found an even greater survival of 70% survival at 45 years.[80]

A consensus expert panel for treatment of neuromuscular scoliosis in association with Rett syndrome was created because of the rarity of disease.[81] Clinical monitoring is recommended every 6 months with increased surveillance in high-risk patients, indicated by hypotonia, abnormal delay or failure to learn to walk, more severe Cobb angle, during growth spurts, and those with genotypes carrying high risk for progression of scoliosis (p.R168X, p.R255, p.R270X). Radiographic monitoring is recommended every 6 months for curves greater than 25 degrees in skeletally immature patients. Yearly full-spine radiographs are recommended after skeletal maturity and until the curve is documented to be stable. Bracing has not been shown to slow the progression of scoliosis but can be helpful in maintaining sitting balance. However, the potential negative consequences of bracing include skin irritation, decrease in trunk strength and activity, respiratory impairment, and exacerbation of gastroesophageal reflux. Ultimately, spinal fusion has been shown to have benefits in terms of ability to sit upright and ease of care from the caregiver standpoint.[82]

Surgical intervention is recommended when the Cobb angle exceeds 45 to 50 degrees. It is not advised to allow a severe curve to worsen while awaiting skeletal maturity before performing fusion. However, crankshaft and decreased trunk height are potential complications if fusion is performed at too young an age. BMI and nutritional status, with adequate nutrition indicated by albumin greater than 3.5 mg/dL, should be considered and hyperalimentation performed preoperatively if weight is less than the 5th percentile.[81]

According to the expert consensus outlined by Downs et al, posterior fusion is the standard treatment for scoliosis in the setting of Rett syndrome.[81] Nonambulatory children with pelvic obliquity may require fusion to the pelvis. However, there is no consensus regarding the degree of pelvic obliquity that necessitates fusion to the pelvis.

Friedreich's Ataxia

Friedreich's ataxia can be associated with scoliosis. The mean age of diagnosis is around the age of 12. Scoliosis is present in about two-thirds (63%) of patients.[83] The curve pattern in these patients is more typical of idiopathic scoliosis, rather than the long C-shaped paralytic curve seen in other types of neuromuscular scoliosis. In a review of 77 patients, Milbrandt et al found double major curves to be the most common (33%), followed by single thoracic curves (29%).[83] Two key findings that differentiate these curves from idiopathic scoliosis are the higher

percentages with left thoracic (22%) curves and hyperkyphosis (24.5%). Others have found rates of hyperkyphosis as high as 45 to 66%.[69,70]

There is debate as to whether the age at diagnosis impacts progression. Milbrandt et al did not find an association, while Labelle et al found that earlier age of onset (before 15 years old) correlated with progression.[83,84] The degree of muscle weakness, ambulatory status, and curve pattern have been shown to not correlate with progression.[84] Brace treatment has been shown to have limited efficacy in these patients. Milbrandt et al were successful in treating only 20% (2/10) of patients with brace therapy alone.[83] Tsirikos and Smith found that only 29% of patients did not require surgery.[85]

Fusion is recommended for curves greater than 40 degrees given the likelihood to progress.[84] Fusion to the pelvis is usually not mandatory but may be necessary in the few patients with pelvic obliquity. Cardiac and pulmonary functions are critical preoperative considerations, as these patients often suffer from cardiomyopathy and restrictive lung disease. Severe hypertrophic cardiomyopathy and left ventricular dysfunction on echocardiogram may preclude surgical intervention.[85]

Familial Dysautonomia (Riley–Day Syndrome)

Scoliosis is the most common orthopaedic manifestation of familial dysautonomia, an autosomal recessive disorder that most commonly affects individuals of the Ashkenazi population. In various studies, incidence of scoliosis varies from 83 to 90%.[86,87,88] Unlike the long C-shaped curve that often occurs with neuromuscular scoliosis, scoliosis in association with familial dysautonomia takes on the form, more typical of idiopathic scoliosis, of single thoracic or double major curves.[89] However, about half of these curves are convex to the left. Scoliosis can occur in isolation but is commonly associated with hyperkyphosis, another key feature that differentiates it from idiopathic scoliosis.[86,87] Scoliosis typically presents at a young age, with just over half of the patients being diagnosed by age 10.[87] Thoracic curves may progress an average 5 degrees per year, lumbar curves average 4 degrees of progression per year, and kyphosis increased an average of 5 degrees per year.[87] Similar rates of progression for scoliosis were found in the review of 51 patients by Kaplan et al, but they found progression of kyphosis up to 9 degrees per year.[88]

The majority of these patients are now surviving into adulthood and thus treatment of scoliosis becomes an increasingly important issue.[87] Of the patients treated with bracing in the retrospective study by Hayek et al, 89% had progression despite bracing. The 11% of patients who did not progress only had small curves to begin with, averaging 21 degrees upon initiation of bracing. Other studies have likewise found that bracing is of minimal benefit in these patients, largely due to poor compliance as a result of pulmonary, emotional, and skin problems (due to insensitivity to pain).[86,88,89]

Historically, spinal fusion has been performed for coronal Cobb angles of 40 to 45 degrees or sagittal Cobb angles measuring 80 degrees or more.[86,88,89] Pulmonary infections are common in these patients; PSF may help avoid further pulmonary complications. Rubery et al, likewise, reported successful posterior-only treatment of 20 of 22 patients.[89] Unlike the constructs needed for many other neuromuscular conditions, shorter fusions may be successful.[88] Regardless of approach or fusion level, great care needs to be taken for preoperative optimization of these patients. In particular, they should have good control over dysautonomic crises, nutrition, psychological issues, and pulmonary infections.[89]

Ataxia-Telangiectasia

Ataxia-telangiectasia (A-T) is a progressive neurodegenerative disorder characterized by autosomal recessive inheritance. Soon after learning to walk, patients develop ataxia and proprioception continues to decrease with age. They are frequently wheelchair bound by age 10.[90] The life span of these patients has been improving, with most living past age 25 years and some surviving into the sixth decade, though earlier studies have reported only 11% living past 30 years.[91,92]

Overall, there is a paucity of literature on scoliosis in association with A-T. In the senior author's experience, gait assistance is often needed by age 9 years with loss of ambulatory ability by age 15 years. Most patients are unable to sit unsupported by age 13 years. There was a 10% prevalence of scoliosis in this group of patients (21 patients). Of the patients with scoliosis, 90% (19) were successfully treated with bracing and observation. The two patients that required surgery had 82- and 70-degree lumbar curves and underwent long construct fusion to the pelvis without complication.

It is important to consider in these patients that they are at risk for leukemia and lymphoma. They are radiation sensitive and therefore radiographs need to be limited when it comes to scoliosis surveillance. During the adolescent growth spurt, when surveillance is most closely needed, annual radiographs are likely sufficient. These patients are also immunocompromised and prone to infection.[90]

3.3 Conclusion

The indications for treatment of neuromuscular deformity are guided by knowledge of the natural history of the specific disorder. Life expectancy, complication rates, and functional limitations are taken into account in the process of shared decision making with families and other medical experts for these patients.

References

[1] Duckworth AD, Mitchell MJ, Tsirikos AI. Incidence and risk factors for postoperative complications after scoliosis surgery in patients with Duchenne muscular dystrophy: a comparison with other neuromuscular conditions. Bone Joint J. 2014; 96-B(7):943–949

[2] Mackenzie WG, Matsumoto H, Williams BA, et al. Surgical site infection following spinal instrumentation for scoliosis: a multicenter analysis of rates, risk factors, and pathogens. J Bone Joint Surg Am. 2013; 95(9):800–806, S1–S2

[3] Murphy NA, Firth S, Jorgensen T, Young PC. Spinal surgery in children with idiopathic and neuromuscular scoliosis. What's the difference? J Pediatr Orthop. 2006; 26(2):216–220

[4] Sharma S, Wu C, Andersen T, Wang Y, Hansen ES, Bünger CE. Prevalence of complications in neuromuscular scoliosis surgery: a literature meta-analysis from the past 15 years. Eur Spine J. 2013; 22(6):1230–1249

[5] Kang GR, Suh SW, Lee IO. Preoperative predictors of postoperative pulmonary complications in neuromuscular scoliosis. J Orthop Sci. 2011; 16(2):139–147

[6] Menga EN, Hirschfeld C, Jain A, et al. Intraoperative cardiopulmonary arrest in children undergoing spinal deformity correction: causes and associated factors. Spine. 2015; 40(22):1757–1762

[7] Verhaert D, Richards K, Rafael-Fortney JA, Raman SV. Cardiac involvement in patients with muscular dystrophies: magnetic resonance imaging phenotype and genotypic considerations. Circ Cardiovasc Imaging. 2011; 4(1):67–76

[8] Sponseller PD, LaPorte DM, Hungerford MW, Eck K, Bridwell KH, Lenke LG. Deep wound infections after neuromuscular scoliosis surgery: a multicenter study of risk factors and treatment outcomes. Spine. 2000; 25(19):2461–2466

[9] Briassoulis G, Zavras N, Hatzis T. Malnutrition, nutritional indices, and early enteral feeding in critically ill children. Nutrition. 2001; 17(7–8):548–557

[10] Lapp MA, Bridwell KH, Lenke LG, Baldus C, Blanke K, Iffrig TM. Prospective randomization of parenteral hyperalimentation for long fusions with spinal deformity: its effect on complications and recovery from postoperative malnutrition. Spine. 2001; 26(7):809–817, discussion 817

[11] Skalsky AJ, Dalal PB. Common complications of pediatric neuromuscular disorders. Phys Med Rehabil Clin N Am. 2015; 26(1):21–28

[12] Gilbert SR, Savage AJ, Whitesell R, Conklin MJ, Fineberg NS. BMI and magnitude of scoliosis at presentation to a specialty clinic. Pediatrics. 2015; 135(6): e1417–e1424

[13] Upasani VV, Caltoum C, Petcharaporn M, et al. Does obesity affect surgical outcomes in adolescent idiopathic scoliosis? Spine. 2008; 33(3):295–300

[14] Hardesty CK, Poe-Kochert C, Son-Hing JP, Thompson GH. Obesity negatively affects spinal surgery in idiopathic scoliosis. Clin Orthop Relat Res. 2013; 471 (4):1230–1235

[15] Sing DC, Yue JK, Metz LN, et al. Obesity is an independent risk factor of early complications after revision spine surgery. Spine. 2016; 41(10):E632–E640

[16] Gutierrez EM, Bartonek A, Haglund-Akerlind Y, Saraste H. Characteristic gait kinematics in persons with lumbosacral myelomeningocele. Gait Posture. 2003; 18(3):170–177

[17] Saito N, Ebara S, Ohotsuka K, Kumeta H, Takaoka K. Natural history of scoliosis in spastic cerebral palsy. Lancet. 1998; 351(9117):1687–1692

[18] Hodgkinson I, Berard C, Chotel F, Berard J. Pelvic obliquity and scoliosis in non-ambulatory patients with cerebral palsy: a descriptive study of 234 patients over 15 years of age [in French]. Rev Chir Orthop Repar Appar Mot. 2002; 88(4):337–341

[19] Majd ME, Muldowny DS, Holt RT. Natural history of scoliosis in the institutionalized adult cerebral palsy population. Spine. 1997; 22(13):1461–1466

[20] Kalen V, Conklin MM, Sherman FC. Untreated scoliosis in severe cerebral palsy. J Pediatr Orthop. 1992; 12(3):337–340

[21] Ginsburg GM, Lauder AJ. Progression of scoliosis in patients with spastic quadriplegia after the insertion of an intrathecal baclofen pump. Spine. 2007; 32(24):2745–2750

[22] Senaran H, Shah SA, Presedo A, Dabney KW, Glutting JW, Miller F. The risk of progression of scoliosis in cerebral palsy patients after intrathecal baclofen therapy. Spine. 2007; 32(21):2348–2354

[23] Shilt JS, Lai LP, Cabrera MN, Frino J, Smith BP. The impact of intrathecal baclofen on the natural history of scoliosis in cerebral palsy. J Pediatr Orthop. 2008; 28(6):684–687

[24] Rushton PR, Nasto LA, Aujla RK, Ammar A, Grevitt MP, Vloeberghs MH. Intrathecal baclofen pumps do not accelerate progression of scoliosis in quadriplegic spastic cerebral palsy. Eur Spine J. 2017; 26(6):1652–1657

[25] Yaszay B, Sponseller PD, Shah SA, et al. Performing a definitive fusion in juvenile CP patients is a good surgical option. J Pediatr Orthop. 2016:(e:-pub ahead of print)

[26] McElroy MJ, Sponseller PD, Dattilo JR, et al. Growing Spine Study Group. Growing rods for the treatment of scoliosis in children with cerebral palsy: a critical assessment. Spine. 2012; 37(24):E1504–E1510

[27] Sponseller PD, Yang JS, Thompson GH, et al. Pelvic fixation of growing rods: comparison of constructs. Spine. 2009; 34(16):1706–1710

[28] Fujimori T, Yaszay B, Bartley CE, Bastrom TP, Newton PO. Safety of pedicle screws and spinal instrumentation for pediatric patients: comparative analysis between 0- and 5-year-old, 5- and 10-year-old, and 10- and 15-year-old patients. Spine. 2014; 39(7):541–549

[29] Abol Oyoun N, Stuecker R. Bilateral rib-to-pelvis Eiffel Tower VEPTR construct for children with neuromuscular scoliosis: a preliminary report. Spine J. 2014; 14(7):1183–1191

[30] Dannawi Z, Altaf F, Harshavardhana NS, El Sebaie H, Noordeen H. Early results of a remotely-operated magnetic growth rod in early-onset scoliosis. Bone Joint J. 2013; 95-B(1):75–80

[31] Cheung KM, Cheung JP, Samartzis D, et al. Magnetically controlled growing rods for severe spinal curvature in young children: a prospective case series. Lancet. 2012; 379(9830):1967–1974

[32] Beckmann K, Lange T, Gosheger G, et al. Surgical correction of scoliosis in patients with severe cerebral palsy. Eur Spine J. 2016; 25(2):506–516

[33] Teli MG, Cinnella P, Vincitorio F, Lovi A, Grava G, Brayda-Bruno M. Spinal fusion with Cotrel-Dubousset instrumentation for neuropathic scoliosis in patients with cerebral palsy. Spine. 2006; 31(14):E441–E447

[34] Imrie MN, Yaszay B. Management of spinal deformity in cerebral palsy. Orthop Clin North Am. 2010; 41(4):531–547

[35] Yaszay B, Scannell BP, Bomar JD, et al. Harms Study Group. Although inconvenient, baclofen pumps do not complicate scoliosis surgery in patients with cerebral palsy. Spine. 2015; 40(8):E504–E509

[36] Alman BA, Raza SN, Biggar WD. Steroid treatment and the development of scoliosis in males with Duchenne muscular dystrophy. J Bone Joint Surg Am. 2004; 86-A(3):519–524

[37] Lebel DE, Corston JA, McAdam LC, Biggar WD, Alman BA. Glucocorticoid treatment for the prevention of scoliosis in children with Duchenne muscular dystrophy: long-term follow-up. J Bone Joint Surg Am. 2013; 95(12):1057–1061

[38] Smith AD, Koreska J, Moseley. CF. Progression of scoliosis in Duchenne muscular dystrophy. J Bone Joint Surg Am. 1989; 71(7):1066–1074

[39] Kinali M, Messina S, Mercuri E, et al. Management of scoliosis in Duchenne muscular dystrophy: a large 10-year retrospective study. Dev Med Child Neurol. 2006; 48(6):513–518

[40] Suk KS, Lee BH, Lee HM, et al. Functional outcomes in Duchenne muscular dystrophy scoliosis: comparison of the differences between surgical and non-surgical treatment. J Bone Joint Surg Am. 2014; 96(5):409–415

[41] Galasko CS, Williamson JB, Delaney CM. Lung function in Duchenne muscular dystrophy. Eur Spine J. 1995; 4(5):263–267

[42] Yamashita T, Kanaya K, Yokogushi K, Ishikawa Y, Minami R. Correlation between progression of spinal deformity and pulmonary function in Duchenne muscular dystrophy. J Pediatr Orthop. 2001; 21(1):113–116

[43] Brook PD, Kennedy JD, Stern LM, Sutherland AD, Foster BK. Spinal fusion in Duchenne's muscular dystrophy. J Pediatr Orthop. 1996; 16(3):324–331

[44] Marsh A, Edge G, Lehovsky J. Spinal fusion in patients with Duchenne's muscular dystrophy and a low forced vital capacity. Eur Spine J. 2003; 12(5):507–512

[45] Kennedy JD, Staples AJ, Brook PD, et al. Effect of spinal surgery on lung function in Duchenne muscular dystrophy. Thorax. 1995; 50(11):1173–1178

[46] Miller F, Moseley CF, Koreska J, Levison H. Pulmonary function and scoliosis in Duchenne dystrophy. J Pediatr Orthop. 1988; 8(2):133–137

[47] Muntoni F, Bushby K, Manzur AY. Muscular Dystrophy Campaign Funded Workshop on Management of Scoliosis in Duchenne Muscular Dystrophy 24 January 2005, London, UK. Neuromuscul Disord. 2006; 16(3):210–219

[48] Manzur AY, Kinali M, Muntoni F. Update on the management of Duchenne muscular dystrophy. Arch Dis Child. 2008; 93(11):986–990

[49] Corrado G, Lissoni A, Beretta S, et al. Prognostic value of electrocardiograms, ventricular late potentials, ventricular arrhythmias, and left ventricular systolic dysfunction in patients with Duchenne muscular dystrophy. Am J Cardiol. 2002; 89(7):838–841

[50] Granata C, Merlini L, Cervellati S, et al. Long-term results of spine surgery in Duchenne muscular dystrophy. Neuromuscul Disord. 1996; 6(1):61–68

[51] Müller EB, Nordwall A, Odén A. Progression of scoliosis in children with myelomeningocele. Spine. 1994; 19(2):147–150

[52] Trivedi J, Thomson JD, Slakey JB, Banta JV, Jones PW. Clinical and radiographic predictors of scoliosis in patients with myelomeningocele. J Bone Joint Surg Am. 2002; 84-A(8):1389–1394

[53] Guille JT, Sarwark JF, Sherk HH, Kumar SJ. Congenital and developmental deformities of the spine in children with myelomeningocele. J Am Acad Orthop Surg. 2006; 14(5):294–302

[54] Khoshbin A, Law PW, Caspi L, Wright JG. Long-term functional outcomes of resected tarsal coalitions. Foot Ankle Int. 2013; 34(10):1370–1375

[55] Mazur J, Menelaus MB, Dickens DR, Doig WG. Efficacy of surgical management for scoliosis in myelomeningocele: correction of deformity and alteration of functional status. J Pediatr Orthop. 1986; 6(5):568–575

[56] Mesfin A, Sponseller PD, Leet AI. Spinal muscular atrophy: manifestations and management. J Am Acad Orthop Surg. 2012; 20(6):393–401

[57] Evans GA, Drennan JC, Russman BS. Functional classification and orthopaedic management of spinal muscular atrophy. J Bone Joint Surg Br. 1981; 63B(4):516–522

[58] McElroy MJ, Shaner AC, Crawford TO, et al. Growing rods for scoliosis in spinal muscular atrophy: structural effects, complications, and hospital stays. Spine. 2011; 36(16):1305–1311

[59] Chiriboga CA, Swoboda KJ, Darras BT, et al. Results from a phase 1 study of nusinersen (ISIS-SMN(Rx)) in children with spinal muscular atrophy. Neurology. 2016; 86(10):890–897

[60] Zebala LP, Bridwell KH, Baldus C, et al. Minimum 5-year radiographic results of long scoliosis fusion in juvenile spinal muscular atrophy patients: major curve progression after instrumented fusion. J Pediatr Orthop. 2011; 31(5):480–488

[61] Fujak A, Raab W, Schuh A, Kreß A, Forst R, Forst J. Operative treatment of scoliosis in proximal spinal muscular atrophy: results of 41 patients. Arch Orthop Trauma Surg. 2012; 132(12):1697–1706

[62] Cirak B, Ziegfeld S, Knight VM, Chang D, Avellino AM, Paidas CN. Spinal injuries in children. J Pediatr Surg. 2004; 39(4):607–612

[63] Mulcahey MJ, Gaughan JP, Betz RR, Samdani AF, Barakat N, Hunter LN. Neuromuscular scoliosis in children with spinal cord injury. Top Spinal Cord Inj Rehabil. 2013; 19(2):96–103

[64] Dearolf WW, III, Betz RR, Vogel LC, Levin J, Clancy M, Steel HH. Scoliosis in pediatric spinal cord-injured patients. J Pediatr Orthop. 1990; 10(2):214–218

[65] Bergström EM, Henderson NJ, Short DJ, Frankel HL, Jones PR. The relation of thoracic and lumbar fracture configuration to the development of late deformity in childhood spinal cord injury. Spine. 2003; 28(2):171–176

[66] Pang D. Spinal cord injury without radiographic abnormality in children, 2 decades later. Neurosurgery. 2004; 55(6):1325–1342, discussion 1342–1343

[67] Mehta S, Betz RR, Mulcahey MJ, McDonald C, Vogel LC, Anderson C. Effect of bracing on paralytic scoliosis secondary to spinal cord injury. J Spinal Cord Med. 2004; 27 Suppl 1:S88–S92

[68] Sison-Williamson M, Bagley A, Hongo A, et al. Effect of thoracolumbosacral orthoses on reachable workspace volumes in children with spinal cord injury. J Spinal Cord Med. 2007; 30 Suppl 1:S184–S191

[69] Parent S, Dimar J, Dekutoski M, Roy-Beaudry M. Unique features of pediatric spinal cord injury. Spine. 2010; 35(21) Suppl:S202–S208

[70] Fassier A, Wicart P, Dubousset J, Seringe R. Arthrogryposis multiplex congenita. Long-term follow-up from birth until skeletal maturity. J Child Orthop. 2009; 3(5):383–390

[71] Herron LD, Westin GW, Dawson EG. Scoliosis in arthrogryposis multiplex congenita. J Bone Joint Surg Am. 1978; 60(3):293–299

[72] Yingsakmongkol W, Kumar SJ. Scoliosis in arthrogryposis multiplex congenita: results after nonsurgical and surgical treatment. J Pediatr Orthop. 2000; 20(5):656–661

[73] Daher YH, Lonstein JE, Winter RB, Moe JH. Spinal deformities in patients with arthrogryposis. A review of 16 patients. Spine. 1985; 10(7):609–613

[74] Astur N, Flynn JM, Flynn JM, et al. The efficacy of rib-based distraction with VEPTR in the treatment of early-onset scoliosis in patients with arthrogryposis. J Pediatr Orthop. 2014; 34(1):8–13

[75] Drummond DS, Mackenzie DA. Scoliosis in arthrogryposis multiplex congenita. Spine. 1978; 3(2):146–151

[76] Greggi T, Martikos K, Pipitone E, et al. Surgical treatment of scoliosis in a rare disease: arthrogryposis. Scoliosis. 2010; 5:24

[77] O'Brien JP, Dwyer AP, Hodgson AR. Paralytic pelvic obliquity. Its prognosis and management and the development of a technique for full correction of the deformity. J Bone Joint Surg Am. 1975; 57(5):626–631

[78] Riise R, Brox JI, Sorensen R, Skjeldal OH. Spinal deformity and disability in patients with Rett syndrome. Dev Med Child Neurol. 2011; 53(7):653–657

[79] Anderson A, Wong K, Jacoby P, Downs J, Leonard H. Twenty years of surveillance in Rett syndrome: what does this tell us? Orphanet J Rare Dis. 2014; 9:87

[80] Tarquinio DC, Hou W, Neul JL, et al. The changing face of survival in Rett syndrome and MECP2-related disorders. Pediatr Neurol. 2015; 53(5):402–411

[81] Downs J, Bergman A, Carter P, et al. Guidelines for management of scoliosis in Rett syndrome patients based on expert consensus and clinical evidence. Spine. 2009; 34(17):E607–E617

[82] Larsson EL, Aaro S, Ahlinder P, Normelli H, Tropp H, Oberg B. Long-term follow-up of functioning after spinal surgery in patients with Rett syndrome. Eur Spine J. 2009; 18(4):506–511

[83] Milbrandt TA, Kunes JR, Karol LA. Friedreich's ataxia and scoliosis: the experience at two institutions. J Pediatr Orthop. 2008; 28(2):234–238

[84] Labelle H, Tohmé S, Duhaime M, Allard P. Natural history of scoliosis in Friedreich's ataxia. J Bone Joint Surg Am. 1986; 68(4):564–572

[85] Tsirikos AI, Smith G. Scoliosis in patients with Friedreich's ataxia. J Bone Joint Surg Br. 2012; 94(5):684–689

[86] Bar-On E, Floman Y, Sagiv S, Katz K, Pollak RD, Maayan C. Orthopaedic manifestations of familial dysautonomia. A review of one hundred and thirty-six patients. J Bone Joint Surg Am. 2000; 82-A(11):1563–1570

[87] Hayek S, Laplaza FJ, Axelrod FB, Burke SW. Spinal deformity in familial dysautonomia. Prevalence, and results of bracing. J Bone Joint Surg Am. 2000; 82-A (11):1558–1562

[88] Kaplan L, Margulies JY, Kadari A, Floman Y, Robin GC. Aspects of spinal deformity in familial dysautonomia (Riley-Day syndrome). Eur Spine J. 1997; 6(1):33–38

[89] Rubery PT, Spielman JH, Hester P, Axelrod E, Burke SW, Levine DB. Scoliosis in familial dysautonomia. Operative treatment. J Bone Joint Surg Am. 1995; 77 (9):1362–1369

[90] Gatti R. Ataxia-Telangiectasia. In: Pagon RA, Adam MP, Ardinger HH, et al., eds. GeneReviews(R). Seattle, WA: University of Washington; 1993

[91] Dörk T, Bendix-Waltes R, Wegner RD, Stumm M. Slow progression of ataxia-telangiectasia with double missense and in frame splice mutations. Am J Med Genet A. 2004; 126A(3):272–277

[92] Morrell D, Cromartie E, Swift M. Mortality and cancer incidence in 263 patients with ataxia-telangiectasia. J Natl Cancer Inst. 1986; 77(1):89–92

4 Intraoperative Issues: Anesthesia, Neuromonitoring, Estimated Blood Loss

Paul D. Kiely, Akhil A. Tawari, Jahangir K. Asghar, and Harry L. Shufflebarger

Abstract

Children with neuromuscular scoliosis pose unique, challenges and a multidisciplinary team approach including the surgeon, pediatrician, experienced anesthesiologist, pediatric respiratory physician, cardiologist, and physical therapist is highly encouraged. Apart from the routine preoperative assessment, nutritional studies, gastrointestinal assessment, pulmonary function testing polysomnogram, and two-dimensional echocardiography must be performed in all cases. Respiratory and cardiac complication rates are higher in patients with neuromuscular spinal, and a respiratory training program comprised of noninvasive positive pressure ventilation may be offered. Intravenous anesthesia offers many benefits to patients with neuromuscular disorders, as the agents are short acting and are usually preferred. Patients are prone to excessive blood loss and thermodysregulation intraoperatively, and the operating room personnel must have appropriate prophylactic and corrective strategies including controlled hypotensive anesthesia, the use of the cell salvage system, intraoperative use of packed red blood cells, fresh frozen plasma, cryoprecipitate, antifibrinolytics, and temperature probe. Intraoperative neuromonitoring might reveal inconsistent signals; however, 50% amplitude reduction of the initial baseline reading should be considered significant.

Keywords: anesthesia, neuromuscular scoliosis, somatosensory evoked potential, tranexamic acid

4.1 Introduction

Neuromuscular scoliosis is the result of disturbed muscle function on the spinal column. The etiology can be either neuropathic or myopathic in origin. In contrast to adolescent idiopathic scoliosis (AIS), neuromuscular spinal often presents at an early age, can rapidly progress during the prepubescent growth phase, and may continue beyond skeletal maturity. Surgical intervention is complex, but quality of life, natural history of the underlying disorder, and the increased complication rate all deserve careful consideration before proceeding with any surgical intervention. This chapter focuses on the intraoperative challenges presented by children with neuromuscular spinal in relation to anesthesia, neuromonitoring, and blood loss during posterior spinal fusion and instrumentation.

The day of surgery likely represents the most dangerous day in the life of a child with neuromuscular spinal. All members of the care team must perform at the peak of their capabilities. A comprehensive plan must be in place well in advance and vigilance must be high. Ongoing discussions about the patient's status throughout the course of surgery are crucial to optimizing outcomes and mitigating untoward events. In spite of excellent planning, the patient's condition often changes during spinal deformity surgery. Skilled team members who communicate effectively can detect such changes early and act to prevent untoward outcomes. Surgeons must be able to make quick, complex decisions as new information emerges. Often, surgical goals and plans must be modified. We strongly encourage the use of dedicated team members who routinely participate in complex spinal deformity surgery—experienced anesthesia, nursing, and radiology personnel, neurophysiology, and surgical assistants.

4.2 Anesthesia

Children with neuromuscular spinal pose many anesthetic challenges and are at greater risk for perioperative complications, particularly of the respiratory and the cardiovascular systems.[1,2] As a consequence, these children require special precautions, including a multidisciplinary approach to optimize their management. The authors employ and recommend the same anesthesia personnel team for all cases. The goals of blood pressure management including hypotensive anesthesia during exposure (generally mean arterial pressure [MAP] < 75 mm Hg), estimated blood loss (EBL) at which blood is to be initiated, and MAP goals greater than 80 mm Hg at rod insertion are discussed at the start of the procedure.

4.2.1 Preoperative Management

Preoperative evaluation and optimization of comorbidities is critical and hence a multidisciplinary team approach is highly recommended. In our center, the multidisciplinary team is composed of a deformity surgeon, pediatrician, pediatric respiratory physician, cardiologist, experienced anesthetist, and physical therapist. Diagnostic studies routinely include complete blood count, basic metabolic panel, coagulation studies, nutritional studies, gastrointestinal assessment, pulmonary function testing if child is cooperative, or polysomnogram and two-dimensional echocardiography.

Particular attention is paid to the respiratory systems of patients with neuromuscular scoliosis, as the Healthcare Cost and Utilization Project Kids' Inpatient Database (HCUP KID) showed that patients with neuromuscular scoliosis were 10 times more likely to aspirate and require mechanical ventilation postoperatively, and 5 times more likely to develop pneumonia than patients with AIS undergoing posterior spinal fusion.[3,4] Pulmonary dysfunction is usually greater in severity and more frequent than in patients with AIS. The high incidence of respiratory complications is due to the frequent involvement of respiratory and pharyngeal musclesas well as the high incidence of sleep apnea in children with neuromuscular scoliosis.[5] Progressive deformities cause restrictive lung disease and aggravate chronic respiratory insufficiency. The administration of anesthetic agents that depress the respiratory system contributes to this decompensation, particularly in patients with disturbed neuromuscular transmission. Preoperative optimization of the respiratory system may also be a useful adjunct in patients with neuromuscular scoliosis awaiting spinal surgery. Khirani et al placed 13 patients with planned spinal surgery in a respiratory training program in which noninvasive positive pressure ventilation and mechanical insufflation/ exsufflation were used for 30 minutes per day for at least 1 to 4 weeks before surgery.[6,7] No postoperative respiratory complications were observed in any of the patients, highlighting the potential role of preoperative optimization prior to spinal surgery.

In patients with neuromuscular scoliosis, cardiac arrest is the second most common reason for perioperative and postoperative mortality.[2,8] Cardiac muscle and conducting pathways are often adversely affected in neuromuscular spinal, even though many patients are asymptomatic.[8] neuromuscular spinal patients are often unaware of this underlying cardiac anomaly, as they are unable to exercise vigorously, owing to the muscle disorder. Understanding their functional cardiac reserve using an echocardiogram is important as perioperative and postoperative stress may induce failure in these vulnerable patients. Volatile anesthetics are cardiodepressive because they reduce the availability of both myoplasmic calcium and also decrease the responsiveness of the contractile filaments to calcium.[9] Volatile anesthetics may also cause arrhythmia due to the sensitization of the heart to catecholamines and from their inhibitory effects on voltage-gated potassium channels, which are essential for membrane repolarization. Prolongation of the QT interval, in addition to hyperkalemia produced by suxamethonium-induced rhabdomyolysis, may contribute to this arrhythmia.[8,10] A cardiology examination, in addition to an electrocardiogram, chest radiograph, and echocardiogram would help identify these susceptible patients preoperatively. Patients with a cardiomyopathy should be optimized preoperatively, with the European Alliance of Muscular Dystrophy Associations recommending treatment for 4 months prior to surgical intervention.[11]

Bowel function requires assessment, as wheelchair-bound patients have bowel dysmotility. A child with neuromuscular spinal who is constipated with a heavily filled bowel will have reduced pulmonary function. Adequate nutrition is also important, as malnutrition often accompanies children with cerebral palsy (CP) and dystrophic dystrophies, due to the dysfunction of the muscles of mastication and swallowing, in addition to reflux esophagitis. Malnutrition is associated with poor wound healing, infection, fatigue, and apathy.

4.2.2 Perioperative Management

A preoperative assessment for lower and upper extremity contractures guides intraoperative patient positioning. Prone positioning on an open Jackson table is performed for all cases. These frame type spine tables are mandatory to accommodate the low positioning of the hips and knees in the presence of flexion contractures that are routine in these patients. In the presence of flexion contractures of the shoulders and elbows, the arms can be tucked at the sides or placed directly on the frame. An ample number of foam and gel pads must be used to avoid pressure sores.

Neuromuscular spinal surgeries are associated with greater blood loss than AIS surgeries. The authors routinely obtain central line, peripheral line, and arterial line accesses for all cases.

Temperature measurement and control is also extremely important, as patients with neuromuscular spinal are susceptible to thermodysregulation.[5] Temperature probe is recommended for all cases. Hypothermia may develop due to reduced heat production from immobile muscles, which may be compounded by the peripheral vasodilation that occurs with general anesthesia. Patients should be normothermic prior to induction, and their temperature maintained with forced air warming systems and warmed fluids, if necessary.[12] In some neuromuscular disorders, hypothermia can exacerbate myotonia and potentially aggravate rhabdomyolysis. Hyperthermia may occur secondary to increased muscle activity, associated with myotonias and malignant hyperthermia. A high index of suspicion should exist for patients with muscular dystrophies and myotonias for concomitant malignant hyperthermia. Unexplained tachycardia with an increase in end tidal carbon dioxide concentration should alert the anesthetist to a potential hyperthermic complication.[13,14]

The use of volatile agents for general anesthesia is controversial. Volatile agents have been contraindicated in the past because of their association with malignant hyperthermia, in conditions such as Duchenne muscular dystrophy (DMD). Although this link is now thought to be tenuous, a total intravenous anesthetic with a clean anesthetic machine is recommended to avoid the development of rhabdomyolysis.[15] Nitrous oxide, potent inhalation agents, and muscle relaxants have been demonstrated to compromise neurophysiological signals.[16,17] In addition to this, cardiovascular decompensation may be caused by volatile agents due to their cardiodepressive and arrhythmogenic properties. Intravenous anesthesia offers many benefits to patients with neuromuscular disorders, as the agents are short acting. However, care must be taken due to the potential for autonomic dysfunction and cardiovascular collapse.

Perioperative antibiotic coverage with clindamycin with repeat doses every 6 hours and changes of gown and gloves after 3 to 4 hours are routinely performed.[18]

4.2.3 Postoperative Management

Patients with neuromuscular disorders in the postoperative period are at an increased risk of cardiorespiratory complications, autonomic dysfunction, myotonias, and rhabdomyolysis.[2,6] Respiratory failure is the most common cause of death in these patients, with bulbar muscle weakness leading to aspiration, poor pharyngeal and respiratory muscle tone, and obstructive sleep apnea all contributing to the development of this problem.[6] Extubation should be achieved as early as possible to prevent further weakening of the respiratory musculature but considered against the risk of atelectasis, aspiration, infection, and respiratory failure. The rate of extubation in the operating room (OR) is variable and highly patient dependent, but it is generally around 70 to 80% at our institution. The decision for immediate postoperative extubation should take into consideration the patient's baseline pulmonary status, the difficulty of intubation at the outset of surgery, and the availability of a team skilled at obtaining an emergent airway. Patients with DMD, preoperative FVC < 30% of predictive, hemodynamic instability and prolonged surgery greater than 8 to 10 hours are more prone to require postoperative ventilator support. Cardiomyopathies and conduction abnormalities may predispose to morbidity and mortality in the postoperative period.[2,3] As a result, a patient with neuromuscular spinal should be treated as a high cardiac risk, with appropriate invasive monitoring in situ, and inotropic drugs administered if required.

Autonomic dysfunction is not uncommon and can be responsible for hypotension on induction. Gastric dysmotility can lead to regurgitation and aspiration during general anesthesia.[19] Sympathomimetic drugs need to be available for use, but the doses modified due to the increased sensitivity of alpha and beta receptors in patients with NMS. Myotonic contractures can occur with the dystrophic and nondystrophic myotonias. The contractures are caused by repeated action potentials that lead to sodium influx and chloride efflux, rendering the neuron hyerexcitable.[10] Myotonic contractures can be caused by a number of agents including opioids, anticholinesterases, and succinylcholine. Environmental factors may also be responsible, including acidosis, alterations in ambient temperature, and shivering. If a myotonia is triggered, agents that block sodium channels, such as antiarrhythmic agents and local anesthetics, should be administered.

Rhabdomyolysis may be associated with volatile agents, myotonias, and depolarizing neuromuscular blocking agents.[15] Signs of rhabdomyolysis include metabolic acidosis, hyperkalemia, myoglobinuria, and elevated creatinine kinase. Treatment involves cessation of the causative agent and correction of the hyperkalemia.

4.3 Neuromonitoring

Iatrogenic spinal cord injury remains the most devastating complication of spinal fusion surgery and ranges from sensory disturbance to paraplegia. The incidence of acute neurological complications during scoliosis surgery varies from 0.5 to 0.72%.[20] The incidence of neurologic injury in neuromuscular spinal is much higher than in AIS[21] and may be related to the greater intraoperative blood loss that compromises the vascularity of the cord, in addition to the distraction techniques adopted occasionally by deformity surgeons to correct the severest and stiffest neuromuscular curves.

Intraoperative neurophysiological monitoring of the spinal cord is essential to reduce the risk of spinal cord injury during deformity surgery. Since Nash et al's seminal paper in 1977 on spinal cord monitoring during operative treatment of the spine, the importance of spinal cord monitoring has increased.[22] Prior to its introduction, the only method for detecting spinal cord injury was the Stagnara wake-up test, which consisted of waking the patient intraoperatively and observing voluntary lower extremity movement.[23] Although the wake-up test is still regarded as the standard to assess global motor function, it is not always practical in patients with neuromuscular spinal who have intellectual disabilities, muscle weakness, or both. In addition, an ischemic spinal cord injury may not present immediately following a correctional maneuver, and the patient may be able to move the lower extremities voluntarily at the time of the wake-up test, only to demonstrate paralysis on emergence from anesthesia.

In contrast to the wake-up test, spinal cord monitoring provides a continuous means to assess the integrity of the cord. Neuromonitoring offers early detection of reversible neurophysiological dysfunction that enables prompt intervention to prevent the occurrence of permanent neurological damage. MacEwen et al have demonstrated that the recovery of a neurological deficit is directly proportional to the speed of removal of malpositioned instrumentation.[24] Intraoperative monitoring using somatosensory evoked potentials (SSEPs) alone is inadequate for monitoring the descending spinal cord motor tracts or the spinal gray matter, as SSEPs are mediated by the posterior sensory column of the spinal cord.[25] Transcranial electric motor evoked potentials (MEPs) are an effective and clinically practical way to monitor spinal cord motor function in real time during corrective spine surgery.[26] Schwartz et al reported that transcranial MEPs were 100% sensitive in detecting evolving neurological injury, whereas SSEPs were only 43% sensitive.[27] In addition to better sensitivities, transcranial MEPs detect emerging spinal cord motor injury at an average of 5 minutes sooner than SSEPs.[27]

The differential sensitivities of transcranial MEPs and SSEPs to evolving spinal cord injury are thought to be related to the vascular supply of the motor pathways. The anterior horn motor neurons within the spinal cord and the spinal motor interneurons have a high metabolic rate and are vulnerable to vascular insult. Since most neurological injuries during deformity surgery are thought to be ischemic in nature, transcranial MEPs are more likely to change first during these corrective maneuvers.[28] Transcranial MEPs have been previously demonstrated to be reliable in identifying cord ischemia during abdominal aortic aneurysm repair and spinal operations.[29]

However, intraoperative neuromonitoring, in neuromuscular spinal is variable and reflects the underlying abnormal neural pathways, particularly in patients with CP or Charcot–Marie–Tooth disease.[6] Hammett et al evaluated 66 patients with CP and were only able to establish reliable baseline SSEPs in 88% of patients.[28] Noordeen et al retrospectively reviewed 99 patients who underwent reconstructive surgery for neuromuscular spinal (55 DMD, 30 spinal muscular atrophy [SMA], and 14 miscellaneous) and obtained SSEP tracings in 98% of patients.[17] Concerns over the perceived potential to initiate epileptic seizures have precluded many authors from the routine use of transcranial MEPs in patients with NMS. Salem et al have, however, recently found that transcranial MEPs do not trigger intraoperative or postoperative seizures in patients with NMS undergoing posterior spinal fusions, nor are they associated with a deterioration in the seizure control of patients who suffer from seizures.[30] While the challenge of obtaining consistently reliable tracing is difficult in patients with NMS, with signal changes being less sensitive and specific, the presence of false-positive SSEPs is usually secondary to hypotension, depth of anesthesia, and temperature changes. A decline in the amplitude of 50% of the initial baseline reading should, however, be considered significant and carries a definitive risk of spinal cord injury.[25,27]

4.4 Blood Loss and Management

Posterior spinal fusion in patients with neuromuscular scoliosis is associated with significantly higher blood loss and transfusion requirements than children with AIS.[30] The increased blood loss is thought to be related to several factors, including the depletion of clotting factors, longer surgical procedures and fusion constructs, malnutrition, and anticonvulsant seizure medication. Kannan et al compared patients with neuromuscular scoliosis and AIS undergoing posterior spinal fusion and found that there was a greater depletion of factor VII clotting in the neuromuscular group.[31] Brenn et al also found a discrepancy in the clotting factors between the two groups, with decreased coagulation factors present in the neuromuscular scoliosis group, in addition to the prolongation of clotting parameters (partial thromboplastin time [PTT] and prothrombin time [PT]).[32] Poor nutritional status and anticonvulsant medication in the NMS group increased intraoperative blood loss by decreasing platelet count and interfering with liver metabolism and the manufacture of clotting factors (factor VIII).[33] Valproic acid has been shown to cause thrombocytopenia and coagulation abnormalities. Chambers et al reported a 26% increase in blood loss in patients on sodium valproate.[34] If feasible, alternative medication may be started in the preoperative period. Furthermore, the clotting profile and especially bleeding time must be closely monitored before, during, and after the surgery.

Strategies such as controlled hypotensive anesthesia, the use of the cell salvage system, intraoperative use of fresh frozen plasma (FFP) and cryoprecipitate, and antifibrinolytics (AF) reduce intraoperative blood loss during spinal fusion. In 1982, Lawhon et al highlighted that controlled hypotensive anesthesia (MAP < 90 mm Hg) was associated with a 49% decrease in blood loss and a 42% decrease in blood product requirement.[35] AF, including aprotinin, tranexamic acid (TXA), and epsilon aminocaproic (EACA), have been shown to reduce operative blood loss but not transfusion rate in both AIS and neuromuscular scoliosis patients.[36,37,38] Verma et al have demonstrated that the maintenance of the mean arterial pressure at or below 75 mm Hg during surgical exposure is critical for maximizing antifibrinolytic effect.[37] Aprotinin is a serine protease inhibitor that inhibits kallikrein, plasmin, and platelet activation factor. Since 2007, the production of aprotinin, however, has been prohibited by the U.S. Food and Drug Administration because of higher mortality rates in patients undergoing cardiac surgery. TXA is a lysine analog that blocks lysine binding sites on plasminogen molecules and inhibits fibrinolysis. EACA is a lysine analog that inhibits fibrinolysis by binding to plasminogen and blocking binding of fibrin.[39]

A multicenter retrospective study in 2012 by Dhawale et al evaluated the safety and efficacy of AF agents in reducing blood loss and transfusions during posterior spinal fusion in children with CP.[40] Forty-four patients received AF (30 TXA and 14 EACA) and 40 received no antifibrinolytics (NAF). The EBL averaged 1,684 mL for the AF group and 2,685 mL for the NAF group (p = 0.002). There was more cell salvage transfusion in the NAF group. There were no significant differences in total transfusion requirements and no adverse effects were seen. There was a trend for decreased inpatient hospital stay in the AF group. TXA was more effective than EACA in decreasing EBL and cell salvage transfusion. In comparison to the NAF, this study demonstrated that AF significantly reduced intraoperative EBL during spinal fusion in children with CP. Interestingly, there has been no randomized controlled trial comparing the efficacy of TXA with other AF in children with neuromuscular scoliosis.

Other novel strategies aimed at reducing blood loss in neuromuscular scoliosis surgery include the use of a single posterior rod instrumentation in patients with DMD.[41] Forty-one patients

with DMD underwent early limited instrumentation to maintain adequate seating posture and facilitate postural control. Cawley et al found that the operative time of 96 minutes and total intraoperative blood loss of 2,300 mL were significantly lower than those of DMD patients who had undergone standard double rod and pedicle screw instrumentation technique.[41]

The authors preoperatively calculate the blood volume that the patient can lose for the hemoglobin to fall to 10 g/dL and packed red blood cells (PRBCs) are initiated to keep the hemoglobin above 10 g/dL throughout the procedure. At least 4 units of cross-matched blood are kept ready for all patients with neuromuscular scoliosis. Massive transfusion trauma protocol including higher ratio of FFP to PRBCs of greater than 0.5 may be used to reduce the amount of blood loss secondary to hypofibrinogenemia.[42]

4.5 Exposure

Posterior spinal fusion in the presence of a baclofen pump can be challenging as well as trying for the surgeon. Although it is usually possible to work around the catheter and preserve it, the path for the catheter should be carefully evaluated on the preoperative films. The authors have frequently encountered loops of the catheter crossing the midline before insertion intrathecally, which renders them prone to disruption. In the event of catheter disruption, it can either be re-anastomosed with other systems or the catheter can be removed and a new catheter placed after spinal fusion.

An incomplete posterior arch in the presence of poor soft-tissue coverage makes dissection very challenging in myelodysplastic cases. A standard midline incision with subperiosteal dissection is commonly utilized, which can also facilitate cord detethering at the same time. The dura is carefully separated from the skin. Since the normal posterior landmarks are lacking, the surgeon should first identify normal bony anatomy and then proceed over absent posterior structures. Some authors have also advocated utilizing an inverted Y-shaped incision; however, cord detethering cannot be performed with this approach.[43] Plastic surgeons may assist in flap closure.

Neuromuscular scoliosis cases are prone to wound complications more than AIS cases, and meticulous wound closure should be performed. The authors use a braided suture for achieving a swift and secure wound closure in all index cases of neuromuscular scoliosis. Some authors also advocate the use of a plastic multilayered closure technique by a plastic surgeon for posterior spinal fusion treatment of neuromuscular scoliosis. Ward et al reported a significantly lower rate of postoperative wound complications (0 vs. 19%; p = 0.007) when multilayered closure was performed by experienced plastic surgeons for nonidiopathic scoliosis.[44]

References

[1] Aboussouan LS. Sleep-disordered breathing in neuromuscular disease. Am J Respir Crit Care Med. 2015; 191(9):979–989

[2] Bianco F, Pane M, D'Amico A, et al. Cardiac function in types II and III spinal muscular atrophy: should we change standards of care? Neuropediatrics. 2015; 46(1):33–36

[3] Fauroux B, Quijano-Roy S, Desguerre I, Khirani S. The value of respiratory muscle testing in children with neuromuscular disease. Chest. 2015; 147 (2):552–559

[4] Witt WP, Weiss AJ, Elixhauser A. Overview of hospital stays for children in the United States, 2012. Healthcare Cost and Utilization Project (HCUP) Statistical Brief #187. Rockville, MD: Agency for Healthcare Research and Quality; 2014

[5] Lee HJ, Kim KS, Jeong JS, Kim KN, Lee BC. The influence of mild hypothermia on reversal of rocuronium-induced deep neuromuscular block with sugammadex. BMC Anesthesiol. 2015; 15:7

[6] Khirani S, Ramirez A, Aubertin G, et al. Respiratory muscle decline in Duchenne muscular dystrophy. Pediatr Pulmonol. 2014; 49(5):473–481

[7] Khirani S, Dabaj I, Amaddeo A, Ramirez A, Quijano-Roy S, Fauroux B. The value of respiratory muscle testing in a child with congenital muscular dystrophy. Respirol Case Rep. 2014; 2(3):95–98

[8] Petri H, Sveen ML, Thune JJ, et al. Progression of cardiac involvement in patients with limb-girdle type 2 and Becker muscular dystrophies: a 9-year follow-up study. Int J Cardiol. 2015; 182:403–411

[9] Latham GJ, Lopez G. Anesthetic considerations in myofibrillar myopathy. Paediatr Anaesth. 2015; 25(3):231–238

[10] Algalarrondo V, Wahbi K, Sebag F, et al. Abnormal sodium current properties contribute to cardiac electrical and contractile dysfunction in a mouse model of myotonic dystrophy type 1. Neuromuscul Disord. 2015; 25(4):308–320

[11] Pruijs JE, van Tol MJ, van Kesteren RG, van Nieuwenhuizen O. Neuromuscular scoliosis: clinical evaluation pre- and postoperative. J Pediatr Orthop B. 2000; 9(4):217–220

[12] Montisci A, Maj G, Zangrillo A, Winterton D, Pappalardo F. Management of refractory hypoxemia during venovenous extracorporeal membrane oxygenation for ARDS. ASAIO J. 2015; 61(3):227–236

[13] Fukushima A, Chazono K, Hashimoto Y, et al. Oseltamivir produces hypothermic and neuromuscular effects by inhibition of nicotinic acetylcholine receptor functions: comparison to procaine and bupropion. Eur J Pharmacol. 2015; 762:275–282

[14] Heytens L, Forget P, Scholtès JL, Veyckemans F. The changing face of malignant hyperthermia: less fulminant, more insidious. Anaesth Intensive Care. 2015; 43(4):506–511

[15] Scalco RS, Gardiner AR, Pitceathly RD, et al. Rhabdomyolysis: a genetic perspective. Orphanet J Rare Dis. 2015; 10(1):51

[16] Ecker ML, Dormans JP, Schwartz DM, Drummond DS, Bulman WA. Efficacy of spinal cord monitoring in scoliosis surgery in patients with cerebral palsy. J Spinal Disord. 1996; 9(2):159–164

[17] Noordeen MH, Lee J, Gibbons CE, Taylor BA, Bentley G. Spinal cord monitoring in operations for neuromuscular scoliosis. J Bone Joint Surg Br. 1997; 79 (1):53–57

[18] Lonstein JE, Koop SE, Novachek TF, Perra JH. Results and complications after spinal fusion for neuromuscular scoliosis in cerebral palsy and static encephalopathy using Luque Galveston instrumentation: experience in 93 patients. Spine. 2012; 37(7):583–591

[19] He Z, Tonb DJ, Dabney KW, et al. Cytokine release, pancreatic injury, and risk of acute pancreatitis after spinal fusion surgery. Dig Dis Sci. 2004; 49(1):143–149

[20] Thuet ED, Winscher JC, Padberg AM, et al. Validity and reliability of intraoperative monitoring in pediatric spinal deformity surgery: a 23-year experience of 3436 surgical cases. Spine. 2010; 35(20):1880–1886

[21] Fehlings MG, Kelleher MO. Intraoperative monitoring during spinal surgery for neuromuscular scoliosis. Nat Clin Pract Neurol. 2007; 3(6):318–319

[22] Nash CL, Jr, Lorig RA, Schatzinger LA, Brown RH. Spinal cord monitoring during operative treatment of the spine. Clin Orthop Relat Res. 1977(126):100–105

[23] Vauzelle C, Stagnara P, Jouvinroux P. Functional monitoring of spinal cord activity during spinal surgery. Clin Orthop Relat Res. 1973(93):173–178

[24] MacEwen GD, Bunnell WP, Sriram K. Acute neurological complications in the treatment of scoliosis. A report of the Scoliosis Research Society. J Bone Joint Surg Am. 1975; 57(3):404–408

[25] Schwartz DM, Sestokas AK, Dormans JP, et al. Transcranial electric motor evoked potential monitoring during spine surgery: is it safe? Spine. 2011; 36 (13):1046–1049

[26] Schwartz DM, Sestokas AK, Hilibrand AS, et al. Neurophysiological identification of position-induced neurologic injury during anterior cervical spine surgery. J Clin Monit Comput. 2006; 20(6):437–444

[27] Schwartz DM, Auerbach JD, Dormans JP, et al. Neurophysiological detection of impending spinal cord injury during scoliosis surgery. J Bone Joint Surg Am. 2007; 89(11):2440–2449

[28] Hammett TC, Boreham B, Quraishi NA, Mehdian SM. Intraoperative spinal cord monitoring during the surgical correction of scoliosis due to cerebral palsy and other neuromuscular disorders. Eur Spine J. 2013; 22 Suppl 1:S38–S41

[29] Tucker SK, Noordeen MH, Pitt MC. Spinal cord monitoring in neuromuscular scoliosis. J Pediatr Orthop B. 2001; 10(1):1–5

[30] Salem KM, Goodger L, Bowyer K, Shafafy M, Grevitt MP. Does transcranial stimulation for motor evoked potentials (TcMEP) worsen seizures in epileptic patients following spinal deformity surgery? Eur Spine J. 2016; 25(10):3044–3048

[31] Kannan S, Meert KL, Mooney JF, Hillman-Wiseman C, Warrier I. Bleeding and coagulation changes during spinal fusion surgery: a comparison of neuromuscular and idiopathic scoliosis patients. Pediatr Crit Care Med. 2002; 3 (4):364–369

[32] Brenn BR, Theroux MC, Dabney KW, Miller F. Clotting parameters and thromboelastography in children with neuromuscular and idiopathic scoliosis undergoing posterior spinal fusion. Spine. 2004; 29(15):E310–E314

[33] Winter SL, Kriel RL, Novacheck TF, Luxenberg MG, Leutgeb VJ, Erickson PA. Perioperative blood loss: the effect of valproate. Pediatr Neurol. 1996; 15 (1):19–22

[34] Chambers HG, Weinstein CH, Mubarak SJ, Wenger DR, Silva PD. The effect of valproic acid on blood loss in patients with cerebral palsy. J Pediatr Orthop. 1999; 19(6):792–795

[35] Lawhon SM, Kahn A, III, Crawford AH, Brinker MS. Controlled hypotensive anesthesia during spinal surgery. A retrospective study. Spine. 1984; 9 (5):450–453

[36] Samdani AF, Belin EJ, Bennett JT, et al. Major perioperative complications after spine surgery in patients with cerebral palsy: assessment of risk factors. Eur Spine JJ. 2016; 25(3):795–800

[37] Verma K, Errico T, Diefenbach C, et al. The relative efficacy of antifibrinolytics in adolescent idiopathic scoliosis: a prospective randomized trial. J Bone Joint Surg Am. 2014; 96(10):e80

[38] Gill JB, Chin Y, Levin A, Feng D. The use of antifibrinolytic agents in spine surgery. A meta-analysis. J Bone Joint Surg Am. 2008; 90(11):2399–2407

[39] Peters A, Verma K, Slobodyanyuk K, et al. Antifibrinolytics reduce blood loss in adult spinal deformity surgery: a prospective, randomized controlled trial. Spine. 2015; 40(8):E443–E449

[40] Dhawale AA, Shah SA, Sponseller PD, et al. Are antifibrinolytics helpful in decreasing blood loss and transfusions during spinal fusion surgery in children with cerebral palsy scoliosis? Spine. 2012; 37(9):E549–E555

[41] Cawley DT, Carmody O, Dodds MK, McCormack D. Early limited instrumentation of scoliosis in Duchenne muscular dystrophy: is a single-rod construct sufficient? Spine J. 2015; 15(10):2166–2171

[42] Sadacharam K, Brenn BR, He Z, Zhang Y. Improving Outcomes after Neuromuscular Scoliosis Surgery: Have We Learned from Massive Transfusion Protocols? The Anesthesiology Annual Meeting; 2014

[43] Mayfield JK. Severe spine deformity in myelodysplasia and sacral agenesis: an aggressive surgical approach. Spine. 1981; 6(5):498–509

[44] Ward JP, Feldman DS, Paul J, et al. Wound closure in nonidiopathic scoliosis: does closure matter? J Pediatr Orthop. 2017; 37(3):166–170

5 Unique Challenges with Scoliosis and Dislocated Hips

Firoz Miyanji and Randal R. Betz

Abstract

The incidence of hip abnormalities in patients with cerebral palsy ranges from 25 to 30%. It is generally agreed that the incidence is higher and associated with the degree of neurological impairment. Classifications have been developed based on the migration index as to whether the hip is subluxed (migration index [MI] > 30%) or is at risk of dislocation (MI > 50%). There is no consensus in the literature or among surgeons as to whether hip subluxation or scoliosis comes first. Parents should be told that correction of the scoliosis and pelvic obliquity will not be "protective" of the potential for developing hip subluxation in the future, nor will it "accelerate" hip subluxation/dislocation. As a general rule, management decisions regarding scoliosis and hip subluxation/dislocation may be considered independent of each other.

Keywords: hip dislocation, pelvic obliquity, neuromuscular scoliosis

5.1 Introduction

Children with cerebral palsy (CP) have a high incidence of spine and hip abnormalities. These deformities are most prevalent in children with more severe involvement. Manifestations of pain, seating difficulties, and pressure ulcers may be the end result of either spine or hip deformity alone or can be the additive result of both deformities. Although many investigators have attempted to evaluate the development, progression, and association between these two most significant musculoskeletal manifestations of CP, no clear consensus exists.

5.1.1 Hip Subluxation in Cerebral Palsy

The incidence of hip abnormalities in patients with CP ranges from 25 to 30%.[1,2] It is generally agreed that the incidence is higher with increasing degree of neurological impairment. Overactivity and muscle imbalance around the hip joint (most commonly flexors, adductors, and medial hamstrings) result in fixed musculotendinous contractures that will ultimately become fixed joint contractures. Muscle imbalances lead to typical posturing of the lower extremities with the hip in a flexed, adducted, and internally rotated position.

Normally the acetabulum and the femoral head develop congruently, which is essential for proper development of both structures. The hip in children with CP is considered normal at birth. Abnormalities in weight-bearing, muscle imbalance, and spasticity cause alterations of the femoral head and acetabular relationship leading to progressive subluxation of the joint. Patients with CP tend to have increase muscular imbalances and tone in the adductors, iliopsoas, and hamstrings, resulting in the proximal femur being directed away from the acetabulum. Excessive pressure on the outer acetabular margin caused by the position of the femoral head may prevent or distort normal acetabular development. The acetabulum becomes dysplastic as subluxation progresses. The process of subluxation includes structural bone deformation in both the acetabulum and the femoral head. The deformation of the acetabulum and femoral head can lead to dislocation of the hip. Posterior dislocation is most common because of the direction of muscle pull in the typical position of hip adduction, flexion, and internal rotation.

Migration percentage or index (MI) is the most commonly used measurement of the hip status in individuals with CP (▶ Fig. 5.1). The measure indicates the amount of ossified femoral head uncovered by the ossified acetabular roof. It is closely

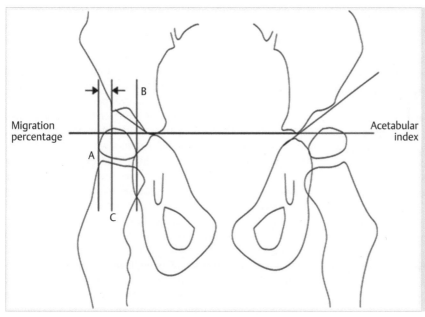

Fig. 5.1 Schematic depiction of migration index measurement of hip subluxation.

Migration percentage

Acetabular index

associated with acetabular index, so that as one measure increases, the other does as well. Miller et al[3] as well as Reimers[4] developed a classification based on the MI as to whether the hip is subluxed (MI > 30%) or is at risk of dislocation (MI > 50%). In the CP population, the MI can increase rapidly at a mean rate of 5.5% per year.[4] The tendency to dislocate is directly related to the degree of impairment. Children who are in a persistent posture of hip adduction with little voluntary movement, unable to weight bear, and have difficulty maintaining head and trunk stability are at greatest risk.

5.1.2 Pelvic Obliquity

Pelvic obliquity refers to a deviation of the pelvis from the horizontal in the frontal plane. Fixed pelvic obliquities can be attributed to contractures either above (suprapelvic) or below (infrapelvic) the pelvis.

Suprapelvic obliquity is secondary to significant scoliosis in which the pelvis acts as an end vertebra. Most authors have shown that as the severity of scoliosis increases, so does the degree of pelvic obliquity.

Infrapelvic obliquity develops because of abnormalities in the position of the hip and imbalances in muscle pull on the pelvis. Both pelvic rotation in the transverse plane and pelvic tilt in the sagittal plane occur with obliquity, and the contribution of each is variable. Hip adduction contractures, weak abductors, iliotibial band contracture, and medial hamstring tightness are all implicated in the development of infrapelvic obliquity.

5.1.3 The Windblown Deformity

Letts et al[5] popularized the concept of the "windblown hip syndrome," which is the triad of hip dislocation, pelvic obliquity, and scoliosis, noting an incidence of 13.3% in their series. The clinical appearance is one in which one hip and femur are pointing toward the midline (adducted), whereas the opposite hip and femur are directed away from the midline (abducted). Letts et al[5] reviewed 22 patients with windblown hip syndrome and noted that in 15 patients the first pathology was subluxation followed by dislocation of the hip. Dislocation of the hip was then followed by the development of pelvic obliquity in 16 patients, and then by scoliosis in 12 patients. The authors concluded that their analysis of the "temporal sequence" was most consistent with hip subluxation, pelvic obliquity, and finally progressive scoliosis. They theorized that spasticity of the iliopsoas muscle led to hip subluxation, then pelvic obliquity, and finally spinal curvature (▶ Fig. 5.2). Although the authors noted that in 12 children scoliosis developed after hip subluxation and pelvic obliquity, in 6 children they found scoliosis on the initial radiographic finding prior to hip subluxation and pelvic obliquity. It is also worth noting that the pelvic obliquity and convexity of the scoliosis were on the opposite side of the hip dislocation in 17 patients; however, in 5 patients these were on the same side as the hip dislocation, challenging their conclusions of the temporal relationship between hip subluxation, pelvic obliquity, and scoliosis. Nonetheless, the authors strongly recommend that hip stability be maintained to prevent subluxation so that the development of pelvic obliquity and scoliosis can be avoided.

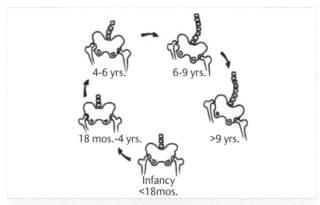

Fig. 5.2 Temporal sequence of hip subluxation, pelvic obliquity, and scoliosis as proposed by Letts et al.[5] (Reproduced with permission from Letts, M., Shapiro, L., Mulder, K., et al. (1984). The windblown hip syndrome in total body cerebral palsy. J Pediatr Orthop. 4(1), 55-62).

Cooperman et al[6] also felt that the deformities of the hip, spine, and pelvis are interrelated. Although the others did note a unilateral hip dislocation with a level pelvis and no scoliosis in 6 patients in their series, they found more commonly unilateral hip dislocations in concert with pelvic obliquity and scoliosis. The authors concluded that successful reduction of a unilateral dislocation increased the likelihood of a level pelvis at maturity and hence decreased the incidence of developing scoliosis.

More recent literature echoes similar findings with authors reporting a positive relationship between hip and spine abnormalities in this patient population.[7,8,9] Porter et al[10] reported a significant relationship between hip dislocation and the emergence of scoliosis. A study by Kalen et al[11] also noted a relationship between hip dislocation and the development of scoliosis.

Others, however, have challenged the temporal sequence of events of the triad of hip subluxation, and pelvic obliquity, followed by the development of scoliosis.[12,13,14,15,16,17] Lonstein et al's[18] cross-sectional study of 464 patients with CP found that hip abnormalities, pelvic obliquity, and scoliosis were most prevalent in severely involved, wheelchair-dependent patients. Although they found a 57% incidence of hip subluxation, a 58% incidence of pelvic obliquity, and an 82% incidence of scoliosis in their cohort, they found no relationship between hip dislocation, windswept direction, and scoliosis. Similarly, Pritchett and colleagues[12] studied 80 institutionalized CP patients with unstable hips. They found 35 had a level pelvis despite unilateral or bilateral unstable hips and none of these patients had severe scoliosis. Of the 45 patients with pelvic obliquity, 32 had severe scoliosis. In 38 of the 45 patients with pelvic obliquity, the dislocated hip was on the high side of the pelvis. The authors felt that the unstable hip was associated with pelvic obliquity and scoliosis but not causal to their development. They concluded that scoliosis and pelvic obliquity were correlated with the severity of neurological involvement rather than with the mechanics of a dislocated hip.

Young et al[19] found evidence of a relationship between tonal asymmetry and direction of windblown deformity in a subgroup of 33 patients, with the hips tending to wind blow toward the side of the lower tone; they found no relationship between direction of tone and direction of scoliosis in another subgroup of 22 patients. In 26 patients who demonstrated both deformities, no relationship was found between direction of windblown deformity and direction of scoliosis.

Abel and colleagues,[20] although hypothesizing that the subluxed hip would be opposite the scoliosis apex and ipsilateral to the high side of the pelvis, were not able to substantiate this in their study of 37 patients with total body involvement CP. They found that hip subluxation strongly correlated with the degree of femoral adduction and weakly with the magnitude of suprapelvic obliquity. They found that at a young age, infrapelvic deformity predominates with asymmetric hip adduction; however, later the windblown position seems to result largely from progressive pelvic obliquity and rotation associated with scoliosis.

Senaran et al's[13] most recent prospective study found that in most patients with unilateral hip dislocation, subluxation occurred on the high side with a significant increase in pelvic obliquity; however, no significant relationship between hip dislocation and the emergence and progression of scoliosis was reported. Others have also shown a poor correlation between the triad of hip subluxation, pelvic obliquity, and scoliosis.[14]

5.1.4 Surgical Implications of the Triad

Despite inconclusive and contrary findings within the literature to date, many investigators still feel the triad of deformity within the hip, pelvis, and spine in this patient population to be interrelated.[6,8,9,21,22] The temporal aspects of the relationship between these deformities are not fully understood; however, earlier authors stressed the importance of maintaining hip congruency and stability to avoid developing pelvic obliquity and subsequent scoliosis.[5,23] More recent data by Garg et al,[24] however, challenge these earlier recommendations. Their study of 98 patients over a 21-year period noted that despite a varus derotation osteotomy (VDRO) of the proximal femur for hip subluxation, a significant increase in maximum Cobb angle continued over time. The average age of the VDRO was 6 years. In addition, they did not find increasing Cobb angle to be a significant predictor of severity of recurrent hip subluxation. The authors therefore concluded that treatment decisions regarding hip subluxation and scoliosis management in CP should be made independent of each other.

The most recent study evaluating the effects of spinal fusion on hip pathology in CP was that of Crawford et al.[21] The authors retrospectively reviewed 47 patients who underwent a posterior spinal fusion over a 6-year period. They found 17% of patients had new-onset hip subluxation/dislocation following spinal arthrodesis and felt that this was secondary to the correction of pelvic obliquity. However, this was not dependent on whether the hip was on the high or low side of the preoperative pelvic obliquity. Although the authors feel that the new-onset hip subluxation/dislocation was the result of correction of the pelvic obliquity, it may simply be the natural history of hip deformity in this patient population.

5.1.5 Authors' Preferred Treatment Algorithm

The decision to intervene surgically in patients with CP should be a collective one with the surgeon, patient, family, and caregivers. Specific goals of either the hip surgery or the spinal deformity surgery should be clearly outlined, and our preference is to make treatment decisions around the hip and spine pathology independent of one another. It is important to express to the family that immediate postoperative changes in the attitude of the lower limbs (i.e., potential for windblown deformity) may be noted following correction of the scoliosis and pelvic obliquity; however, correction of the scoliosis and pelvic obliquity will not be "protective" of the potential for developing hip subluxation in the future, nor will it "accelerate" hip subluxation/dislocation. In the presence of an increased Reimer's MI with a hip at risk in a patient without significant scoliosis, moving forward with hip surgery should be a strong consideration and the patient should be followed with serial X-rays and clinical examination to determine whether scoliosis will develop. In the presence of a hip at risk concomitant with significant pelvic obliquity and scoliosis, we prefer to stabilize the spine and correct the pelvic obliquity ideally prior to surgery around the hip. This would help make the pelvis *horizontal*, providing a stable *foundation* around which femoral-acetabular procedures can be carried out to stabilize the hip at risk and treat any lower limb positioning concerns (i.e., windblown deformity).

Patients with significant adduction and flexion contractures around the hips may require soft-tissue-release procedures prior to stabilization of the spine if positioning for spine surgery may not be possible due to the soft-tissue contractures around the hip. Although some authors have suggested that soft-tissue releases (specifically hip flexion contractures) can help with correction of pelvic deformity and excessive lumbar lordosis, we have not found this to be an absolute necessity in this setting and have moved in the direction of treating hip and spine abnormalities independent of one another in this patient population.

Patient positioning for spine surgery in the presence of hip contractures can be facilitated by positioning the lower extremities in a sling to accommodate the flexion contractures of the hips and knees common in this patient population. It is important to keep the patient from sliding down the table by securing a strap around the ischium (▶ Fig. 5.3a, b). We now use intraoperative halo-femoral traction in this patient population more liberally and have found this to help significantly in correcting the pelvic obliquity and also aid in positioning for spine surgery despite the presence of significant hip contractures (▶ Fig. 5.4). Traction is also very effective in correcting the significant lumbar lordosis seen in many of these patients.

It is also worth noting that screw trajectory for iliac wing fixation follows a path aimed at obtaining screw length to be as far *anterior* to the lumbosacral pivot point as possible without violating the hip joint and approximately 15 mm above the sciatic notch where the thickness of the ilium is greatest. This, however, may inhibit future acetabular procedures if required and either a shorter screw length and/or a more horizontal trajectory (if possible) may need to be considered at the time of pelvic fixation for the spinal deformity procedure. Alternatively, removal of the iliac screw may be considered concomitant with the pelvic osteotomy once hip surgery is deemed necessary (▶ Fig. 5.5a–g).

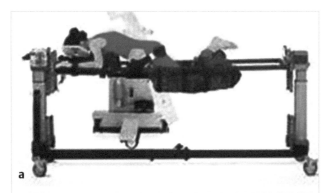

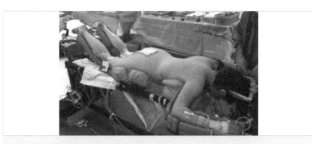

Fig. 5.4 Intraoperative *static* halo-femoral traction.

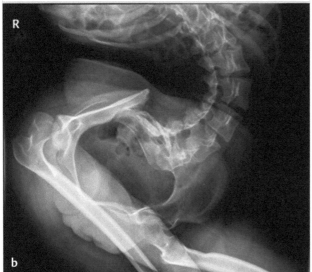

Fig. 5.3 (a) Traditional positioning of patient on Jackson table with significant hip flexion contractures. **(b)** Preoperative anteroposterior pelvis X-ray emphasizing significant hip flexion deformity.

5.2 Conclusion

Despite studies reporting an association, findings on the relationship between hip dislocation, pelvic obliquity, and the emergence or progression of scoliosis in CP remain inconclusive. The temporal relationship of the triad is unclear and does not follow a predictable relationship. Although earlier studies stressed the importance of preventing hip subluxation/dislocation in this patient population to prevent the windblown syndrome and the development of significant scoliosis, more recent data have not supported this prior dogma. The natural history of the "terrible triad" of hip subluxation, pelvic obliquity, and scoliosis in CP may be more independent than once thought and is likely related to the degree of neurological impairment and spasticity in these patients; hence, management decisions regarding scoliosis and hip subluxation/dislocation may be considered independent of each other.

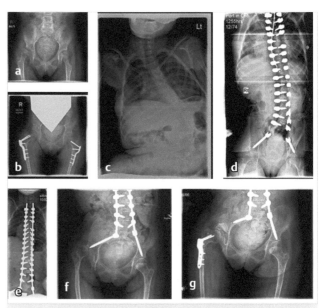

Fig. 5.5 12-year-old patient with CP noted to have right hip subluxation **(a)** who had femoral and pelvic osteotomies **(b)**. At the age of 14 years, her scoliosis progressed significantly despite hips being stabilized **(c)**; she underwent anterior and posterior procedures to correct her spinal deformity **(d,e)**; 2 years post spinal fusion, she had recurrence of right hip subluxation **(f)** and the right iliac wing screw was changed for smaller length to allow for pelvic osteotomy **(g)**.

References

[1] Cornell MS. The hip in cerebral palsy. Dev Med Child Neurol. 1995; 37 (1):3–18

[2] Onimus M, Allamel G, Manzone P, Laurain JM. Prevention of hip dislocation in cerebral palsy by early psoas and adductors tenotomies. J Pediatr Orthop. 1991; 11(4):432–435

[3] Miller F, Bagg MR. Age and migration percentage as risk factors for progression in spastic hip disease. Dev Med Child Neurol. 1995; 37(5):449–455

[4] Reimers J. The stability of the hip in children. A radiological study of the results of muscle surgery in cerebral palsy. Acta Orthop Scand Suppl. 1980; 184:1–100

[5] Letts M, Shapiro L, Mulder K, Klassen O. The windblown hip syndrome in total body cerebral palsy. J Pediatr Orthop. 1984; 4(1):55–62

[6] Cooperman DR, Bartucci E, Dietrick E, Millar EA. Hip dislocation in spastic cerebral palsy: long-term consequences. J Pediatr Orthop. 1987; 7(3):268–276

[7] Flynn JM, Miller F. Management of hip disorders in patients with cerebral palsy. J Am Acad Orthop Surg. 2002; 10(3):198–209

[8] Terjesen T. The natural history of hip development in cerebral palsy. Dev Med Child Neurol. 2012; 54(10):951–957

[9] Hägglund G, Andersson S, Düppe H, Lauge-Pedersen H, Nordmark E, Westbom L. Prevention of dislocation of the hip in children with cerebral palsy. The first ten years of a population-based prevention programme. J Bone Joint Surg Br. 2005; 87(1):95–101

[10] Porter D, Michael S, Kirkwood C. Patterns of postural deformity in non-ambulant people with cerebral palsy: what is the relationship between the direction of scoliosis, direction of pelvic obliquity, direction of windswept hip deformity and side of hip dislocation? Clin Rehabil. 2007; 21(12):1087–1096

[11] Kalen V, Conklin MM, Sherman FC. Untreated scoliosis in severe cerebral palsy. J Pediatr Orthop. 1992; 12(3):337–340

[12] Pritchett JW. The untreated unstable hip in severe cerebral palsy. Clin Orthop Relat Res. 1983(173):169–172

[13] Senaran H, Shah SA, Glutting JJ, Dabney KW, Miller F. The associated effects of untreated unilateral hip dislocation in cerebral palsy scoliosis. J Pediatr Orthop. 2006; 26(6):769–772

[14] Loeters MJ, Maathuis CG, Hadders-Algra M. Risk factors for emergence and progression of scoliosis in children with severe cerebral palsy: a systematic review. Dev Med Child Neurol. 2010; 52(7):605–611

[15] Cooke PH, Cole WG, Carey RP. Dislocation of the hip in cerebral palsy. Natural history and predictability. J Bone Joint Surg Br. 1989; 71(3):441–446

[16] Gu Y, Shelton JE, Ketchum JM, et al. Natural history of scoliosis in nonambulatory spastic tetraplegic cerebral palsy. PM R. 2011; 3(1):27–32

[17] Hodgkinson I, Bérard C, Chotel F, Bérard J. Pelvic obliquity and scoliosis in non-ambulatory patients with cerebral palsy: a descriptive study of 234 patients over 15 years of age. Rev Chir Orthop Repar Appar Mot. 2002; 88(4):337–341

[18] Lonstein JE, Beck K. Hip dislocation and subluxation in cerebral palsy. J Pediatr Orthop. 1986; 6(5):521–526

[19] Young NL, Wright JG, Lam P, et al. Windswept hip deformity in spastic quadriplegic cerebral palsy. Pediatr Phys Ther. 1998; 10(3)

[20] Abel MF, Blanco JS, Pavlovich L, Damiano DL. Asymmetric hip deformity and subluxation in cerebral palsy: an analysis of surgical treatment. J Pediatr Orthop. 1999; 19(4):479–485

[21] Crawford L, Herrera-Soto J, Ruder JA, Phillips J, Knapp R. The fate of the neuromuscular hip after spinal fusion. J Pediatr Orthop. 2015:[Epub ahead of print]

[22] Ko PS, Jameson PG, II, Chang TL, Sponseller PD. Transverse-plane pelvic asymmetry in patients with cerebral palsy and scoliosis. J Pediatr Orthop. 2011; 31(3):277–283

[23] Persson-Bunke M, Hägglund G, Lauge-Pedersen H. Windswept hip deformity in children with cerebral palsy. J Pediatr Orthop B. 2006; 15(5):335–338

[24] Garg S, Engelman G, Yoshihara H, McNair B, Chang F. The relationship of gross motor functional classification scale level and hip dysplasia on the pattern and progression of scoliosis in children with cerebral palsy. Spine Deform. 2013; 1(4):266–271

6 Predicting Complications: When to Operate or Not

Mark F. Abel and Anuj Singla

Abstract

Spinal deformities, including scoliosis and severe sagittal deformities, are common in patients with neuromuscular conditions, yet the indications for surgical intervention can be controversial. Patients with cerebral palsy, muscle diseases, and myelomeningocele often have impairments of major organ systems including cardiac, pulmonary, genitourinary, and gastrointestinal systems. Their fragile medical condition and the high rates of reported complications in this group of patients, coupled with the paucity of data on the impact of interventions on quality of life, make decision making particularly challenging. This ethical dilemma is presented in this chapter. Also, this chapter discusses the various neuromuscular conditions commonly occurring in patients with spinal deformities. The risk assessment is coupled with information on complication rates. Some guidelines are provided to mitigate risks, and medical thresholds are provided when the risks may be too high to embark on surgery.

Keywords: complications, kyphosis, neuromuscular, outcomes, risks, scoliosis

6.1 Introduction

The general principle of the Hippocratic Oath suggests that physicians should withhold treatments that are likely to produce harm to the patient. This dictum is highly relevant for many patients with neuromuscular spinal deformities such as kyphosis and scoliosis. This group of patients includes those with cerebral palsy (CP), muscle diseases, and myelomeningocele as well as a range of genetic syndromes. Many of these patients are totally dependent on a parent or other caregiver for all their daily needs including hygiene and feeding. Furthermore, the patients often have multiple comorbid conditions including intellectual disabilities, joint contractures, seizure disorders, oral-motor dysfunction requiring supplemental tube feedings or gastrostomies, cardiac disease (especially in the muscular dystrophy group), and pulmonary deficits of a restrictive and/or obstructive nature. Furthermore, the spinal deformities are progressive and difficult to control with nonoperative methods, yet the impact of surgical interventions on overall quality of life has only recently been investigated.

Surgical correction may involve anterior, posterior, or combined approaches with intraoperative or preoperative traction depending on the configuration and magnitude of the spinal deformity. Whichever surgical techniques are chosen, the complication rate still remains highest in this category of patient because of the previously mentioned comorbid conditions, magnitude of the deformities, and poor bone quality. The existing medical literature clearly defines the high rate and severity of complications (between 25 and 75%),[1] yet absolute contraindications to surgical correction are not well documented or defined. Thus, the relative contraindications of surgery are subjective at best. The decision to perform the surgery and the

ability to correct these challenging deformities should be carefully weighed based on the patient's medical condition (and the natural history thereof), associated comorbidities, curve characteristics, surgeon's experience, and the resources available at the treating institution.

This chapter will review presurgical risk assessment in patients with neuromuscular conditions undergoing spinal correction surgery. The first goal of the chapter is to provide parameter thresholds to consider in determining if spinal reconstructive surgery should be done, keeping in mind that the prime goal of our intervention is to improve the patient's quality of life, which essentially means avoiding a complication that leaves the patient in a worse condition than they were preoperatively. ▶ Table 6.1 lists medical parameters that should make the surgeon particularly wary of surgical interventions. When these conditions are present, the patient is much more likely to have a serious complication.

The second goal of the chapter is to provide guidelines for decision making used by the authors. Our role as physicians is to educate patients and their families as best as we can with incomplete data on risks, benefits, and alternatives to empower them to share in the choice for their child. Families vary in their willingness to assume risk or to accept intensive interventions for a modicum of perceived benefit for their child. Before undertaking life-threatening surgery, the surgeon and care team must forge a collaborative partnership with the family. In pediatric neuromuscular spinal deformity, the process of informed consent is as potentially complex as the procedure itself.

6.2 Risk Assessment

6.2.1 Multidisciplinary Input

The medical complexity and variety of pediatric patients with spinal deformities secondary to neuromuscular disorders

Table 6.1 Warning parameters of increasing risk of complication from long fusions (> 13 levels)

1. BMI < 5% or > 95%

2. PFTs with VC < 40%; VC < 1 L

3. Cyanotic cardiac disease pO_2 sat < 90%

4. Cardiac output of < 50%

5. Clotting deficiency: INR > 1.7; platelet < 100,000

6. Coronal Cobb > 90 degrees (traction > 70 degrees)

7. Kyphosis > 100 degrees (maximum correction with bolster extension > 90 degrees)

8. Lumbar lordosis > 120 degrees (maximum correction with flexion > 100 degrees)

Abbreviations: BMI, body mass index; INR, international normalized ratio; PFTs, pulmonary function tests; VC, vital capacity.

Table 6.2 Factors in the authors' current practice guidelines to avoid complications

1. Preoperative assessment of cardiac, pulmonary, and nutrition

2. Assess IV access

3. Preanesthesia assessments

4. Tranexamic acid: 30 mg/kg loading; running 10 mg/kg/h intraoperatively

5. Antibiotics (vancomycin powder) in bone graft

6. Consideration to intraoperative traction. By using intraoperative traction, less invasive techniques such as vertebral resections, multiple osteotomies, and anterior releases can be avoided[2]

7. Intraoperative monitoring of blood parameters: CBC, fibrinogen, platelets, electrolytes

8. ICU monitoring as needed

9. Setting realistic correction goals: limit the extent of surgery; avoid going to the pelvis

10. Use growth constructs if possible with postoperative bracing

Abbreviations: CBC, complete blood count; ICU, intensive care unit.

necessitates that multiple medical specialists get involved in the presurgical examination and analysis. These specialists collaborate to define the risks of the proposed spine surgery and the interventions needed to mitigate those risks. The spine surgeon should not be expected to understand and acquire all of the multisystem medical data alone. Most hospital systems, including the authors', have standardized care pathways for preoperative, intraoperative, and postoperative management. ▶ Table 6.2 lists some elements that are a standard part of our pathway. Chapter 1 addresses preoperative assessment more fully. Ideally, the team of specialists can assist not only in the assessment and care, but also in the counseling and decision making. For complex cases, a multidisciplinary preoperative case conference or e-mail communications can facilitate decision making.

6.2.2 Disease-Specific Risk

Cerebral Palsy

CP, the leading cause of physical disability in childhood, is a static encephalopathy occurring in the developing, immature brain producing a range of motor, cognitive, and neurological deficits. The Gross Motor Function Classification System (GMFCS) is an international classification system, with five categories, developed to differentiate patients by their ability to move.[3] Those in class 4 or 5 require assistance to move, underscoring their poor muscle function and the severity of their neuromuscular impairment. The literature related to "complication rates for spinal deformity surgery" is heavily weighted toward patients with CP because of the high prevalence of CP among neuromuscular conditions and the high incidence of spinal deformities in this group.[4] Despite the static nature of the brain lesion, these same patients in GMFCS 4 and 5 have the highest incidence of spinal deformities, approaching 50%, due to the absence of trunk balance and the presence of excessive high or low muscle tone.[5] Furthermore, the majority of these patients, particularly those in GMFCS level 5, have other significant medical disabilities including seizures, oral motor dysfunction, and reactive airway disease to name a few.[6,7] Not

unexpectedly, given these conditions, surgical complication rates after spine surgery are 25 to 50% in patients with CP compared to rates of 1 to 3% in idiopathic scoliosis.[8] Also the more severe and complex curves in these patients (Cobb > 90 degrees) require a longer total operative time and result in an increased total blood loss, all resulting in a propensity for major complications.[8] Furthermore, the complications encountered in some of these patients can be potentially life-threatening.[9] The rate of mortality ranges from 1 to 4% in some recent series.[9,10, 11,12] Where patient/parent satisfaction with treatment has been assessed, the occurrence of a complication requiring prolonged hospital stay, reoperation, or death results in dissatisfaction with the intervention.[13]

When taken on whole, surgical intervention for patients with spinal deformity does lead to improved scores on the CPCHILD (Caregiver Priorities and Child Health Index of Life with Disabilities) questionnaire, a validated HRQL (Health-Related Quality of Life) instrument.[14] The major area of improvement was in the "Transfer & Basic Mobility" domain, and on average no domain saw deterioration.[14,15] Unfortunately, despite the positive change reported from surgery, the lack of randomization casts some doubt on the relevance of these outcomes.[16]

Muscle Diseases

Of patients with muscle disease, those with Duchenne muscular dystrophy (DMD) account for the largest prevalence; thus, we have the most information on spinal deformity surgery in this group. DMD is a progressive muscle disease caused by an X-linked recessive gene, altering a structural protein, dystrophin, critical for muscle function. The disease progression involves cardiac and pulmonary function with cardiomyopathy and, most commonly, respiratory failure as the main causes of death. Spinal deformities occur in virtually all patients with DMD after their disease progresses to the point they are no longer ambulatory.[17] The popular use of steroids has markedly altered the natural history of spinal deformity in DMD in that spinal deformities are occurring at a later age and with less severity.[17, 18,19] However, reduced life expectancy and progressive cardiopulmonary decline are still inevitable, even if spinal surgery is performed.[20] However, the purported benefits from spinal surgery include improved sitting tolerance,[21] ease of nursing requirement, and less pain. The effect of spinal stabilization on pulmonary function, motor function, and survival is controversial, in large part because there are no clinical trials or randomized studies on this question. The Cochrane review published by Cheuk et al[22] reported the controversial results. Some studies report deterioration of pulmonary function and no improvement in life expectancy,[17,18] while others found improved outcomes compared with those not treated with spinal surgery.[23] Furthermore, the trunk lengthening and mobility loss following spinal fusion can impede upper extremity function.[23]

A recent prospective, observational report by Suk et al[24] compared 32 patients selecting nonsurgical treatment to 45 surgically treated patients with DMD using functional tests (modified Rancho scale and manual muscle test), a validated HRQL questionnaire (the Muscular Dystrophy Spine Questionnaire) and pulmonary function tests (PFTs). The authors found that surgical patients, as expected, had better radiographic alignment and significantly higher scores on the MDSQ, which was only given at final follow-up. There was no difference in strength or pulmonary function, but the rate of decline in PFTs was less in the surgically treated group. Based on these outcomes, the authors concluded that surgical intervention was beneficial.

In addition to these uncertain outcomes from spinal surgery, we know that complications from surgery can occur in up to 44% (20–68%) of cases,[25,26] and include cardiac arrest, massive bleeding, spinal cord injury, pneumonia, wound dehiscence, infections, severe ileus, pseudarthrosis, pain, and difficulty with hand-to-mouth functions,[22] and these complications generally increase with curve severity.

Thus, the general treatment philosophy for patients with flaccid muscular dystrophies has not changed drastically since the publication of the classic report by Kurz et al,[27] suggesting that surgery should be done early, before a decline in forced vital capacity (FVC) of less than 40% (▶ Table 6.1). A clear change from that era is the use of glucocorticoids in DMD, which has resulted in longer survival and a slower rate of spine deformity progression.[17] Consequently, in the present era, spine surgery in DMD is deferred until scoliosis is greater than 40 degrees,[18,28] though agreement on a threshold Cobb angle has not been reached. Also, advancements in ICU (intensive care unit) care including the use of bilevel positive airway pressure (BiPap) and aggressive pulmonary therapies and mobilization have made survival from surgery more likely even if the FVC is less than 40%; clearly the risks are much higher as pulmonary function declines. Thus, multiple factors need to be considered with families as one discusses the question of surgical or nonsurgical treatment.

The authors begin the assessment by inquiring about the occurrence of back pain and looking at the sitting balance. The past history of pulmonary illness and hospitalizations is considered along with the serial PFTs. Then the sitting sagittal and coronal radiographs are considered. The presence of scoliosis with pelvic obliquity seems to be most associated with back and buttock pain and poor sitting posture. Patients with these characteristics tend to benefit most from spinal surgery.

Myelomeningocele

Myelomeningocele, a complex congenital spinal anomaly, results from a neural tube defect during the first 4 weeks of gestation. Spinal deformity (kyphosis and scoliosis) in patients with myelomeningocele is common with greater than 80% eventually developing significant spinal deformity.[29,30] However, many patients with myelomeningocele and spinal deformity do have functional capacities for performing activities of daily living, such as eating and dressing, and they often can independently transfer or propel themselves in a wheelchair. These functional capabilities set this group apart from those children with DMD or CP in whom functional capacity is severely restricted. Thus, functional decline as a result of spinal fusion is a relevant consideration in patients with myelomeningocele. The aims of spinal deformity surgery in patients with myelomeningocele are to stop progression (as many times the deformity occurs at a young age) and to improve sitting alignment.[31] Often the pelvic obliquity or gibbus deformity can lead to areas of pressure concentration and ulceration so that a secondary goal may be to alleviate these skin problems.

The dilemma created with the surgical approach is the high complication rate, which is related to the ubiquitous association with other medical impairments. Comorbid conditions in patients with myelomeningocele include intellectual impairments (although many have normal IQ), hydrocephalus requiring shunting, and tethering of the spinal cord or progressive Chiari malformations. Insensate skin, latex allergy, renal anomalies, bacterial colonization of the urinary tract, bowel and bladder incontinence, and lower extremity malalignment are other factors that often require evaluation and impact spinal surgery decisions.[29] These patients may also display a reduced FVC with the average cited at 59% of predicted, and the impaired pulmonary function may be independent of severity of scoliosis.[32]

Singh et al[33] analyzed the anesthetic concerns and perioperative complications in patients with myelomeningocele. This retrospective review of 135 cases shows a high incidence of intraoperative cardiac and respiratory problems in 15.6 and 11.1% of cases, respectively, including two cases (1.5%) of cardiac arrest. They also reported a high incidence of other anomalies to be considered including hydrocephalus (67.4% of cases), Chiari II malformation (58.4% of cases), and renal anomalies (9% of cases). This study highlights the importance of a thorough preoperative evaluation and treatment of associated Chiari malformation and/or hydrocephalus prior to spinal surgery to avoid major surgical complications. Mortality in these patients is often related to acute elevation of the intracranial pressure with hydrocephalus, or shunt insufficiency with herniation.[31,34] The importance of confirming the patency of shunt prior to deformity correction cannot be overemphasized.[31,33] Another study[35] analyzed the risk factors for sudden death in these patients. Six patients, all of whom were young women, had experienced sudden death in this series. In multivariate analysis of 106 patients, this study reported female sex, sleep apnea, and midbrain elongation 15 mm or greater on magnetic resonance (MR) imaging to be of significantly higher risk of sudden death.[35] Careful attention should be paid to the evaluation and treatment of associated anomalies, especially hydrocephalus and shunt status as well as sleep apnea.

Poor skin coverage, high frequency of bacteremias, and absence of protective sensation collectively lead to high surgical rate of complications, such as pseudarthrosis, implant failure, and infection.[35] Instrumentation problems, such as broken rods or displacement of anchors, were seen in 29% of all patients. Furthermore, the poor skin coverage over the original myelomeningocele, coupled with a lack of protective sensation, leads frequently to wound breakdown and implant infections. Management of infection, especially for the commonly associated gram negative organism, is fraught with difficulty and can lead to renal damage in patients who have compromised renal function. Nevertheless, positive urine culture and poor nutritional status are known to be strongly correlated with high risk of surgical site infection, and their correction before surgery is highly recommended.[36]

Thus, the surgical correction of deformities in patients with myelomeningocele is a high-risk undertaking, and outcomes of studies with quality-of-life metrics suggest that improvement is difficult to achieve. Wai et al developed a valid and reliable questionnaire to evaluate the impact of spinal deformity on patients with meningomyelocele.[37,38] Studies have found little association between the presence of spinal deformity and functional capacity.[23,38,39] Of greater concern was the finding of Schoenmakers et al[40] showing that function can be lost following spinal surgery including the ability to perform transfers or to perform catheterizations. These adverse outcomes have called into question the advisability of performing surgery on patients with myelomeningocele unless sitting or skin problems are particularly recalcitrant to management through nonsurgical means such as adjusting the seating system.

The authors tend to avoid surgery except in cases where a gibbus deformity can be managed with a vertebral column resection and relatively short fusion. The gibbus deformity is frequently associated with repeated skin breakdown, severe hip flexion contractures, and obstruction of diaphragm excursion. For patients having a balanced scoliosis, surgery is not recommended.

6.3 Predicting Complications: Mixed Population Results

Several reports have analyzed patient and surgeon factors in an attempt to predict complications from spinal deformity surgery. Most recently Basques et al[4] used the National Surgical Quality Improvement Program (NSQIP) database to analyze 147 variables and determine predictors of short-term morbidity in 940 patients with neuromuscular conditions undergoing posterior spinal fusion (PSF) surgery. In this survey, the authors found that 14% of patients had a an adverse event (10.5% had severe adverse events). The only independent risk factor for adverse event, among the many factors analyzed, was an American Society of Anesthesiologists (ASA) classification of greater than 3. The authors also found that an extended length of stay (> 7 days), which occurred in 27% of cases, was correlated with ASA > 3, presence of seizure disorder, previous cardiac surgery, operative time of greater than 470 minutes and greater than 13 levels in the fusion. Infections were associated with body mass index (BMI) > 95th percentile, ASA > 3, and instrumentation to

the pelvis. Finally, 8.1% were readmitted within 30 days, with infection as the most common reason, and the only significant predictor was BMI > 95th percentile. The takeaway points from this report are intuitively obvious: the more complex the surgery, the more levels fused and the longer the fusion and, especially in obese patients, the more chance of an infection or extended hospital stay. The relationship between ASA > 3 and an adverse event serves to underscore that patients with neuromuscular scoliosis are generally ill as the majority of patients in GMFCS 5 would be in the ASA > 3 class. Thus, the ASA classification is not discriminating enough to help predict complications.

To better discriminate those at risk for complications, Jain et al[41] reported their analysis of 199 patients with CP (all GMFCS 5 undergoing spinal fusion for neuromuscular spinal deformity). The researchers subclassified the patients based on the number of comorbid conditions that they believed would predispose to complications. The following conditions were considered in the subclassification: presence of a gastrojejunostomy tube (G-tube), tracheostomy, history of seizures, and nonverbal status with patients divided into three groups for comparison based on whether they had one, two, or three of these conditions. The authors found a highly significant increase in complication rate as the number of these medical conditions coexisted. In fact, 49% of those with three of these conditions were found to have a major complication and five of seven who expired following surgery were in the GMFCS 5.3 subclass. Unfortunately, this was a retrospective study, so details of the subclassification were not validated or planned in advance of the analysis. However, this study does provide a strategy for subclassification and risk assessment going forward.

Nishnianidze et al[42] retrospectively analyzed 18 different complications with preoperative conditions in 10 physical and functional domains in an attempt to determine predictors of complications in 303 patients with CP undergoing a spinal fusion. A preoperative and postoperative scoring system was devised to perform the analysis. The data came from one center and one surgeon, so its generalizability may be questioned. Three patients (1%) died of "cardiovascular issues" during the surgery. The authors could not find any correlation between preoperative score and postoperative complication score. The major finding from this study was that patients with G-tube dependency had a greater number of complications, especially infections and pancreatitis.

Nutritional status has been assessed to determine its impact on recovery and complications in patients with CP undergoing PSF. A preoperative level of serum albumin of less than 3.5 mg %, and a total blood-lymphocyte count of less than 1,500 cells per cubic millimeter were found to be associated with higher rate of infections and perioperative complications.[2] However, other studies have failed to duplicate this finding.[42]

Curve size has also been correlated with complication rate, but a threshold value has not been determined.[9] Furthermore, comparison of studies is also hampered by the lack of standards for position of radiographs and assessment of flexibility. A Cobb angle of 70 degrees was often used to indicate the necessity for anterior surgery, but with the introduction of traction[43] and osteotomies, evidence suggests that anterior releases can often be avoided (► Table 6.2).

6.3.1 Pulmonary Complications

Pulmonary complications are the most common complications among patients with neuromuscular scoliosis, particularly those with muscle and paralytic conditions, because of comparatively poor baseline pulmonary function.[44] Abnormal hypopharyngeal tone, weaker ventilatory muscle, reduced lung volumes and excessive secretions, and elements of bronchospasm all contribute to decreased breathing reserve in these patients. Spinal deformity surgery results in acute declines in pulmonary function, especially when an anterior approach is used to access the spine. Yuan et al[8] looked at preoperative and daily postoperative bedside pulmonary function in 24 patients. The authors reported that the pulmonary function declined up to 60% after surgery on the third postoperative day and remained 50% below baseline for a week, only returning to baseline 1 to 2 months after surgery.[8,9] This decline can further potentiate preexisting poor respiratory reserve, which could become clinically significant leading to respiratory arrest and death.[9] In a separate study, Yuan et al[46] found an increased risk of requiring mechanical ventilation beyond 3 days after scoliosis surgery correlated with preoperative forced expiratory volume at the end of the first second (FEV1) < 40% of predicted. Other predictors of patients requiring prolonged mechanical ventilation in their study included vital capacity (VC) < 60% predicted, inspiratory capacity (IC) < 30 mL/kg, total lung capacity (TLC) < 60% predicted, and/or maximal inspiratory pressure (MIP) < 60 cm.[46]

A limited number of studies have tried to objectively define the pulmonary function that increases risk of complications. Padman and McNamara[46] analyzed postoperative complications in 38 patients with neuromuscular scoliosis patients treated with PSF and reported that the increased risk of postoperative pulmonary edema in patients with preoperative VC of 44%, atelectasis in patients with VC of 49% as compared to no major respiratory complications in patients with average VC of 64%. Historically, patients with FVC of less than 40% are considered to be at particularly high risk for perioperative complications.[44] Payo et al[44] reviewed the outcome of surgical management of spinal deformities in patients whose FVC was below this threshold. Twenty four patients were treated with instrumented spinal fusions. These patients had a mixture of neurological causes for the deformities including spinal cord atrophy and muscle diseases. Thirteen of 24 patients (58%) sustained complications, including one death, despite extensive preparations to minimize adverse complications. Preoperative interventions included preoperative BiPAP, tracheostomy (1), volumetric ventilation (1), nutritional support (9), and traction. Thus, patients with severe deformity and poor baseline pulmonary function are at high risk of prolonged intubation and mechanical ventilation. Preoperative pulmonary function assessment can be helpful in anticipating the risks and also in avoiding the complications.

6.3.2 Cardiovascular Complications

Patients with neuromuscular scoliosis are reported to have an inherent risk of significant bleeding, coagulopathy, and electrolyte derangements leading to cardiac arrest.[9,10,12] These patients can have an almost seven times higher risk of extensive blood loss (defined as > 50% of estimated total blood volume) during surgery in comparison with patients with idiopathic scoliosis.[9,47] Osteopenic bone, decreased coagulation factor reserve as well as changes in the mitochondrial structure of vascular smooth muscle and increased fibrinolytic activity may affect the quality of hemostasis and lead to increased blood loss without frank coagulopathy. Higher prevalence of seizure disorders and use of valproic acid are also additional risk factors for major blood loss.[12,48] Major intraoperative factors leading to cardiac arrest included significant blood loss with resultant anemia (hemoglobin 5 g% or less), hyperkalemia (potassium > 5.5 mEq/L), and hypocalcemia (ionized calcium was less than or equal to 1 mmol/L). The risk of intraoperative cardiac arrest was reported to increase with more extensive spinal fusion, low BMI, significant blood loss, and proportion of blood volume lost. Finally, patients with intrinsic cardiac muscle dysfunction, particularly those with muscle diseases, are at high risk of cardiac failure in the perioperative periods. Diligent preoperative assessment including cardiac function and perioperative management is required in these patients.

6.3.3 Surgical Site Infections

Surgical site infections are a known complication of spinal surgery with a spectrum ranging from superficial wound healing delay to significant systemic infection and sepsis.

Master et al[49] reported their analysis of 151 patients with neuromuscular scoliosis and reported an overall incidence of deep wound infections as 5.3%. The presence of a ventriculoperitoneal shunt, patients with cognitive impairment, severe neurologic involvement, nonambulatory status, and a history of seizure disorder are significant risk factors for wound infection after corrective surgery for neuromuscular scoliosis.[9,49,50]

Sponseller et al[50] studied the incidence and risk factors associated with deep wound infections in patients with neuromuscular scoliosis after spinal fusion, and reported an overall incidence of 6.4% deep wound infection. The infection is reported to be significantly higher in patients with the presence of a gastrostomy/gastrojejunostomy tube. G-tube may be a reflection of underlying poor nutritional status and overall health. The other risk factors associated with higher infection rate include older age, larger curve size, higher preoperative serum white blood cell count, and longer operative time.

Another study looked at unplanned hospital readmissions and reoperations after pediatric spinal fusion in 1,002 patients[51] and reported surgical site infections and wound complications to be the most common reason for readmission within 90 days and reoperation. Surgical site infections and related complications were noted to be three of the four most common causes for readmission and reoperation. The most common causes of readmission were wound dehiscence (1.8%), deep wound infection (1.5%), pulmonary complications (1%), and superficial wound infection (0.9%). Associated risk factors include large and rigid curves, higher number of levels fused, combined approaches,[43] greater estimated blood loss, and longer length of stay.

6.4 Case Example

A 2.5-year-old patient with severe neuromuscular scoliosis (▶ Fig. 6.1) was considered for surgical management due to the severity and progression of the spinal deformity. Underlying medical comorbidities included nemaline myopathy, G-tube dependence, tracheostomy, and a history of multiple chest and ear infections. The planned surgical procedure included proximal and distal fixation and fusion with spanning rods to minimize operative time. Intraoperatively, the patient experienced two episodes of asystole requiring resuscitation and a breach of the sterile field. Postoperatively, the patient developed a deep instrumentation infection that required surgical drainage and broad spectrum antibiotics. The patient was discharged home after 2 weeks but arrested at home 2 months postoperatively, sustaining extensive anoxic brain injury that led to a decision for withdrawal of ventilator support, and the patient expired.

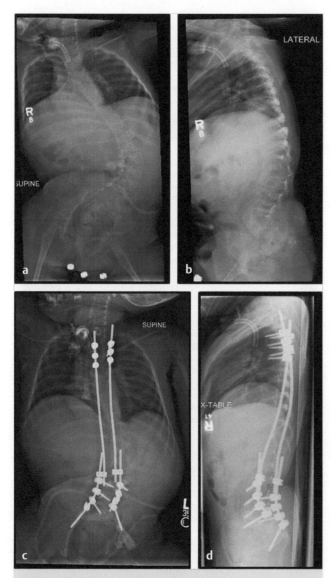

Fig. 6.1 (a,b) Supine frontal and lateral images of neuromuscular scoliosis secondary to underlying nemaline myopathy. **(c,d)** Surgical correction using growing rod constructs (pedicle screws and a side-to-side connector).

6.5 Ethical Considerations for Spinal Fusion in Severe Neuromuscular Conditions

As can be discerned from the preceding paragraphs, patients developing neuromuscular spinal deformities are typically medically fragile. Outcome studies are observational, and quality-of-life parameters are obtained from parents or caregivers. Thus, some argue that decisions for high-risk interventions like spinal reconstruction require a consideration of an ethical framework.[16] Whitaker et al[16] proposed a four-topic model to assist in the clinical decision making in which the domains of medical indications, patient preferences, quality of life, and contextual factors are innumerate and considered in the decision.[16] While medical indications in favor of surgery include improved alignment for sitting, the high complication rate and equivocal impact on natural history may tilt against surgical intervention. Quality-of-life considerations have only recently been reported in a prospective study with concurrent controls.[50] In this study, patients with CP undergoing spinal surgery reported higher quality-of-life scores than a comparison group that did not have surgery during the time interval considered. However, uncertainty persists because this was not a randomized comparison and, while the questionnaires used have been validated, they are completed by the parent or caregiver, not the patient. The fourth and final domain includes contextual features such as the social, economic, and legal considerations; thus, they are external to the patient. Although funding models are changing, there is a tradition of treating patients aggressively; despite the risks, withholding treatment is seen as callous and uncaring. Furthermore, while funding models in medicine are in flux, we still practice in a fee-for-service environment, which by design motivates to treat. Therefore, in the absence of strong randomized studies, the treatment team in conjunction with the family must transparently consider the indications and risks as best as possible. This process of shared decision making is particularly important given the heterogeneity of the neuromuscular population and the lack of standard pathways. However, within each institution, one should strive toward consistent care teams and treatment pathways, which continually improve in an iterative manner with new insights, to guide the treatment discussion. ▶ Table 6.2 shows the elements of the care pathways used at the authors' institution.

6.6 Conclusion

Despite major advances in the medical management and the surgical techniques, the complication rate remains highest (24–75%) in patients with neuromuscular scoliosis.[1,9] Furthermore, many have progressive disorders for which spinal surgery will not have a long-term impact on life expectancy. The goals of surgery are to improve quality of life as many of these patients have little functional ability, yet our ability to measure this effect is subjective and relies on proxy evaluators. Thus, as surgeons, we must be extremely cautious when embarking on the surgical treatment of neuromuscular scoliosis. Surgical complications are a great disappointment to the parents and caregivers and they drastically increase the cost of the care.[13] Often the patients are worse off after surgery than before the surgery. Even in the successful cases, despite satisfaction in many domains of care, such as positioning, personal care, and comfort, overall improvement in quality of life can be small.[15] Therefore, avoiding surgery may be a more prudent approach; in the most severe cases, opting instead for nonoperative measures such as wheelchair modification and bracing may be a better decision.[52] ▶ Table 6.2 shows some medical parameters that, if present in the patient, should make the surgeon pause before proceeding with spinal reconstruction. This chapter provides only guidelines to help in the decision making as absolute contraindications to surgery are relative and depend on the expertise of the surgical team, the skill of the consultants, and the capacity of the hospital system to manage these complicated patients.

References

[1] Mohamad F, Parent S, Pawelek J, et al. Perioperative complications after surgical correction in neuromuscular scoliosis. J Pediatr Orthop. 2007; 27(4):392–397

[2] Jevsevar DS, Karlin LI. The relationship between preoperative nutritional status and complications after an operation for scoliosis in patients who have cerebral palsy. J Bone Joint Surg Am. 1993; 75(6):880–884

[3] Rosenbaum PL, Palisano RJ, Bartlett DJ, Galuppi BE, Russell DJ. Development of the Gross Motor Function Classification System for cerebral palsy. Dev Med Child Neurol. 2008; 50(4):249–253

[4] Basques BA, Chung SH, Lukasiewicz AM, et al. Predicting short-term morbidity in patients undergoing posterior spinal fusion for neuromuscular scoliosis. Spine. 2015; 40(24):1910–1917

[5] Persson-Bunke M, Hägglund G, Lauge-Pedersen H, Wagner P, Westbom L. Scoliosis in a total population of children with cerebral palsy. Spine. 2012; 37 (12):E708–E713

[6] Barsdorf AI, Sproule DM, Kaufmann P. Scoliosis surgery in children with neuromuscular disease: findings from the US National Inpatient Sample, 1997 to 2003. Arch Neurol. 2010; 67(2):231–235

[7] Blackmore AM, Bear N, Blair E, et al. Factors associated with respiratory illness in children and young adults with cerebral palsy. J Pediatr. 2016; 168:151–157

[8] Yuan N, Fraire JA, Margetis MM, Skaggs DL, Tolo VT, Keens TG. The effect of scoliosis surgery on lung function in the immediate postoperative period. Spine. 2005; 30(19):2182–2185

[9] Master DL, Son-Hing JP, Poe-Kochert C, Armstrong DG, Thompson GH. Risk factors for major complications after surgery for neuromuscular scoliosis. Spine. 2011; 36(7):564–571

[10] Tsirikos AI, Lipton G, Chang WN, Dabney KW, Miller F. Surgical correction of scoliosis in pediatric patients with cerebral palsy using the unit rod instrumentation. Spine. 2008; 33(10):1133–1140

[11] Menga EN, Hirschfeld C, Jain A, et al. Intraoperative cardiopulmonary arrest in children undergoing spinal deformity correction: causes and associated factors. Spine. 2015; 40(22):1757–1762

[12] Modi HN, Hong JY, Mehta SS, et al. Surgical correction and fusion using posterior-only pedicle screw construct for neuropathic scoliosis in patients with cerebral palsy: a three-year follow-up study. Spine. 2009; 34(11):1167–1175

[13] Watanabe K, Lenke LG, Daubs MD, et al. Is spine deformity surgery in patients with spastic cerebral palsy truly beneficial?: a patient/parent evaluation. Spine. 2009; 34(20):2222–2232

[14] Sewell MD, Malagelada F, Wallace C, et al. A preliminary study to assess whether spinal fusion for scoliosis improves carer-assessed quality of life for children with GMFCS level IV or V cerebral palsy. J Pediatr Orthop. 2016; 36 (3):299–304

[15] Difazio RL, Vessey JA, Zurakowski D, Snyder BD. Differences in health-related quality of life and caregiver burden after hip and spine surgery in non-ambulatory children with severe cerebral palsy. Dev Med Child Neurol. 2016; 58 (3):298:305

[16] Whitaker AT, Sharkey M, Diab M. Spinal fusion for scoliosis in patients with globally involved cerebral palsy: an ethical assessment. J Bone Joint Surg Am. 2015; 97(9):782:787

[17] Kinali M, Main M, Eliahoo J, et al. Predictive factors for the development of scoliosis in Duchenne muscular dystrophy. Eur J Paediatr Neurol. 2007; 11 (3):160–166

[18] Kinali M, Messina S, Mercuri E, et al. Management of scoliosis in Duchenne muscular dystrophy: a large 10-year retrospective study. Dev Med Child Neurol. 2006; 48(6):513–518

[19] Biggar WD, Harris VA, Eliasoph L, Alman B. Long-term benefits of deflazacort treatment for boys with Duchenne muscular dystrophy in their second decade. Neuromuscul Disord. 2006; 16(4):249–255

[20] Cervellati S, Bettini N, Moscato M, Gusella A, Dema E, Maresi R. Surgical treatment of spinal deformities in Duchenne muscular dystrophy: a long term follow-up study. Eur Spine J. 2004; 13(5):441–448

[21] Bridwell KH, Baldus C, Iffrig TM, Lenke LG, Blanke K. Process measures and patient/parent evaluation of surgical management of spinal deformities in patients with progressive flaccid neuromuscular scoliosis (Duchenne's muscular dystrophy and spinal muscular atrophy). Spine. 1999; 24(13):1300–1309

[22] Cheuk DK, Wong V, Wraige E, Baxter P, Cole A. Surgery for scoliosis in Duchenne muscular dystrophy. Cochrane Database Syst Rev. 2015; 10(10): CD005375

[23] Mercado E, Alman B, Wright JG. Does spinal fusion influence quality of life in neuromuscular scoliosis? Spine. 2007; 32(19) Suppl:S120–S125

[24] Suk KS, Lee BH, Lee HM, et al. Functional outcomes in Duchenne muscular dystrophy scoliosis: comparison of the differences between surgical and nonsurgical treatment. J Bone Joint Surg Am. 2014; 96(5):409–415

[25] Mehta SS, Modi HN, Srinivasalu S, et al. Pedicle screw-only constructs with lumbar or pelvic fixation for spinal stabilization in patients with Duchenne muscular dystrophy. J Spinal Disord Tech. 2009; 22(6):428–433

[26] Modi HN, Suh SW, Yang JH, et al. Surgical complications in neuromuscular scoliosis operated with posterior- only approach using pedicle screw fixation. Scoliosis. 2009; 4:11

[27] Kurz LT, Mubarak SJ, Schultz P, Park SM, Leach J. Correlation of scoliosis and pulmonary function in Duchenne muscular dystrophy. J Pediatr Orthop. 1983; 3(3):347–353

[28] Arun R, Srinivas S, Mehdian SM. Scoliosis in Duchenne's muscular dystrophy: a changing trend in surgical management: a historical surgical outcome study comparing sublaminar, hybrid and pedicle screw instrumentation systems. Eur Spine J. 2010; 19(3):376–383

[29] Guille JT, Sarwark JF, Sherk HH, Kumar SJ. Congenital and developmental deformities of the spine in children with myelomeningocele. J Am Acad Orthop Surg. 2006; 14(5):294–302

[30] Iorio JA, Jakoi AM, Steiner CD, et al. Minimally invasive lateral interbody fusion in the treatment of scoliosis associated with myelomeningocele. Surg Technol Int. 2015; 26:371–375

[31] Carstens C, Schmidt E, Niethard FU, Fromm B. Spinal surgery on patients with myelomeningocele. Results 1971–1990. Z Orthop Ihre Grenzgeb. 1993; 131 (3):252–260

[32] Patel J, Walker JL, Talwalkar VR, Iwinski HJ, Milbrandt TA. Correlation of spine deformity, lung function, and seat pressure in spina bifida. Clin Orthop Relat Res. 2011; 469(5):1302–1307

[33] Singh D, Rath GP, Dash HH, Bithal PK. Anesthetic concerns and perioperative complications in repair of myelomeningocele: a retrospective review of 135 cases. J Neurosurg Anesthesiol. 2010; 22(1):11–15

[34] Geiger F, Parsch D, Carstens C. Complications of scoliosis surgery in children with myelomeningocele. Eur Spine J. 1999; 8(1):22–26

[35] Jernigan SC, Berry JG, Graham DA, et al. Risk factors of sudden death in young adult patients with myelomeningocele. J Neurosurg Pediatr. 2012; 9(2):149–155

[36] Hatlen T, Song K, Shurtleff D, Duguay S. Contributory factors to postoperative spinal fusion complications for children with myelomeningocele. Spine. 2010; 35(13):1294–1299

[37] Wai EK, Owen J, Fehlings D, Wright JG. Assessing physical disability in children with spina bifida and scoliosis. J Pediatr Orthop. 2000; 20(6):765–770

[38] Wai EK, Young NL, Feldman BM, Badley EM, Wright JG. The relationship between function, self-perception, and spinal deformity: implications for treatment of scoliosis in children with spina bifida. J Pediatr Orthop. 2005; 25 (1):64–69

[39] Khoshbin A, Vivas L, Law PW, et al. The long-term outcome of patients treated operatively and non-operatively for scoliosis deformity secondary to spina bifida. Bone Joint J. 2014; 96-B(9):1244–1251

[40] Schoenmakers MA, Gulmans VA, Gooskens RH, Pruijs JE, Helders PJ. Spinal fusion in children with spina bifida: influence on ambulation level and functional abilities. Eur Spine J. 2005; 14(4):415–422

[41] Jain A, Sponseller PD, Shah SA, et al. Harms Study Group. Subclassification of GMFCS level-5 cerebral palsy as a predictor of complications and health-related quality of life after spinal arthrodesis. J Bone Joint Surg Am. 2016; 98 (21):1821–1828

[42] Nishnianidze T, Bayhan IA, Abousamra O, et al. Factors predicting postoperative complications following spinal fusions in children with cerebral palsy scoliosis. Eur Spine J. 2016; 25(2):627–634

[43] Keeler KA, Lenke LG, Good CR, Bridwell KH, Sides B, Luhmann SJ. Spinal fusion for spastic neuromuscular scoliosis: is anterior releasing necessary when intraoperative halo-femoral traction is used? Spine. 2010; 35(10):E427–E433

[44] Payo J, Perez-Grueso FS, Fernandez-Baillo N, Garcia A. Severe restrictive lung disease and vertebral surgery in a pediatric population. Eur Spine J. 2009; 18 (12):1905–1910

[45] Yuan N, Skaggs DL, Dorey F, Keens TG. Preoperative predictors of prolonged postoperative mechanical ventilation in children following scoliosis repair. Pediatr Pulmonol. 2005; 40(5):414–419

[46] Padman R, McNamara R. Postoperative pulmonary complications in children with neuromuscular scoliosis who underwent posterior spinal fusion. Del Med J. 1990; 62(5):999–1003

[47] Edler A, Murray DJ, Forbes RB. Blood loss during posterior spinal fusion surgery in patients with neuromuscular disease: is there an increased risk? Paediatr Anaesth. 2003; 13(9):818–822

[48] Winter SL, Kriel RL, Novacheck TF, Luxenberg MG, Leutgeb VJ, Erickson PA. Perioperative blood loss: the effect of valproate. Pediatr Neurol. 1996; 15 (1):19–22

[49] Master DL, Poe-Kochert C, Son-Hing J, Armstrong DG, Thompson GH. Wound infections after surgery for neuromuscular scoliosis: risk factors and treatment outcomes. Spine. 2011; 36(3):E179–E185

[50] Sponseller PD, Jain A, Shah SA, et al. Deep wound infections after spinal fusion in children with cerebral palsy: a prospective cohort study. Spine. 2013; 38(23):2023–2027

[51] Jain A, Puvanesarajah V, Menga EN, Sponseller PD. Unplanned hospital readmissions and reoperations after pediatric spinal fusion surgery. Spine. 2015; 40(11):856–862

[52] Terjesen T, Lange JE, Steen H. Treatment of scoliosis with spinal bracing in quadriplegic cerebral palsy. Dev Med Child Neurol. 2000; 42(7):448–454

Part II

Diagnosis Specific

7　Scoliosis in Cerebral Palsy　　　　　　　*40*

8　Surgical Treatment of Spinal Deformity
　in Myelomeningocele　　　　　　　　　*49*

9　The Patient with Spinal Cord Injury:
　Surgical Considerations　　　　　　　　*59*

10　The Spine in Duchenne Muscular
　　Dystrophy　　　　　　　　　　　　　*66*

11　Spinal Muscular Atrophy　　　　　　　*71*

12　Other Neuromuscular Conditions: Rett
　　Syndrome, Charcot–Marie–Tooth
　　Disease, and Friedreich's Ataxia　　　　*78*

13　Neurosurgical Causes of Scoliosis　　　　*88*

14　Sagittal Plane Spinal Deformity in
　　Patients with Neuromuscular Disease　　*95*

15　Spinal Deformity Associated with
　　Neurodegenerative Disease in Adults　　*104*

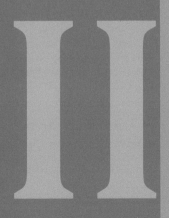

7 Scoliosis in Cerebral Palsy

Paul D. Sponseller and Stuart L. Mitchell

Abstract

Surgical treatment of spinal deformity in patients with cerebral palsy is complex and has one of the highest complication rates of any spinal deformity surgery. Most profoundly affected patients with Gross Motor Function Classification System level IV or V develop neuromuscular scoliosis that can be characterized using the Lonstein classification. It is safest to use a proactive approach when deciding the optimal time to proceed with surgery. During fusion surgery, the spine can be instrumented using a number of options, including a precontoured "unit" rod or segmental pedicle screw and custom-contoured rods. Pelvic fixation can be accomplished best with the unit rod or sacral–alar–iliac screws in custom-contoured rod constructs. Recent outcome data have shown modest but statistically significant improvements in caretaker satisfaction measures after surgical treatment of spinal deformity.

Keywords: cerebral palsy, kyphosis, Lonstein classification, neuromuscular, pedicle screw instrumentation, pelvic fixation, sacral–alar–iliac screws, scoliosis, spinal deformity, unit rod instrumentation

7.1 Characteristics of Scoliosis Specific to Patients with Cerebral Palsy

Cerebral palsy (CP) is a static encephalopathy affecting the immature brain that leads to secondary consequences, including permanent motor dysfunction. There are multiple subtypes of CP and variable degrees of impairment, as indicated by the Gross Motor Function Classification System (GMFCS), which often follow different clinical courses and require unique clinical management. The GMFCS is a classification tool developed by Palisano et al.[1] to categorize patients with CP into one of five levels on the basis of activities such as sitting and ambulatory ability.[2] Patients who are more severely affected also tend to have more medical and physical problems, including spinal deformity. Scoliosis is the most frequently occurring spinal deformity in patients with CP. Kyphosis may occur separately or in conjunction with scoliosis. Often, the severity of the spinal deformity in these patients is associated with the severity and type of CP. Spinal deformity in these patients is a complex problem that requires consideration of multiple factors when choosing to proceed with surgical treatment.

7.1.1 Incidence

CP is one of the most common chronic childhood disabilities in the developed world, with an incidence of 2 to 2.5 per 1,000 live births.[2] Reported scoliosis prevalence rates range from approximately 15 to 80% depending on the severity of neurologic involvement (i.e., GMFCS level), patient age, and functional status.[3,4,5,6,7] There is an association between increasing incidence

and severity of scoliosis and degree of involvement of neurologic impairment as it relates to the GMFCS level. However, this may represent a confounding effect, which can be explained by the findings of Persson-Bunke et al.[8] They analyzed the association between the development of scoliosis, GMFCS level, CP subtype, and age at diagnosis of scoliosis in a population of children with CP.[8] They found that the proportion of patients with scoliosis increased with GMFCS level, but that there was no significant association with scoliosis and CP subtype independent of GMFCS level. In their series, only children with GMFCS levels IV and V developed scoliosis of greater 40 degrees. There is value in subclassifying GMFCS level V on the basis of axial motor functions. Jain et al[9] has shown that additional motor impairments in feeding (presence of gastrostomy tube), airway control (presence of tracheostomy), speech (nonverbal status), and cortical instability (seizures) may be tabulated to produce subscores from 5.0 to 5.4. These predict health-related quality-of-life scores and risk of complications and death in surgically treated patients.

7.1.2 Natural History

The cause of neuromuscular scoliosis in CP is related to muscle weakness, spasticity, impaired motor control, truncal imbalance, and impaired sensory feedback.[10,11,12,13] These factors may lead to asymmetric spinal forces, and, initially, children will present with flexible, postural curves.[11,13] Persson-Bunke et al[8] found that the prevalence and risk of developing moderate or severe scoliosis was related to age and GMFCS level. They found that children at GMFCS level IV or V have approximately 50% risk of clinically moderate or severe scoliosis at 18 years of age. Although most children are diagnosed after 8 years of age, many children develop substantial curves in the juvenile or infantile period (▶ Fig. 7.1a, b).

More severely involved children (GMFCS levels IV and V) tend to have long, C-shaped curves, which lead to imbalance of the pelvis.[11,14] Curves that occur earlier (before 15 years of age) tend to progress more rapidly and result in larger, stiffer curves.[6,15] The rate of progression may increase dramatically to as much as 2 to 4 degrees per month during the adolescent growth phase.[6,16] As a patient's curve becomes larger with age, a structural component develops. One must also consider that patients with CP may begin puberty much earlier or later than typically developing children, and the age of skeletal maturity may also vary widely.[5,7,17,18] In addition, spinal deformity in patients with CP may progress after maturity. Thometz and Simon[7] found that patients with the largest curves (> 50 degrees) at the time of skeletal maturity had the largest curve progression.

7.1.3 Functional Effects of Scoliosis in Children with Cerebral Palsy

Scoliosis in patients with CP may contribute to major limitations in function, activity, sitting, standing, comfort, self-image,

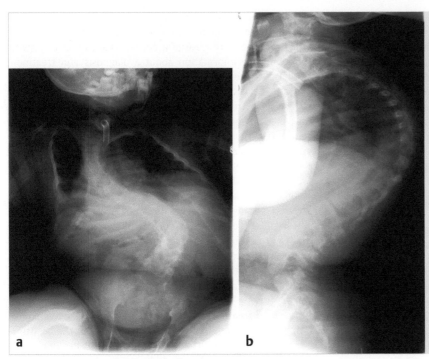

Fig. 7.1 A 6-year-old girl with profound intellectual disability and cerebral palsy from anoxic brainstem injury at birth who presented for evaluation of rigid kyphoscoliosis. She was found to have a 64-degree thoracic curve and a right-sided, 85-degree thoracolumbar curve on anteroposterior radiograph **(a)**. The lateral view **(b)** showed thoracic kyphosis of 112 degrees.

and social perceptions. The concept of form following function is useful in understanding some of the physical impairments of patients with CP. Patients with a single, long spinal curvature tend to experience trunk decompensation, limiting the ability to sit upright without support.[12] Pelvic obliquity can result from unbalanced curvature and can lead to abnormal pressure distribution.[12,14] A balanced, erect sitting position is essential for improved health and activity in patients with CP because it maximizes use of the upper extremities, communication, vision, and feeding. Upright position optimizes gastrointestinal function by decreasing aspiration and reflux with gravitational assistance.[12]

An unbalanced seating position leads to excessive pressure on the skin overlying the ischial tuberosity or, in more severe cases, over the greater trochanter.[12] This alteration in pressure distribution can cause decubitus ulceration of soft tissues, especially if the child is unable to communicate.[14] Patients with rib prominences resulting from scoliotic rotational deformities often experience discomfort at contact points with the iliac crest, as well as with chairs and braces.[12,13] The resultant pressure ulcer and abnormal contact points may produce severe discomfort and pain. Furthermore, the ability to perform basic functions, such as looking forward or at keyboards, swallowing without aspiration, and communicating, depends on an upright sitting position.[11] Nonambulatory patients also have decreased functional capacity as a consequence of their increased reliance on their upper extremities for balance and physical support.[10,11,13]

The degree and nature of spinal deformity can affect the overall health status and comorbidities of patients with CP. Several studies have suggested that substantial scoliosis also leads to impairment in cardiopulmonary function. However, Kalen et al[4] compared patients with CP and untreated scoliosis of Cobb angles greater than 45 degrees to those CP patients with mild

or no scoliosis and found no significant difference in pulse, oxygen saturation, functional loss, or incidence of decubiti. They noted that adult CP patients without scoliosis had no better cardiopulmonary function than those with scoliosis and lost as much functional ability over time. It is important to consider that the scoliosis itself may not be the cause of the functional impairments but may simply represent an additional symptom of the neuromuscular dysfunction in patients with CP.[4]

7.2 Classification of Scoliotic Curves in Cerebral Palsy

Curve types vary in number (single or double), the balance between them, the degree of pelvic obliquity, and the degree of kyphosis. Lonstein and Akbarnia[19] published the most widely used classification system in 1983. It classifies patients with spinal deformities and CP or intellectual disability as group 1 if they have a double curve with thoracic and lumbar components and further subclassifies them as "A" if the curve is well balanced or "B" if the thoracic curve is more severe with a fractional, partially compensatory curve below it. Group 2 patients have large lumbar or thoracolumbar curves with marked pelvic obliquity and are further subclassified as "C" if there is a short fractional curve between the end of the curve and the sacrum (providing some degree of compensation) or "D" if the major curve continues into the sacrum (leading to the most substantial pelvic obliquity). For example, a patient with a large lumbar curve that continues into the sacrum leading to marked pelvic obliquity would be classified as group 2D. However, this classification does not capture all of the key elements needed for surgical planning and therefore does not fully drive modern surgical decision-making.

7.3 Nonoperative Management

Nonoperative treatment may be chosen on the basis of multiple factors, including the curve type, the patient's functional level, and how the curvature is affecting other aspects of the patient's care. The three general types of nonoperative management are observation, bracing, and seating modification (for patients who rely on wheelchairs). The purpose of a brace or seating modification is to support comfortable upright posture and aid the functional use of the upper extremities. The use of a spinal orthosis and seating modifications are not mutually exclusive.

7.3.1 Spinal Orthoses

Bracing is used in patients with CP with the goal of providing postural support and potentially delaying curve progression to allow for optimal timing of definitive spinal surgery. There is conflicting evidence regarding the efficacy of bracing, with some authors supporting the idea that brace use may slow curve progression[16] and others refuting this claim.[11] Most authors recommend the use of a soft brace given that the goal of bracing is to provide postural support, not correction of the curve. Rigid orthoses can lead to problems with skin integrity, pulmonary function, and gastrointestinal function.[9,10,12] Braces are still widely used for children with curves in the 30- to 60-degree range with the hope of providing periods of support or comfort, or of slowing the curve.[11,16] However, experience has shown that children can rarely tolerate bracing for periods longer than 8 hours per day. Most experienced orthopaedists still use orthoses as part of nonoperative care.

7.3.2 Seating Modification

Supportive features of a wheelchair can help enable better sitting. These include lateral supports, head rests, chin supports, vests, variable-angle seatbacks, custom-molded backs and seats, and tilt-in-space systems. These features can optimize function and delay or even prevent the need for surgery.[13] Prescribing these modifications is a technical specialty, best done in combination with a physical therapist and technician.

7.4 Surgical Management

The goals of surgical treatment of spinal deformity in patients with CP are a combination of reactive and proactive ones that vary among patients. Existing problems that may improve after spinal arthrodesis include pain, feeding tolerance, respiratory health, self-image, social perceptions, sitting position and endurance, pelvic obliquity, and coronal and sagittal balance.[13,14] Surgical correction of spinal deformity has the benefit of helping prevent or reduce the likelihood of the organic and social problems mentioned previously and to halt progression of the deformity.

7.4.1 Indications

There is no definitive set of criteria for when to proceed with surgical treatment. Surgical decision-making involves multiple factors, including current and future problems. It is best done as a shared decision-making process with the patient's medical decision-maker, surgeon, and other important members of the health care team. The use of a decision aid (a tool to provide comprehensive information about a diagnosis and treatment options) has been shown to improve knowledge gain, satisfaction, and decisional conflict when deciding to proceed with surgery in the treatment of neuromuscular scoliosis.[20]

Factors to consider when choosing to proceed with surgery include patient age, functional capacity, comorbidities, curve type, curve severity, curve flexibility, response to and tolerance of nonoperative treatments, and desires expressed by caregivers. Surgery should be delayed as close to maturity as possible but should be performed before the risk of complications increases because of the greater difficulty of treating larger, more rigid curves. Delaying surgery allows more time for the child to grow and can help minimize the risks associated with anesthesia and complex spine surgery at a young age. However, this must be balanced against the progression of the curve. Smaller curves are associated with lower complication rates after surgery.[11,21] Thus, there is justification for this "proactive" approach to treatment with surgery before the likelihood of complications increases. Most experts agree that the best time to proceed with surgery is during early adolescence in patients with well-compensated comorbidities and curves of 50 to 75° degrees.[6,10,11,19]

7.4.2 Technique

Type of Instrumentation

The two most commonly used instrumentation systems are the unit rod and segmental pedicle screws with custom-contoured rods. Compared with older instrumentation, the unit rod (▶ Fig. 7.2a–d) is able to accomplish better correction of spinal curvature and pelvic obliquity with relatively low complication rates.[7,19,22] Many surgeons feel that the unit rod remains the standard of care in patients with CP because of the ease of use, low cost, excellent deformity correction, and low loss of correction.[23] However, some caution its use in the presence of hyperkyphosis due to the increased risk of proximal and distal loss of fixation in this setting.[24] Segmental pedicle screw fixation is considerably more expensive than unit rod systems but has the benefit of using custom-bent rods, which provide more adaptability. Additionally, pedicle screws are able to achieve three-column fixation and thus have the potential to avoid anterior release and may provide a greater degree of correction of the major curve.[22,25,26] Patients with CP often have marked osteopenia, limiting the strength of pedicle screw fixation at a given level, which may limit the degree of curve correction that can be performed.[13] Many studies have compared the use of the unit rod versus the custom-bent rod and pedicle screw fixation. In a multicenter series of 157 patients treated with unit rod or pedicle screws with pelvic fixation, Sponseller et al[26] found that both groups had a comparable degree of curve correction, but the unit rod had significantly greater pelvic obliquity correction (74 vs. 22%). The unit rod group had a significantly shorter operative time and better maintenance of pelvic correction at 2 years but had longer intensive care unit and overall hospital stays, required more allogeneic blood transfusions, and had a higher rate of infection (15 vs. 5%). The unit rod may be difficult

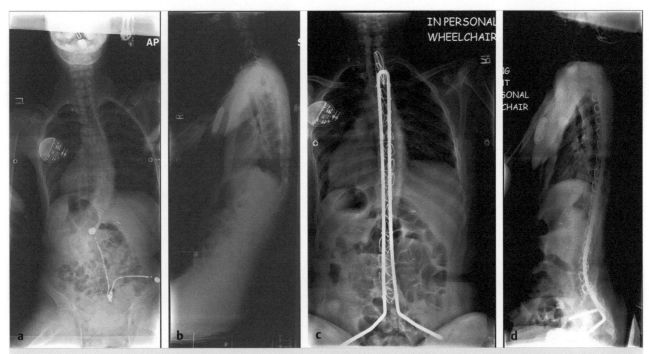

Fig. 7.2 Adolescent boy with cerebral palsy who has lumbar major and thoracic minor curves seen on the anteroposterior view (**a**) and focal thoracolumbar kyphosis seen on a lateral radiograph (**b**). Anteroposterior image (**c**) obtained 1 year after posterior spinal fusion and instrumentation with unit rod construct showing well-maintained correction. Lateral radiograph (**d**) showing excellent improvement of his preoperative thoracolumbar kyphosis.

or impossible to insert in patients with substantial asymmetry of the pelvis in the right versus the left side.

Extent of Fusion

Choice of fusion levels primarily depends on the functional status of the patient and the type of spinal deformity. In patients with good trunk balance and well-compensated curves, the deformity can be fused short of the pelvis. In other cases, the deformity requires much more extensive treatment with fusion proximally to the upper thoracic spine and distally to the pelvis. Proximally, the fusion should extend to T1 or T2 and no lower than T3 because of the increased risk of developing proximal junctional kyphosis.[13,14] Arthrodesis ending in the midthoracic spine is associated with increased risk of proximal junctional kyphosis because of the normal anatomic kyphosis of the thoracic spine.[14]

Pelvic Fixation

The choice of distal extent of the fusion depends on the same factors as the choice of proximal extent. Most cases require fixation to the pelvis to correct pelvic obliquity.[27] Patients with Lonstein group 2, long C-shaped, decompensated curves frequently have pelvic obliquity, but it is important to consider that pelvic obliquity can be the result of multiple factors. Spinal deformity and asymmetric contractures in the musculature about the hip can be independent or coexistent causes of pelvic obliquity.[13] If the fusion is terminated short of the pelvis, there is an increased risk of recurrent deformity that would require revision surgery.[13,28] However, certain circumstances allow the surgeon to end the arthrodesis and instrumentation proximal

to the pelvis (▶ Fig. 7.3**a–d**). They include the following: presence of upright balance such as standing or independent sitting, curve apex at or above T12, and no preoperative pelvic obliquity above 10 degrees.

In cases that require fixation to the pelvis, multiple methods are available. The goals of pelvic fixation are to provide adequate correction of pelvic obliquity and to facilitate arthrodesis. This should be achieved with minimal implant prominence and no implant failure. The Galveston technique was the earliest form of pelvic fixation available, which was later incorporated into the development of the unit rod. The Galveston technique (also used with the unit rod) provides fixation to the pelvis through rods inserted into the iliac wings. These rods can fail by loosening in the ilium (seen as a "windshield wiper effect") or by pulling out of the inferior aspect of the construct.[23] Pedicle screws placed in S1 and S2 are another option for fixation, but this not commonly used because of less robust bony purchase. Iliac screws placed directly into the ilium posteriorly have the benefit of increased modularity compared with the Galveston technique; however, they tend to be prominent. More recently described sacral–alar–iliac (SAI, also called S2AI) screw fixation is similar to iliac screws in terms of modularity but requires less surgical dissection for placement, has a lower implant profile, and provides greater correction of pelvic obliquity (▶ Fig. 7.4**a–d**).[29] Shabtai et al[30] recently showed that pelvic fixation fails 75% less frequently when SAI screws are used compared with iliac screws. Regardless of the type of fixation, at least three pairs of anchors are needed from L4 to the pelvis to reduce the risk of fixation failure.[30] Myung et al[31] found that when bilateral L5 and S1 pedicle screws were not placed in conjunction with two iliac screws, there was a 35% rate of early failure of pelvic fixation.

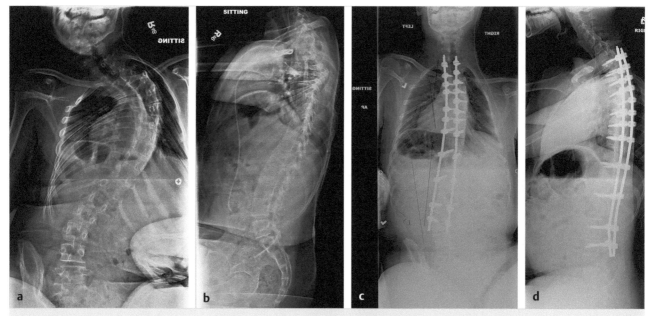

Fig. 7.3 A 15-year-old boy with cerebral palsy who presented with a 117-degree, right-sided, thoracic curve on anteroposterior view **(a)** with loss of thoracic kyphosis on lateral radiograph **(b)**. Anteroposterior **(c)** and lateral **(d)** radiographs obtained 1 year after posterior spinal fusion with segmental pedicle screw and custom-contoured rod instrumentation with fusion short of the pelvis.

Anterior Approach

Spinal fusion through a posterior approach can provide adequate correction in most cases but occasionally, large (Cobb > 100 degrees), stiff, or lordotic curves will require anterior release to increase the flexibility of the curve before posterior fusion. Anterior instrumentation is not always indicated in cases with planned anterior and posterior approaches because the rigidity of the anterior instrumentation limits the degree of correction made posteriorly.[13] Anterior release and posterior instrumentation can be performed in a staged manner with the anterior and posterior procedures occurring on two separate days, or in a combined, single-stage procedure on the same day. Staged and combined procedures have been shown to produce comparable correction of spinal deformity, but combined surgery was associated with increased mortality rate, morbidity rate, and risk of technical complications in a comparative study of only patients with CP.[32] (For further information, refer to Chapter 21).

Use of Perioperative Traction

Traction can be used preoperatively, intraoperatively, and to assess curve flexibility on radiographs before surgery. Preoperative traction is rarely used because patients with totally involved CP do not tolerate immobilization in traction well, and their curves tend to be greatest distally where traction has less effect. Intraoperative traction can be useful to safely improve postoperative alignment and correction of pelvic obliquity.[33,34] Traction can also be used to externally distract the spine to assess curve flexibility with traction radiographs for the purpose of surgical planning (▶ Fig. 7.5a–d).

Bleeding and Antifibrinolytics

Bleeding during spinal fusion can be a major cause of morbidity and death. Patients with CP are particularly susceptible to risks associated with increased blood loss for several reasons. In a recent study, Jain et al[35] showed that among patients undergoing posterior spinal fusion for deformity correction, patients with CP had significantly higher normalized blood loss than any other diagnostic group. In a subsequent study, Jain et al[36] found that patients with less body mass lose a larger proportion of their total blood volume during posterior spinal fusion. This is particularly important because patients with CP tend to have smaller body size for a number of reasons. Other factors that may contribute to increased blood loss in patients with CP include use of valproic acid, depletion of clotting factors, and poor nutritional status.[37] In addition to standard blood conservation measures, one method for safely reducing intraoperative blood loss is antifibrinolytic therapy. Antifibrinolytic agents have been shown to reduce blood loss by at least one-third. Tranexamic acid is most commonly used, but epsilon-aminocaproic acid is another option.[37]

Intraoperative Neuromonitoring

The monitoring of motor evoked potentials and somatosensory evoked potentials can be technically challenging in patients with CP and less reliable than when used in patients with idiopathic scoliosis. Reliability can be limited by factors such as hydrocephalus, periventricular leukomalacia, and encephalomalacia.[38] Although many patients with CP are nonambulatory, intraoperative spinal cord injury is important to avoid because it can lead to intraoperative hypotension, increased spasticity, pain, incontinence, and pressure sores. Despite its lower reliability and technical challenges, attempted intraoperative neuromonitoring is still recommended.[38] Direct stimulation of the cervical cord may provide signals if transcranial stimulation does not. (For further information, refer to Chapter 4).

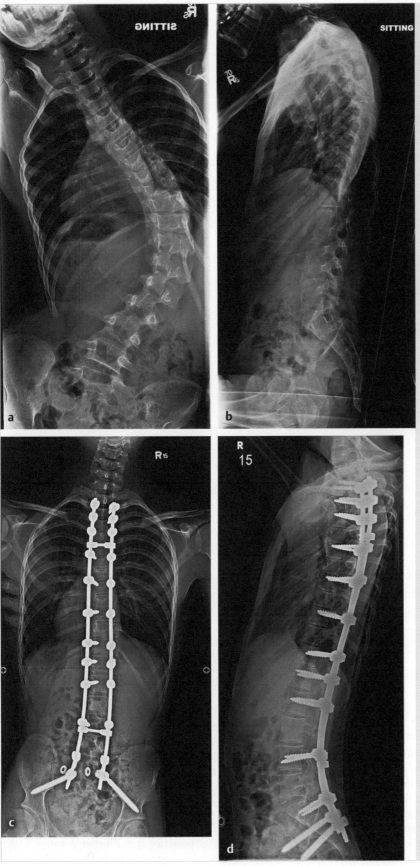

Fig. 7.4 Anteroposterior (**a**) and lateral (**b**) radiographs of a 15-year-old boy with cerebral palsy who presented with a Lonstein Group 2-C curve with 89-degree thoracolumbar major curve and 30 degrees of pelvic obliquity. Follow-up anteroposterior (**c**) and lateral (**d**) radiographs obtained 2 years after posterior spinal fusion from T2 to the pelvis with sacral–alar–iliac pelvic fixation showing excellent correction that is well maintained.

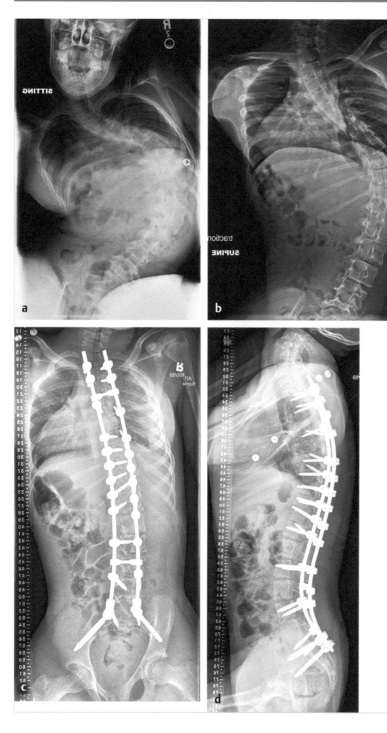

Fig. 7.5 An 11-year-old girl with totally involved cerebral palsy evaluated for spinal fusion. She has a 119-degree thoracolumbar curve shown on this sitting anteroposterior view (**a**). Anteroposterior (AP) traction view (**b**) was obtained to assess rigidity of the curve, which showed improvement of the curve to 75 degrees, leading to the decision to perform the procedure all posteriorly. The postoperative AP (**c**) and lateral (**d**) views show excellent curve correction.

7.4.3 Complications

The surgical treatment of spinal deformity has inherent risks, and in patients with CP with neuromuscular spinal deformity the rate of complications is even higher. A review of the literature shows complication rates ranging from 40 to 80%.[12] In a recent, prospective, multicenter cohort study of 127 patients with CP who underwent spinal fusion surgery, the authors observed 87 major perioperative complications within 90 days of surgery in 50 patients, for a major perioperative complication rate of 39% (50/127).[39] Pulmonary complications occurred most frequently (30%), consistent with previous data.[11] Other complications were gastrointestinal (19%), other medical (12%), wound infection (4.7%), instrument related (1.6%), unplanned staged surgery (0.8%), and neurologic (0.8%). (For information on complications discussed elsewhere in this text, refer to Chapters 22 and 25.)

Wound Infections

Wound infection after posterior spinal fusion in patients with neuromuscular spinal deformity is much more common than in patients with idiopathic scoliosis. Patients with CP have a 6.1 to 15% rate of surgical site infection after spinal fusion,[40,41,42,43,44,]

[45] and presence of a gastrostomy/gastrojejunostomy tube has also been associated with a higher rate of infection. Gram-positive organisms are causal in greater than 50% of all orthopaedic and neurosurgical surgical site infections.[46] However, the causal organism in patients with CP is typically gram-negative; thus, it is reasonable to consider using perioperative antibiotic prophylaxis targeting gram-positive and gram-negative organisms.[42] (For information regarding management of postoperative infections, refer to Chapter 23).

Postoperative Survival

In addition to overall health effects and infection, it is important to consider how spinal fusion affects survival rates in patients with CP. Reported postoperative mortality rates vary considerably, from 0 to 7%.[25] In one uncontrolled, observational study of life expectancy in 288 severely affected patients with spastic CP and neuromuscular scoliosis who underwent spinal arthrodesis, the authors reported a postoperative mortality rate of 1% (3/288).[47] The mean age of the patients at the time of surgery was 13.9 years (SD: 3.3 years), and they found a mean long-term predicted survival of 11.2 years after surgery. They found that only preoperative thoracic hyperkyphosis and number of days spent in the intensive care unit after surgery were significantly associated with decreased life expectancy. However, they found no association between preoperative comorbidities and postoperative length of stay in the intensive care unit.

7.5 Outcomes

In assessing and treating patients with CP and spinal deformities, the best objective measure of health-related quality of life is the Caregiver Priorities and Child Health Index of Life with Disabilities (CPCHILD) scoring system developed by Narayanan et al,[2] which quantifies the degree of activity limitation, overall health, and well-being of children with the most severe involvement with CP as assessed by caregivers. It measures the ease of caring for these children, and because it measures all of these domains, it can be a useful tool to measure outcomes after treatment. A recent prospective study found that small but statistically significant improvements in CP-CHILD scores can be observed from preoperatively to postoperatively and also when compared with controls treated nonoperatively.[48] (For more information regarding outcomes, refer to Chapter 26.)

References

[1] Palisano R, Rosenbaum P, Walter S, Russell D, Wood E, Galuppi B. Development and reliability of a system to classify gross motor function in children with cerebral palsy. Dev Med Child Neurol. 1997; 39(4):214–223

[2] Narayanan UG, Fehlings D, Weir S, Knights S, Kiran S, Campbell K. Initial development and validation of the Caregiver Priorities and Child Health Index of Life with Disabilities (CPCHILD). Dev Med Child Neurol. 2006; 48 (10):804–812

[3] McCarthy JJ, D'Andrea LP, Betz RR, Clements DH. Scoliosis in the child with cerebral palsy. J Am Acad Orthop Surg. 2006; 14(6):367–375

[4] Kalen V, Conklin MM, Sherman FC. Untreated scoliosis in severe cerebral palsy. J Pediatr Orthop. 1992; 12(3):337–340

[5] Madigan RR, Wallace SL. Scoliosis in the institutionalized cerebral palsy population. Spine. 1981; 6(6):583–590

[6] Saito N, Ebara S, Ohotsuka K, Kumeta H, Takaoka K. Natural history of scoliosis in spastic cerebral palsy. Lancet. 1998; 351(9117):1687–1692

[7] Thometz JG, Simon SR. Progression of scoliosis after skeletal maturity in institutionalized adults who have cerebral palsy. J Bone Joint Surg Am. 1988; 70 (9):1290–1296

[8] Persson-Bunke M, Hägglund G, Lauge-Pedersen H, Wagner P, Westbom L. Scoliosis in a total population of children with cerebral palsy. Spine. 2012; 37 (12):E708–E713

[9] Jain A, Sponseller PD, Shah SA, Samdani A, Cahill PJ, Yaszay B, et al. Subclassification of GMFCS level-5 cerebral palsy as a predictor of complications and health related quality of life after spinal arthrodesis. J Bone Joint Surg. 2016; 98(21):1821–1828

[10] Allam AM, Schwabe AL. Neuromuscular scoliosis. PM R. 2013; 5(11):957–963

[11] Imrie MN, Yaszay B. Management of spinal deformity in cerebral palsy. Orthop Clin North Am. 2010; 41(4):531–547

[12] Koop SE. Scoliosis in cerebral palsy. Dev Med Child Neurol. 2009; 51 Suppl 4:92–98

[13] Tsirikos AI, Spielmann P. Spinal deformity in paediatric patients with cerebral palsy. Curr Orthop. 2007; 21(2):122–134

[14] Chan G, Miller F. Assessment and treatment of children with cerebral palsy. Orthop Clin North Am. 2014; 45(3):313–325

[15] Gu Y, Shelton JE, Ketchum JM, et al. Natural history of scoliosis in nonambulatory spastic tetraplegic cerebral palsy. PM R. 2011; 3(1):27–32

[16] Miller A, Temple T, Miller F. Impact of orthoses on the rate of scoliosis progression in children with cerebral palsy. J Pediatr Orthop. 1996; 16(3):332–335

[17] Gilbert SR, Gilbert AC, Henderson RC. Skeletal maturation in children with quadriplegic cerebral palsy. J Pediatr Orthop. 2004; 24(3):292–297

[18] Whitaker AT, Sharkey M, Diab M. Spinal fusion for scoliosis in patients with globally involved cerebral palsy: an ethical assessment. J Bone Joint Surg Am. 2015; 97(9):782–787

[19] Lonstein JE, Akbarnia A. Operative treatment of spinal deformities in patients with cerebral palsy or mental retardation. An analysis of one hundred and seven cases. J Bone Joint Surg Am. 1983; 65(1):43–55

[20] Shirley E, Bejarano C, Clay C, Fuzzell L, Leonard S, Wysocki T. Helping families make difficult choices: creation and implementation of a decision aid for neuromuscular scoliosis surgery. J Pediatr Orthop. 2015; 35(8):831–837

[21] Hasler CC. Operative treatment for spinal deformities in cerebral palsy. J Child Orthop. 2013; 7(5):419–423

[22] Tsirikos AI, Lipton G, Chang WN, Dabney KW, Miller F. Surgical correction of scoliosis in pediatric patients with cerebral palsy using the unit rod instrumentation. Spine. 2008; 33(10):1133–1140

[23] Tsirikos AI, Chang WN, Dabney KW, Miller F. The outcome of spinal fusion using the unit rod instrumentation in pediatric patients with cerebral palsy and spinal deformity. J Bone Joint Surg Br. 2004; 86:118

[24] Sink EL, Newton PO, Mubarak SJ, Wenger DR. Maintenance of sagittal plane alignment after surgical correction of spinal deformity in patients with cerebral palsy. Spine. 2003; 28(13):1396–1403

[25] Sarwark J, Sarwahi V. New strategies and decision making in the management of neuromuscular scoliosis. Orthop Clin North Am. 2007; 38(4):485–496

[26] Sponseller PD, Shah SA, Abel MF, et al. Harms Study Group. Scoliosis surgery in cerebral palsy: differences between unit rod and custom rods. Spine. 2009; 34(8):840–844

[27] Gau YL, Lonstein JE, Winter RB, Koop S, Denis F. Luque-Galveston procedure for correction and stabilization of neuromuscular scoliosis and pelvic obliquity: a review of 68 patients. J Spinal Disord. 1991; 4(4):399–410

[28] Dias RC, Miller F, Dabney K, Lipton GE. Revision spine surgery in children with cerebral palsy. J Spinal Disord. 1997; 10(2):132–144

[29] Sponseller PD, Zimmerman RM, Ko PS, et al. Low profile pelvic fixation with the sacral alar iliac technique in the pediatric population improves results at two-year minimum follow-up. Spine. 2010; 35(20):1887–1892

[30] Shabtai L, Andras LM, Portman M, et al. Sacral alar iliac (SAI) screws fail 75% less frequently than iliac screws in neuromuscular scoliosis. J Pediatr Orthop. 2016

[31] Myung KS, Lee C, Skaggs DL. Early pelvic fixation failure in neuromuscular scoliosis. J Pediatr Orthop. 2015; 35(3):258–265

[32] Tsirikos AI, Chang WN, Dabney KW, Miller F. Comparison of one-stage versus two-stage anteroposterior spinal fusion in pediatric patients with cerebral palsy and neuromuscular scoliosis. Spine. 2003; 28(12):1300–1305

[33] Takeshita K, Lenke LG, Bridwell KH, Kim YJ, Sides B, Hensley M. Analysis of patients with nonambulatory neuromuscular scoliosis surgically treated to the pelvis with intraoperative halo-femoral traction. Spine. 2006; 31 (20):2381–2385

[34] Vialle R, Delecourt C, Morin C. Surgical treatment of scoliosis with pelvic obliquity in cerebral palsy: the influence of intraoperative traction. Spine. 2006; 31(13):1461–1466

[35] Jain A, Njoku DB, Sponseller PD. Does patient diagnosis predict blood loss during posterior spinal fusion in children? Spine. 2012; 37(19):1683–1687

[36] Jain A, Sponseller PD, Newton PO, et al. Harms Study Group. Smaller body size increases the percentage of blood volume lost during posterior spinal arthrodesis. J Bone Joint Surg Am. 2015; 97(6):507–511

[37] Dhawale AA, Shah SA, Sponseller PD, et al. Are antifibrinolytics helpful in decreasing blood loss and transfusions during spinal fusion surgery in children with cerebral palsy scoliosis? Spine. 2012; 37(9):E549–E555

[38] Mo AZ, Asemota AO, Venkatesan A, Ritzl EK, Njoku DB, Sponseller PD. Why no signals? Cerebral anatomy predicts success of intraoperative neuromonitoring during correction of scoliosis secondary to cerebral palsy. J Pediatr Orthop. 2015

[39] Samdani AF, Belin EJ, Bennett JT, et al. Major perioperative complications after spine surgery in patients with cerebral palsy: assessment of risk factors. Eur Spine J. 2016; 25(3):795–800

[40] Borkhuu B, Borowski A, Shah SA, Littleton AG, Dabney KW, Miller F. Antibiotic-loaded allograft decreases the rate of acute deep wound infection after spinal fusion in cerebral palsy. Spine. 2008; 33(21):2300–2304

[41] Cahill PJ, Warnick DE, Lee MJ, et al. Infection after spinal fusion for pediatric spinal deformity: thirty years of experience at a single institution. Spine. 2010; 35(12):1211–1217

[42] Sponseller PD, Jain A, Shah SA, et al. Deep wound infections after spinal fusion in children with cerebral palsy: a prospective cohort study. Spine. 2013; 38(23):2023–2027

[43] Sponseller PD, Shah SA, Abel MF, Newton PO, Letko L, Marks M. Infection rate after spine surgery in cerebral palsy is high and impairs results: multicenter analysis of risk factors and treatment. Clin Orthop Relat Res. 2010; 468 (3):711–716

[44] Li Y, Glotzbecker M, Hedequist D. Surgical site infection after pediatric spinal deformity surgery. Curr Rev Musculoskelet Med. 2012; 5:111–119

[45] Mohamed Ali MH, Koutharawu DN, Miller F, et al. Operative and clinical markers of deep wound infection after spine fusion in children with cerebral palsy. J Pediatr Orthop. 2010; 30(8):851–857

[46] Hidron AI, Edwards JR, Patel J, et al. National Healthcare Safety Network Team, Participating National Healthcare Safety Network Facilities. NHSN annual update: antimicrobial-resistant pathogens associated with healthcare-associated infections: annual summary of data reported to the National Healthcare Safety Network at the Centers for Disease Control and Prevention, 2006–2007. Infect Control Hosp Epidemiol. 2008; 29(11):996–1011

[47] Tsirikos AI, Chang WN, Dabney KW, Miller F, Glutting J. Life expectancy in pediatric patients with cerebral palsy and neuromuscular scoliosis who underwent spinal fusion. Dev Med Child Neurol. 2003; 45(10):677–682

[48] Sewell MD, Malagelada F, Wallace C, et al. A preliminary study to assess whether spinal fusion for scoliosis improves carer-assessed quality of life for children with GMFCS level IV or V cerebral palsy. J Pediatr Orthop. 2016; 36 (3):299–304

8 Surgical Treatment of Spinal Deformity in Myelomeningocele

Peter G. Gabos

Abstract

The term "neuromuscular scoliosis" encompasses many unique and distinct diagnoses in which spine deformity can have a major impact. While some generalizations and treatment principles may exist across diagnoses, each specific condition lends itself to considerations that are quite unique to that patient population. Certainly, this is no better elucidated than in the treatment of spine deformity associated with myelomeningocele. A thorough knowledge of the underlying complexities of this patient population is required and will impact all levels of surgical and nonsurgical decision-making. The goal of this chapter is to elucidate the complexities present in myelomeningocele specifically as they relate to decision-making in the treatment of spinal deformity, and to highlight management principles to optimize the safe and successful execution of surgical care.

Keywords: kyphosis, myelomeningocele, neuromuscular spine deformity, scoliosis, spinopelvic fixation

8.1 Introduction

Surgical treatment of spinal deformity in myelomeningocele presents complex challenges that are unique to this patient population. The combined effects of severe multiplanar spinal deformity that can include scoliosis, kyphosis, and lordosis along with congenital vertebral malformations, absent posterior elements, abnormal pedicle anatomy, subcutaneous dura, compromised skin, and disuse osteopenia can challenge all aspects of surgical care. A number of confounding medical conditions can also have a major impact on perioperative morbidity (see text box below), all of which in combination make the surgical treatment of spinal deformity in myelomeningocele highly complex with the potential for significant complications.

Confounding Conditions That Can Impact Instrumented Spinal Fusion in Myelomeningocele
- Shunted hydrocephalus
- Chiari malformation
- Tethered cord
- Neurogenic bowel and bladder
- Bladder augmentation procedures
- Thoracic insufficiency syndrome
- Latex allergy
- Truncal obesity
- Lower extremity contractures
- Insensate skin

8.2 Treatment Guidelines

In general, scoliotic curves less than 40 to 50 degrees can be managed nonoperatively. Bracing can be utilized in select cases to assist in truncal stabilization and hands-free sitting but would not typically be used for curve management.[1] Compromised and insensate skin, anterior genitourinary and bowel appliances, truncal obesity, and respiratory compromise can render bracing difficult at best.

Surgical treatment of spine deformity may be indicated with curve progression as well as other functional problems that may be associated with increasing curvature. The impact of scoliosis on "hands-free" sitting can result in profound loss of functional independence. Altered pressure distribution across the ischial tuberosities, greater trochanters, or coccyx due to increasing pelvic obliquity can lead to ulceration over insensate skin. Signs of respiratory decline due to progressing spinal deformity may increase the work of breathing and lead to increasing fatigue. In the presence of kyphosis, pressure ulceration over the apex of the kyphus can be a lifelong struggle, and chronic ulceration and vertebral osteomyelitis can occur (▶ Fig. 8.1).

8.3 Preoperative Evaluation

8.3.1 Radiographic Imaging

Preoperative evaluation should involve comprehensive characterization of all aspects of the spinal deformity. Knowledge of

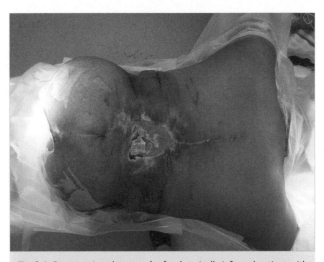

Fig. 8.1 Preoperative photograph of a chronically infected patient with myelomeningocele who sustained skin breakdown over an area of untreated severe lumbar kyphosis. There is a draining wound, loss of skin coverage, spinal osteomyelitis, and exposed, necrotic vertebral bone.

the location of bifid or open bony segments and subcutaneously located dural elements is critical to avoid dural tearing or further neurologic injury, as posterior deficiencies cephalad to the frankly obvious level of the myelomeningocele can also exist. Pelvic and sacral anatomy must also be rigorously defined, as the majority of patients will require stabilization and fusion to the pelvis. Plain imaging should include posteroanterior and lateral sitting spine and anteroposterior pelvic radiographs. Flexibility evaluation can include supine bending, fulcrum bending, and/or spinal traction films to assess the need for anterior spinal release, spinal osteotomies, and/or vertebral column resection (VCR). Computed tomography (CT) scan and the use of three-dimensional (3D) CT technology can facilitate preoperative planning of surgical approach, correction techniques, and spinal and pelvic anchor placements, especially in cases involving multiple congenital malformations where plain radiography alone may not be sufficient. Magnetic resonance imaging (MRI) should be considered in cases of rapidly progressing curvature as spinal cord tethering, undiagnosed Arnold–Chiari malformation, syrinx, or progressive hydrocephaly from ventriculoperitoneal (VP) shunt malfunction may be present.[2,3]

If the patient has a preexisting VP shunt, a preoperative shunt evaluation should include radiographic confirmation of the structural integrity of any shunts from point of exit from the skull, with particular attention to the cervical region where shunt fracture is most common. Preoperative brain CT or MRI can be invaluable as a comparison tool for assessing postoperative hydrocephalus should shunt failure after deformity correction occur. This is of particular importance if a structural failure (separation) of a shunt is noted preoperatively, as arrested hydrocephalus should not be assumed.[4,5] Postoperatively, radiographic confirmation of shunt integrity along its entire length should be immediately obtained. Symptoms of hydrocephalus due to shunt failure can include headache, nausea, emesis, lethargy, extraocular movement abnormalities, cognitive changes, neurologic deterioration, and even respiratory arrest and death.

8.3.2 Medical Management

A multidisciplinary approach, including consultation with neurosurgery (for shunt management and consideration for detethering), plastic surgery (for assistance with incisional planning, skin closure, and wound management), urologic surgery (for placement of preoperative urinary catheters if bladder reconstruction or diversion procedures have been performed), and rehabilitative medicine colleagues (for optimizing postoperative rehabilitation and functional outcome) can solidify decisions regarding timing of surgery and plans for postoperative recovery.

Signs of impaired pulmonary function due to thoracic insufficiency syndrome (TIS) from increasing loss of thoracic volume due to scoliosis, thoracic lordosis, and/or diaphragmatic intrusion of the abdominal contents into the thorax should be recognized. On physical examination, this may present as labored breathing, including the presence of the "Marionette sign of Campbell."[6] Pulmonary function testing may be useful to quantify the degree of pulmonary insufficiency. Radiographic measures of the space available for lung (SAL) may not adequately

characterize the degree of thoracic insufficiency in spina bifida, as a constricted hemithorax may not be present.[7] A more useful measurement may be the Diaphragm Intrusion Index (DII), which quantifies the SAL after upward displacement of the diaphragm by the abdominal cavity is accounted for (▶ Fig. 8.2).[8] The DII can be calculated for each side of the thorax and so is independent of the presence of scoliosis and a constricted hemithorax.

Preoperative nutritional parameters including serum albumin and white blood cell count, urinalysis, and urinary cultures should be obtained, and treatment of urinary tract infection should be completed prior to surgery.[9] The choice of intraoperative and postoperative antibiotics should be based on sensitivities of preoperatively cultured urinary organisms.[10] Intraoperatively, verification of the patency of a Foley catheter placed into the urethra or a urinary diversion site is critical throughout the procedure to avoid catheter occlusion. This is particularly critical at bladder augmentation sites where mucous plugging of the catheter is problematic. Catheter occlusion during prolonged surgery can lead to kidney damage as well as overwhelming urosepsis, which can lead to patient

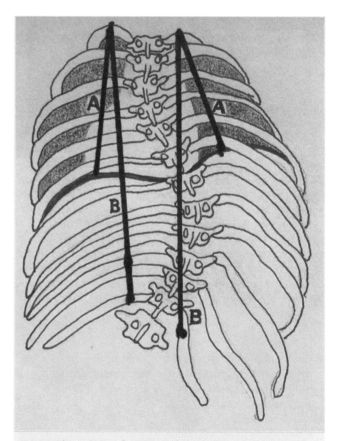

Fig. 8.2 The technique for measuring the Diaphragm Intrusion Index (DII). The space available for the lung is defined as the distance from the middle of the most cephalad rib down to the center of the hemidiaphragm (line A). The height of the hemithorax is defined as the distance from the middle of the most cephalad rib to a point equidistant from the spine along the most inferior rib (line B). The DII, expressed as a percentage, is derived by dividing the space available for the lung (line A) by the height of the hemithorax (line B). It can be calculated for each side of the thorax, and so is independent of the presence of scoliosis and a constricted hemithorax.

demise postoperatively. A urinary protocol (see text box below) should be in place and strictly adhered to.[8]

Alfred I. DuPont Hospital for Children Perioperative Urologic Protocol for Spine Fusion in Myelomeningocele[5]

- Urology consult preoperatively.
- Urine analysis and culture/sensitivity 14 days prior to procedure; if positive, treat with antibiotics according to organism sensitivities up until day of surgery. Repeat culture 3 days prior to surgery. If still positive but asymptomatic, continue to treat until surgery. If symptomatic, surgery is postponed until fully treated.
- Incorporate organism sensitivity into selection of intraoperative and postoperative antibiotic regimen.
- At surgery, urologist places urinary catheter preoperatively if bladder reconstruction has been performed. Irrigates bladder with Gentamicin solution (480 mg gentamicin in 1 L of normal saline solution; instill 30 mL into bladder, then remove 10 mL to verify backflow). Foley secured.
- After final prone positioning of patient, prior to prepping and draping, urologist verifies patency of Foley catheter by re-irrigating bladder. Catheter adjustments made if necessary.
- Bladder is re-irrigated during surgery if there is any reduction in urine output, or once every hour.

Meticulous inspection of the entire skin envelope is critical, including the skin overlying the feet and pelvic prominences. This also includes anterior stoma and any other anterior abdominal incisions. The posterior scar from previous neurosurgical closure over the neural placode should be carefully evaluated for capillary refill, hypertrophic scar, overall mobility, and adhesions to underlying bony structures (typically the posterior superior iliac spines [PSIS]; ▶ Fig. 8.3). Areas of deep pitting may be present and difficult to sterilize. Scar configuration (midline, off-centered, cruciate, inverted "Y," etc.) will greatly impact incisional planning. Trunk obesity, dentition, and overall hygiene should also be assessed.

Functional assessments should include detailed evaluation of motor and sensory level, upper and lower extremity use, ambulatory function and adaptive equipment where applicable, technique of independent or caregiver self-catheterization, and overall level of desired postoperative independence. Careful preoperative assessment of reliance on upper extremity and shoulder girdle function for mobility is important in counseling the patient or family regarding the potential effects of the use of muscle transfer flaps (if needed) on crutch, walker, or wheelchair propulsion. Range of motion of all major upper and lower extremity joints should be recorded. In ambulatory patients, hip contractures and lower limb alignment may affect ambulation postoperatively and may require treatment prior to or after any spinal surgery. Hip extension contractures can place undue tension on the spinal implants when the child is in a sitting position and lead to loss of fixation.

The social environment to which the child will be returning after surgery can also greatly impact the overall success of the procedure, and evaluation of family structure and dynamics by a Social Work team is essential.

8.3.3 Surgical Planning

Surgical approach will vary based on curve stiffness and severity, procedural goals, and surgeon preference, and may include single- or two-stage anterior and/or posterior surgery. There is literature support for almost any surgical approach in myelomeningocele, with theoretical and real advantages and disadvantages for each.

Historically, combined anterior and posterior arthrodesis and instrumentation provide the best chance to achieve a durable fusion.[1,2,3,4,5,6,7,8,9,10,11,12,13,14,15,16] Anterior diskectomy improves the flexibility and correctability of the curve, and anterior

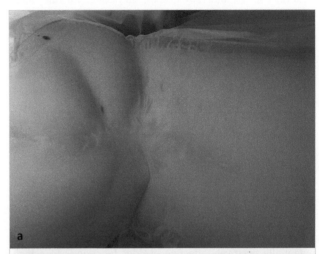

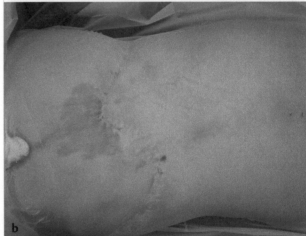

Fig. 8.3 Residual skin incisions over the area of previous myelomeningocele repairs can pose a substantial risk for skin dehiscence, skin flap necrosis, infection, and lack of adequate coverage of spinal implants after deformity correction. **(a)** Diffuse, paper-thin and poorly vascularized skin overlying the lower lumbar spine and sacrum of a patient with myelomeningocele undergoing posterior deformity correction. The skin is adherent to the PSIS bilaterally. **(b)** Cruciate incisions with offset closures from previous gluteal flaps may pose a risk for loss of a large area of peri-incisional skin from flap necrosis after instrumented deformity correction. Careful planning of the surgical incision is critical and may require consultation with a plastic surgeon prior to the procedure.

interbody fusion increases the stability and surface area for fusion, especially in areas of deficient posterior elements. Anterior fusion and instrumentation alone can be considered for select curves. There may also be a role for spinal fusion without extension to the sacrum and/or pelvis in select cases, but this has received little attention in the literature,[18] with most authors overwhelmingly advocating spinopelvic fusion and instrumentation.

Preoperative halo traction may be indicated for markedly stiff and/or severe scoliosis or kyphosis. If a halo is to be placed, the location of preexisting VP shunts must be considered.

Single-stage, posterior-only approaches have become increasingly popular due to the availability of improved implants. In cases of severe rigid deformity, advanced posterior osteotomy techniques, including VCR, can allow for single-stage surgery. Posterior lumbar interbody fusion (PLIF) using structural interbody support may help improve circumferential surface area and construct strength, especially in those areas where posterior elements are absent or deficient.[19]

Spinal cord untethering prior to spinal deformity correction should be considered if some degree of useful lower extremity function is present and/or if the patient shows symptoms from tethering. Untethering may not be necessary in all asymptomatic patients, although selection criteria for performing scoliosis surgery without detethering is lacking.[20] Historically, untethering has been performed prior to surgical correction of spinal deformity but can be performed concurrently in a safe and effective manner.[21] Cordotomy is considered in select patients with high-level lesions and must be performed cephalad to dural sac closure at the selected level to avoid disruption of cerebrospinal fluid (CSF) flow. Cordotomy can allow for better deformity correction, potentially decreasing spasticity and potentially positively affecting bladder function.[22] In a high-level patient with a focal spine infection, such as over a severe kyphosis with overlying skin breakdown, cordotomy proximal to the site of infection may help decrease the chance of dural tear and catastrophic risk of CSF contamination (▶ Fig. 8.4).

Neuromonitoring is considered on a case-by-case basis depending on underlying neurologic deficit. In the nonambulatory child with little or no lower extremity function, intraoperative upper extremity monitoring may be useful to prevent brachial plexopathy or peripheral nerve compression in the arms, especially in cases where prolonged surgical time is anticipated.

Consultation with a plastic surgeon for incision planning and wound closure may be helpful in optimizing wound management and may include the use of preoperatively placed soft-tissue expanders.

Latex allergy is assumed in all patients, and a latex-free environment is standard.

8.4 Surgical Techniques

Careful attention to body positioning on the spinal operating table must incorporate adequate padding and positioning of all soft-tissue and bony prominences to avoid pressure ulceration. Lower extremity positioning may be difficult in the face of significant extremity deformity or contracture and may be time-consuming, but its importance cannot be overemphasized to optimize the surgery and recovery. Extending or flexing the hips can be helpful in achieving more or less lumbar lordosis, respectively. Patency of the Foley catheter must be confirmed after patient positioning is finalized and is facilitated by bladder irrigation (with a gentamicin solution). Patency is verified throughout the spine procedure, as a mucous plug is common, and can lead to overwhelming urosepsis. Skin incisions must take into account preexisting skin scarring, and the skin quality must be assessed over the ilia bilaterally if pelvic fixation will incorporate the PSIS. If fluoroscopic imaging will be utilized for placement of pelvic fixation, taking the necessary images prior to prepping and draping will confirm unobstructed radiographic access to the pelvis (▶ Fig. 8.5). Wide prepping and draping should allow access to all areas of planned (or unplanned) muscle flaps and/or skin flaps or grafts needed for wound closure, including the posterior thighs and gluteal skin.

Meticulous handling of the skin and subcutaneous tissues is attended to at all times. Frequent repositioning of retractors can help avoid tissue damage and necrosis. As the skin and soft-tissue dissection proceeds, definitive knowledge of the location of exposed dura and posterior bony deficiencies must be taken into account to avoid dural tearing or spinal cord injury.

Fixation options for the spine and sacropelvic region will vary based on surgeon experience and corrective goals. For the majority of patients, surgical goals will include restoration of spinopelvic balance for wheelchair use, and so strategizing for reduction of pelvic obliquity and pelvic-to-shoulder (truncal) rotation is important. Restoring the center sacral line to a neutral position to bring the head back over the pelvis in both the sagittal and coronal planes also allows for better weight distribution from the ischial tuberosities to the posterior thighs to avoid skin breakdown and pressure ulceration. Coccygeal morphology should also be noted, as surgical lordosis may impact ulceration over this prominence in thinner children. Whichever sacropelvic and spine instrumentation options are selected, adherence to the principles of firm and stable fixation that is not prominent and allows for maximizing restoration of spinopelvic balance is essential.

Anchors based within the posterior elements, such as sublaminar wires or laminar hooks, cannot be utilized in regions of frank posterior element deficiency. Pedicle screws can offer improved versatility and strength of fixation in the spine.

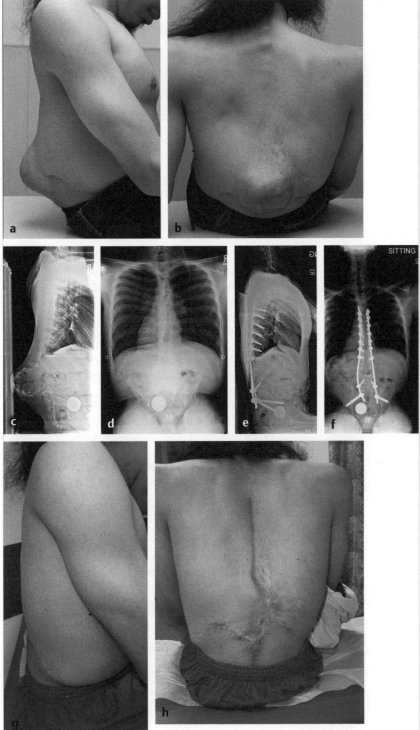

Fig. 8.4 **(a,b)** Clinical photographs of a patient with high lumbar level myelomeningocele and a deteriorating lumbar kyphosis. He has chronic purulent drainage from skin breakdown directly over the apex of his kyphotic segment. Skin breakdown initially occurred during a prolonged urologic operative procedure that required supine positioning. Adequate padding and, ideally, donut padding that suspends the kyphosis entirely may have avoided this complication. Progressive deformity has led to loss of hands-free sitting. **(c,d)** Preoperative sitting lateral and posteroanterior plain radiographs demonstrating the severe lumbar kyphosis and loss of vertical height of the lumbar spine that can lead to crowding of the abdominal contents and diaphragmatic intrusion. **(e,f)** Postoperative sitting lateral and posteroanterior plain radiographs obtained 1 year after spinal cord transection above the infected region, apical kyphectomy and instrumented spinopelvic fusion. **(g, h)** Photographs obtained 1 year after surgery. He has achieved hands-free sitting and improved sitting tolerance. He has a well-healed surgical scar.

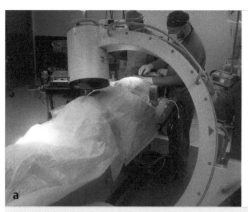
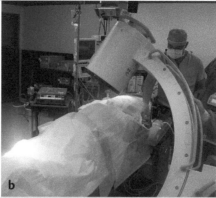
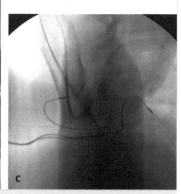

Fig. 8.5 **(a,b)** Prior to prepping and draping for the deformity correction procedure, fluoroscan imaging is obtained to assure unobstructed radiographic visualization of the pelvic landmarks for iliac or sacral–alar–iliac (SAI) screw fixation. **(c)** The iliac teardrop presents a clearly definable and robust channel for secure screw placement within the ilia.

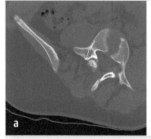
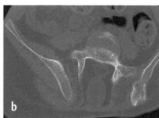

Fig. 8.6 **(a)** Axial computed tomography (CT) image of a normal patient demonstrating the anatomic relationships of the pedicle and posterior iliac wing at the fifth lumbar level (L5). **(b)** Corresponding axial CT image of a patient with myelomeningocele. Note the absence of posterior elements with wide splaying of the spinous processes, markedly abnormal lateral to medial pedicle trajectory, midline-exposed dura, and posteriorly positioned dural sac, and obstruction to the pedicle starting point by the posterior superior iliac spine.

Temporary stabilization rods placed into pedicle screws around destabilizing osteotomies and areas of VCR can help avoid abrupt spinal translation, typically that which occurs from the distal spinal segment translating anteriorly. Reduction screws and polyaxial screws allow for easier and more gradual rod capture into the screw heads, especially in osteopenic bone. Uniplanar screws can enhance spinal derotation, typically at curve apices and at upper and lower construct foundations. In regions of posterior element absence, disk excision, bone grafting, and placement of structural interbody supports from an anterior or posterior (PLIF) approach can add stability and surface area for fusion. When performed posteriorly, these supports are placed prior to rod insertion.

The pedicles in the lower vertebral segments may be difficult to access secondary to marked lateral-to-medial trajectory (▶ Fig. 8.6). Obese body habitus combined with increased lumbar lordosis can pose a particularly difficult problem to cannulating the pedicles. Osteotomy of the iliac wings can allow better access and trajectory for pedicle screw placement into the lower lumbar vertebral bodies and sacral promontory (▶ Fig. 8.7). In regions where dense scarring and compromised

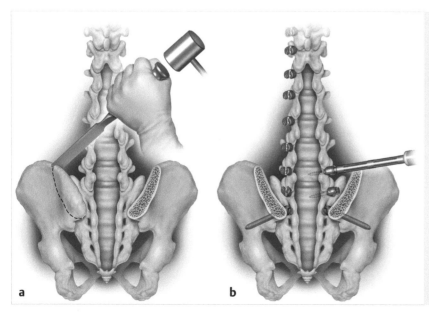

Fig. 8.7 Osteotomy of the iliac wings **(a)** can allow better access and trajectory for pedicle screw placement into the lower lumbar vertebrae and sacral promontory **(b)**.

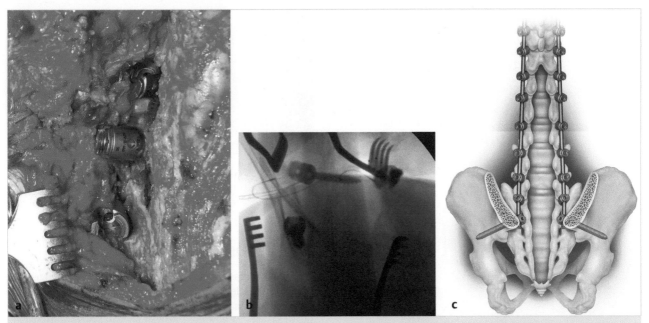

Fig. 8.8 Placing lower lumbar and sacral screws prior to the sacral–alar–iliac (SAI) screws can help accommodate in-line seating of the spinal fixation rods. **(a)** In this photo, the most proximal screw is in L5 and was placed first (after completing a PLIF at L5–S1), the middle screw is in S1, and the most distal screw is the SAI screw, placed last. **(b)** Intraoperative fluoroscan image demonstrating the final placement of the SAI screw into the lower quadrant of the iliac teardrop. **(c)** Image shows the straight alignment of the L5 pedicle screws, S1 promontory screws, and SAI pelvic screws. The screws were placed in that sequence to allow rod seating directly from the spine to the pelvis without the need for any type of lateral or offset connector to the pelvic fixation.

skin overlie the posterior iliac spines, osteotomizing the posterior iliac crest and leaving a thin rim of crest cartilage (if present) can also serve to prevent skin tearing in compromised and adherent areas. Iliac osteotomy should be performed with caution if PSIS screw placement is desired as it may compromise fixation.

Multiple surgical techniques have been described for sacropelvic fixation, including Galveston, Dunn–McCarthy, and Warner–Fackler.[23,24,25,26] Iliac screws provide strong pelvic fixation and may avoid some of the complications of S-hook or Dunn–McCarthy fixation.[27] Second sacral–alar–iliac (SAI) screw fixation allows deeper seating of the iliac screws to avoid skin breakdown over the screw heads and caudal spinal rods and is not compromised by iliac crest osteotomy. In most cases, the SAI screw allows rod seating directly from the spine to pelvis without the need for offsets or other lateral connectors to link up the rod, which may eliminate an area of potential fixation failure.[28] Placement of the caudal lumbar screws and/or sacral promontory screws (if utilized) prior to selection of the start point for SAI screw insertion is helpful if in-line seating of the rod is desired (▶ Fig. 8.8). If more standard iliac screw placement from a PSIS starting point is desired, recession of the

screw head into a surgically created iliac slot in the PSIS should be performed to avoid implant prominence (▶ Fig. 8.9). Other fixation options would include sacral fixation utilizing S1 promontory screws and screws directed cephalad and lateral from S2 to the sacral ala if the pelvis cannot be cannulated for some reason (▶ Fig. 8.10).

Techniques of rod placement for deformity correction will vary depending on surgical goals and surgeon preference. Principles of load-sharing across multiple points of fixation and gradual rod reduction should be adhered to in order to prevent pullout of implants in osteopenic bone. Rod reduction techniques can vary from sequential versus simultaneous dual rod placement. When placing dual rods simultaneously, a surgeon-contoured or precontoured set of rods can be linked proximally with a cross-connector similar to unit rod instrumentation utilizing cantilever correction. In this case, the pelvic screws are captured first, followed by caudal to cephalad gradual rod capture maintaining constant manual pressure on the rods as they are reduced to the spine. En bloc versus segmental rotational correction can be achieved with uniplanar screw fixation, typically utilized at curve apices. Other corrective techniques can include translational correction, distraction (to restore kyphosis

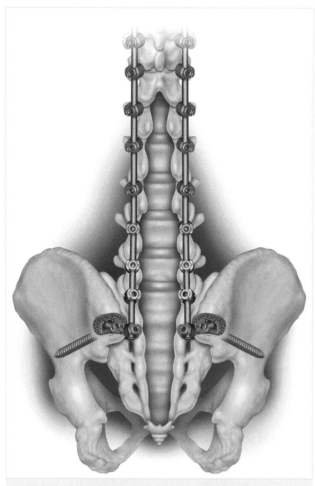

Fig. 8.9 If posterior superior iliac spine fixation is chosen, a surgically created iliac slot will help avoid implant prominence. A lateral connector or offset is needed to link up the spinal fixation rods to the pelvic implants.

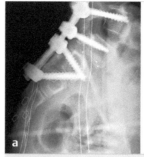
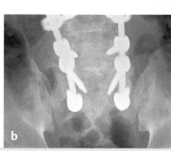

Fig. 8.10 (a,b) S1 promontory screws and screws directed cephalad and lateral from S2 to the sacral ala can be utilized if the pelvis cannot be cannulated for some reason.

8.5 Wound Management

Operative success is critically impacted by wound management. Skin and muscle closure in these patients can be extremely complex, and inability to gain stable coverage over the spine and implants can lead to catastrophic deep infection. The use of preoperative skin expanders may be considered in some cases. Careful skin and soft-tissue handling during the entire procedure is important. Mobilization of large soft-tissue flaps, muscle rotation flaps from the latissimus dorsi or abdominal obliques, and skin grafting may be necessary. Use of perioperative deep and superficial drains may help alleviate swelling and its subsequent effect on skin tension. Occlusive dressings must be skillfully applied, especially around the gluteal fold, where fecal contamination can undermine the dressing. Specialized air mattresses for use during postoperative recovery are utilized. Frequent inspection of the dressing for soiling or liftoff must be performed, and the wound must be inspected closely for signs of dehiscence, infection, or contamination.

8.6 Postoperative Care

The majority of patients will recover in an intensive care unit (ICU) setting until they are medically stabilized. The patient is mobilized as soon as possible. If a dural repair was required, they are managed flat in bed for 48 hours to protect the repair. Their existing wheelchair may need modifications and should be evaluated. Daily inspections of the dressing are performed, and the lower portion is always kept resealed with a waterproof occlusive dressing to prevent soiling. Any surgical drains are kept in place until output totals less than approximately 50 to 100 mL of fluid per day. Aggressive postoperative nutrition via hyperalimentation may be utilized to support wound healing. Weightbearing, if applicable, and transfer training are started as tolerated.

and/or gain concave curve correction) and compression (to restore lordosis and/or convex curve correction), and in situ rod bending, although this must be weighed against the overall quality of the bone and the strength of the fixation. After initial correction is completed, intraoperative fluoroscan images allow for assessment of any residual pelvic obliquity, which can be further improved utilizing compression or distraction across the lumbosacral and pelvic fixation points. A full-length lateral spinal plain radiograph is also performed to assess overall sagittal contour prior to wound closure. Addition of antibiotics to the spinal wound at the time of surgical closure or directly into the bone graft utilized for fusion may decrease infection rates[29] (▶ Fig. 8.11).

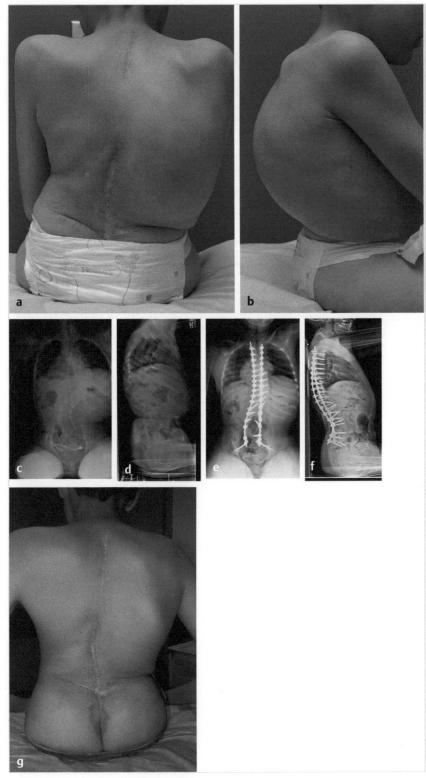

Fig. 8.11 Case example of a midlumbar level, nonambulatory patient referred with myelomeningocele and a progressive kyphoscoliosis that was previously managed with spinal growing rods which fractured and were removed. **(a,b)** Clinical photos demonstrating a significant kyphoscoliosis. The patient has a healed cruciate incision over the lower lumbosacral spine that is densely adherent to the posterior iliac crests. **(c,d)** Preoperative sitting posteroanterior and lateral radiographs demonstrate significant kyphoscoliosis. **(e,f)** Postoperative sitting posteroanterior and lateral radiographs 4 years after instrumented spinopelvic fusion using the techniques described in this chapter. **(g)** Clinical photo demonstrates a well-balanced spine and pelvis. There were no postoperative complications.

References

[1] Olafsson Y, Saraste H, Al-Dabbagh Z. Brace treatment in neuromuscular spine deformity. J Pediatr Orthop. 1999; 19(3):376–379

[2] Hall PV, Lindseth RE, Campbell RL, et al. Myelodysplasia and developmental scoliosis. Spine. 1976; 1(1):48–56

[3] Müller EB, Nordwall A, Maggio WM, et al. Brace treatment of scoliosis in children with myelomeningocele. Spine. 1994; 19(2):151–155

[4] Abu-Sneineh K, Lipton GE, Gabos PG, Miller F. Dysfunction of a ventriculoperitoneal shunt after posterior spinal fusion in children with cerebral palsy: a report of two cases. J Bone Joint Surg Am. 2003; 85-A(6):1119–1124

[5] Geiger F, Parsch D, Carstens C. Complications of scoliosis surgery in children with myelomeningocele. Eur Spine J. 1999; 8(1):22–26

[6] Campbell RM, Jr, Smith MD, Mayes TC, et al. The effect of opening wedge thoracostomy on thoracic insufficiency syndrome associated with fused ribs and congenital scoliosis. J Bone Joint Surg Am. 2004; 86-A(8):1659–1674

[7] Campbell RM, Jr, Smith MD, Mayes TC, et al. The characteristics of thoracic insufficiency syndrome associated with fused ribs and congenital scoliosis. J Bone Joint Surg Am. 2003; 85-A(3):399–408

[8] Gabos PG. Surgical correction of scoliosis in myelomeningocele. Scoliosis Research Society (SRS) Half-Day Course, Lyon, France, September 19, 2013

[9] Hatlen T, Song K, Shurtleff D, Duguay S. Contributory factors to postoperative spinal fusion complications for children with myelomeningocele. Spine. 2010; 35(13):1294–1299

[10] Núñez-Pereira S, Pellisé F, Rodríguez-Pardo D, et al. Individualized antibiotic prophylaxis reduces surgical site infections by gram-negative bacteria in instrumented spinal surgery. Eur Spine J. 2011; 20(3) Suppl 3:397–402

[11] Banit DM, Iwinski HJ, Jr, Talwalkar V, Johnson M. Posterior spinal fusion in paralytic scoliosis and myelomeningocele. J Pediatr Orthop. 2001; 21(1):117–125

[12] Banta JV. Combined anterior and posterior fusion for spinal deformity in myelomeningocele. Spine. 1990; 15(9):946–952

[13] McMaster MJ. Anterior and posterior instrumentation and fusion of thoracolumbar scoliosis due to myelomeningocele. J Bone Joint Surg Br. 1987; 69(1):20–25

[14] Parsch D, Geiger F, Brocai DR, Lang RD, Carstens C. Surgical management of paralytic scoliosis in myelomeningocele. J Pediatr Orthop B. 2001; 10(1):10–17

[15] Stella G, Ascani E, Cervellati S, et al. Surgical treatment of scoliosis associated with myelomeningocele. Eur J Pediatr Surg. 1998; 8 Suppl 1:22–25

[16] Ward WT, Wenger DR, Roach JW. Surgical correction of myelomeningocele scoliosis: a critical appraisal of various spinal instrumentation systems. J Pediatr Orthop. 1989; 9(3):262–268

[17] Sponseller PD, Young AT, Sarwark JF, Lim R. Anterior only fusion for scoliosis in patients with myelomeningocele. Clin Orthop Relat Res. 1999(364):117–124

[18] Wild A, Haak H, Kumar M, Krauspe R. Is sacral instrumentation mandatory to address pelvic obliquity in neuromuscular thoracolumbar scoliosis due to myelomeningocele? Spine. 2001; 26(14):E325–E329

[19] Rodgers WB, Williams MS, Schwend RM, Emans JB. Spinal deformity in myelodysplasia. Correction with posterior pedicle screw instrumentation. Spine. 1997; 22(20):2435–2443

[20] Samdani AF, Fine AL, Sagoo SS, et al. A patient with myelomeningocele: is untethering necessary prior to scoliosis correction? Neurosurg Focus. 2010; 29(1):E8

[21] Mehta VA, Gottfried ON, McGirt MJ, Gokaslan ZL, Ahn ES, Jallo GI. Safety and efficacy of concurrent pediatric spinal cord untethering and deformity correction. J Spinal Disord Tech. 2011; 24(6):401–405

[22] Lalonde F, Jarvis J. Congenital kyphosis in myelomeningocele. The effect of cordotomy on bladder function. J Bone Joint Surg Br. 1999; 81(2):245–249

[23] McCall RE. Modified Luque instrumentation after myelomeningocele kyphectomy. Spine. 1998; 23(12):1406–1411

[24] McCarthy RE, Bruffett WL, McCullough FL. S rod fixation to the sacrum in patients with neuromuscular spinal deformities. Clin Orthop Relat Res. 1999 (364):26–31

[25] McCarthy RE, Dunn H, McCullough FL. Luque fixation to the sacral ala using the Dunn-McCarthy modification. Spine. 1989; 14(3):281–283

[26] Thomsen M, Lang RD, Carstens C. Results of kyphectomy with the technique of Warner and Fackler in children with myelodysplasia. J Pediatr Orthop B. 2000; 9(3):143–147

[27] Walick KS, King JT, Johnston CE, Rathjen KE. Neuropathic lower extremity pain following Dunn-McCarthy instrumentation. Spine. 2008; 33(23):E877–E880

[28] Chang TL, Sponseller PD, Kebaish KM, Fishman EK. Low profile pelvic fixation: anatomic parameters for sacral alar-iliac fixation versus traditional iliac fixation. Spine. 2009; 34(5):436–440

[29] Borkhuu B, Borowski A, Shah SA, Littleton AG, Dabney KW, Miller F. Antibiotic-loaded allograft decreases the rate of acute deep wound infection after spinal fusion in cerebral palsy. Spine. 2008; 33(21):2300–2304

9 The Patient with Spinal Cord Injury: Surgical Considerations

Joshua M. Pahys, Amer F. Samdani, and Randal R. Betz

Abstract

The incidence of the development of scoliosis in young patients with spinal cord injury (SCI) is essentially 100% if they are injured before the age of 10 years and 67% if they are injured prior to skeletal maturity. Patients with scoliosis secondary to SCI can benefit from different strategies such as prophylactic bracing, especially if started immediately following the injury, as this has been shown to delay or even eliminate the need for spinal fusion. Aligning the spine during a fusion in a sitting posture with a level pelvis and proper sagittal alignment to maximize the patient's independence and function as well as reduce the potential for decubitus ulcerations is critical. Relatively early fusion to minimize the surgical complication risks should also be considered. Failure to recognize the compensatory movement patterns that the patient with SCI may be utilizing prior to a spinal fusion may result in unanticipated postoperative challenges in management. A comprehensive team approach with physical/occupational therapy, wheelchair specialists, orthotists, rehabilitation medicine physicians, and orthopaedic surgeons is therefore highly recommended to provide optimal global care for this patient population. When a surgical treatment is recommended by the team, patients with scoliosis secondary to SCI can continue to lead full and active lives after spinal fusion.

Keywords: paralytic scoliosis, pelvic obliquity, sagittal balance, spinal cord injury, spinal fusion

9.1 Etiology

Spinal deformity as a result of spinal cord injury (SCI) most commonly affects children and adolescents, but may also impact adults. The coronal and/or sagittal plane deformity typically develops secondary to muscle weakness and/or imbalance. The development of progressive kyphosis alone can also present as a residual deformity following a fracture or iatrogenic injury secondary to a laminectomy possibly performed at the time of initial surgical decompression/stabilization.[1]

9.2 Prevalence

The prevalence of scoliosis in SCI is quite high, especially when an injury occurs in a younger patient. Lancourt et al[2] reported that the prevalence of scoliosis was 100% in patients with SCI under the age of 10 years, 19% in patients from 11 to 16 years, and 12% in patients over 16 years of age. Dearolf et al[3] found that the risk of surgery for spinal deformity resulting from SCI was 67% if the injury occurred prior to maturity. Mulcahey et al[4] reported that children injured before the age of 12 years were 3.7 times more likely to require a spinal fusion as compared to those injured after the age of 12 years in a study of 217 children with SCI.

A multitude of problems can be incurred as a result of spinal deformity in a patient with SCI. Most notably, the spinal deformity may lead to significant pelvic obliquity that results in poor sitting balance; this puts the patient at risk for pressure ulcerations from asymmetrical sitting and increased unilateral ischial weight bearing. Further, poor sitting ability can inhibit upper extremity function and lead to difficulties with fitting and using lower extremity orthotics. It has been shown that gastrointestinal dysfunction can result from severe pelvic obliquity, while a patient's cardiopulmonary status can be negatively impacted when the spinal deformity progresses above 80 to 90 degrees (▶ Fig. 9.1a, b).

9.3 Management

9.3.1 Nonoperative

Bracing

Historically, the timing and efficacy of bracing for paralytic scoliosis has been debated. The standard bracing protocols for idiopathic scoliosis were often followed for patients with SCI, and bracing was initiated only after the curves progressed to greater than 25 degrees in growing children. However, more recently, Mehta et al[5] evaluated a more aggressive bracing regimen at Shriners Hospitals for Children—Philadelphia. The study demonstrated a significant reduction in the need for surgery when brace treatment was initiated on curves less than 20 degrees. There was a trend toward a reduction in the need for surgery if bracing was started when the curves measured 21 to 40 degrees, although this was not statistically significant ($p = 0.08$). There was minimal to no effect on risk of surgery when bracing was initiated on curves greater than 40 degrees. The timing of surgery was also evaluated in the study and demonstrated similar trends with regard to earlier bracing. There was a significantly prolonged delay in the need for surgery of over 4 years when patients were braced with a curve measuring less than 10 degrees. A 3-year delay was noted when bracing was initiated for curves between 11 and 20 degrees. Finally, only a 1-year delay in surgery was identified when bracing was started for curves between 21 and 40 degrees.

Compliance with brace wear can be a challenge with any pediatric patient.[6] However, this hurdle is increased for children with preexisting functional limitations secondary to SCI. A study of pediatric patients with SCI demonstrated a 28% reduction in the reachable workspace when the children were wearing a thoracolumbosacral orthosis (TLSO).[7] These potential limitations in upper extremity range of motion can compromise a patient's independence and may hinder their compliance. Preliminary studies performed at the author's institution have unfortunately been underpowered to provide sufficient evidence on brace wear compliance in this patient population. However, given that approximately two-thirds of all patients who sustain an SCI prior to maturity will require a spinal fusion, the practitioner must aggressively pursue and

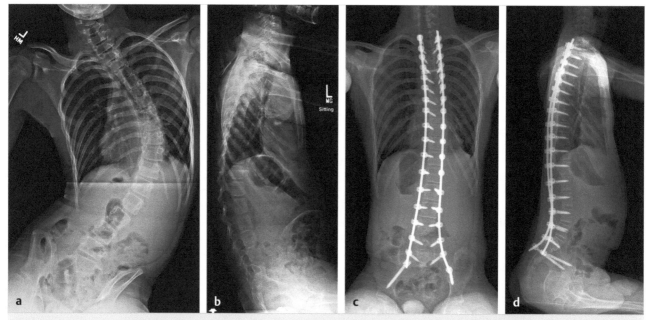

Fig. 9.1 (a) A 13-year-old male patient sustained a complete spinal cord injury (SCI) at an early age and subsequently developed severe, progressive spinal deformity. His scoliosis measured greater than 80 degrees, with 22 degrees of pelvic obliquity. (b) The lateral radiograph demonstrates kyphosis across the thoracolumbar junction, which commonly develops in patients with SCI who are skeletally immature. Postoperative posteroanterior (c) and lateral (d) images demonstrate excellent correction of the spinal deformity in both the sagittal and the coronal planes after a posterior spinal fusion from T2 to the sacrum/pelvis. The preoperative pelvic obliquity has been corrected to achieve a well-balanced, level pelvis.

encourage nonoperative management to potentially diminish and/or delay this unacceptably high risk of surgery.

Wheelchair Modification

Additional and/or alternative options do exist that attempt to prevent or delay the progression of spinal deformity. Lateral supports on a wheelchair may or may not affect curve progression but can be useful to improve sitting balance and allow use of the arms. The patient's wheelchair should be intermittently pressure mapped to identify areas of increased dependence due to pelvic obliquity. Variations can be made in seating materials and custom molding to attempt to reduce the development of pressure ulcerations.

Lower Extremity Orthotics

Ambulation for patients with incomplete SCI should be encouraged if motor strength allows. While not specifically evaluated in the pediatric SCI population, it has been shown that maintaining some upright mobility can diminish the risk for significant curve development and progression in patients with Duchenne muscular dystrophy.[8,9] The spinal orthosis can be utilized as the pelvic portion of a hip–knee–ankle–foot orthosis (HKAFO). Alternatively, the pelvic portion of the HKAFO can be modified to fit over the spinal orthosis to allow concomitant wear of both braces.

9.3.2 Surgical

Indications for Surgery

Surgical intervention is recommended for progressive spinal deformity secondary to SCI when the curvatures progress to greater than 40 degrees in a growing child and/or significant functional limitations are encountered related to the deformity. The nature of the procedure is contingent on the patient's age and skeletal maturity. Typically, standard spinal fusions can be performed on children older than 10 years of age, whereas specialized instrumentation allowing for continued spine and chest wall growth is considered for patients younger than 10 years who have significant deformities.

The threshold curve magnitude of greater than 40 degrees for surgical intervention in skeletally immature patients was derived in part from the study of patients with spina bifida. Müller et al[10] reported an average progression of 13 degrees per year once the curve exceeded 40 degrees in patients with spina bifida. Complication rates have also been reported to be significantly higher for surgical intervention with larger spinal deformities (> 70 degrees).[11] Despite this, for some younger patients with flexible curves, surgical intervention may be delayed beyond 40 degrees in hopes of reaching enough growth to warrant a definitive fusion, avoiding the challenges of "growth friendly" systems.

Spinal fusion may also be considered for scoliosis in a skeletally mature patient with SCI if the deformity leads to significant functional limitations. Poor sitting balance can result in pressure ulcerations on the dependent buttocks and hip. Further, sitting imbalance can restrict the maximal capacity of the patient's upper extremities if the leaning requires an arm for stabilization. Lastly, cardiopulmonary function has also been shown to be negatively impacted by severe spinal deformity. There are no objective studies of the indications for recommending spinal fusion to mature patients with SCI.

Growing Instrumentation

Standard spinal fusion is typically avoided in patients under the age of 10 years, as significant spinal height and chest wall growth remain in this age group. Two posterior distraction–based options for progressive curves in this age group are growing rods and the vertical expandable prosthetic titanium rib (VEPTR), each of which can be lengthened at regular intervals during a child's growth. The growing rods are connected to the spine at the proximal and distal aspects of the construct with hooks and/or pedicle screws. The VEPTR differs in part from growing rods in that its proximal fixation point is laterally on the rib rather than on the spine. These systems have rods/connectors, which allow progressive lengthening at regular intervals, typically every 6 months, to keep up with the patient's spinal growth. Externally driven, magnetically controlled growing rods and growth guidance rod systems are also an option for those with early onset scoliosis. Anterior vertebral growth modulation with a tethering implant may also be considered for some in the juvenile age group.

However, there are no studies to date that specifically evaluate the use of growing systems in patients with SCI. Unfortunately, these constructs carry a significantly high complication rate of 25 to 72% in the able-bodied population.[12,13,14] In the authors' experience, this risk is much higher in the SCI population. Children with SCI are already prone to urinary tract and respiratory infections. This risk is increased with the need for surgical lengthening procedures of the growing instrumentation every 6 months. Typically, most patients with growing systems will eventually undergo a spinal fusion.

Preoperative Workup

The preoperative evaluation includes a rigorous medical and anesthesia workup. We recommend a 30-minute chlorhexidine gluconate solution back scrub starting 3 days preoperatively. Many of these patients are on an every-other-day bowel program, and we ensure a bowel movement the day prior to surgery. Patients with SCI may develop deep venous thrombosis (DVT), and preoperative ultrasound of all four extremities is performed. These often reveal clinically insignificant, chronic superficial vein thrombosis, which then provides a baseline for comparison postoperatively. However, there have been reports of patients having clots in deep veins that may require treatment before surgery.[15]

A preoperative evaluation by physical and occupational therapy is also valuable. The purpose of this evaluation is multifold: first, the therapist can educate the patient and family about the potential positive and negative functional consequences of a straighter, yet stiffer, spine. They emphasize the effect on activities of daily living (ADLs) that the patient currently performs. Part of this evaluation may include placing a rigid TLSO on the patient to emulate the lost motion anticipated following a spinal fusion. In addition, the TLSO trial on patients with high tetraplegia can predict what happens with loss of compensatory movement patterns that may affect upper extremity function following a spinal fusion. The preoperative physical therapy evaluation also reinforces the postoperative restrictions. Generally, patients are not allowed to self-propel their wheelchair, assist in transfers, or flex their hips past 90 degrees for a period of 6 months. Power wheelchairs may aid in maintaining independence in mobility.

The preoperative evaluation includes standard posteroanterior/lateral sitting full-spine radiographs (▶ Fig. 9.1**a, b**) and supine full-spine bend or traction films. An X-ray of the hips and pelvis is essential to understand the status of the hip joints with regard to dysplasia/dislocation. In particular, a high-quality sitting lateral radiograph is imperative, as these patients rely on an exaggerated kyphosis to permit the performance of ADLs, including self-catheterization and feeding. We analyzed the sagittal profile in 30 patients with SCI at our center and found that the usually neutral T10–L2 region measured a kyphosis of 19.8 degrees (▶ Fig. 9.1**b**). Similarly, the lumbar lordosis averaged 9.8 degrees.[16] Thus, fusing these patients with a "normal" sagittal thoracic kyphosis and lumbar lordosis may represent substantial change and prevent them from performing many activities at their preoperative level. This is particularly true of patients with cervical-level injuries and limited upper extremity functioning. It is very instructive for the surgeon to observe these patients performing ADLs to truly appreciate the importance of maintaining their kyphosis. When a patient with tetraplegia cannot sit up, the authors will make a temporary TLSO and see how the patient can function. If the patient does well in the TLSO, then a lateral radiograph in the TLSO is obtained and the rods are bent to match.

Intraoperative Management

Similar to other patients with neuromuscular scoliosis, these patients may benefit from the use of antifibrinolytics, although this should be weighed against the potential increased risk of DVT. The surgeon should also consider the use of a central line, as patients with cervical-level injuries may demonstrate hemodynamic instability secondary to autonomic dysfunction.[17] Furthermore, the anesthesia team should refrain from the use of succinylcholine, as it may cause release of potassium and sudden cardiac arrest.[18]

The infection rate for scoliosis surgery in patients with SCI has been reported to be 16% in a recent large-volume retrospective study.[19] Intraoperative antibiotics, therefore, should include coverage of gram-positive and gram-negative bacteria. We prefer cefazolin and gentamicin, with vancomycin substituting when there is a penicillin allergy. In addition, many have begun to mix vancomycin with the bone graft and/or use vancomycin powder spread on the wound surfaces prior to closure to decrease the incidence of infection.[20,21]

Intraoperative neuromonitoring is typically feasible in the paralytic and neuromuscular scoliosis population, with the exception of monitoring neurologic function below the level of a complete SCI.[22,23] As such, intraoperative neuromonitoring with somatosensory evoked potentials and motor evoked potentials is recommended for all cases with any neurologic function distal to the levels of planned surgery. Neurologic injury is a potentially devastating complication to an already impaired population. Neuromonitoring can also provide information for the upper extremities that may require repositioning after being in a prolonged, static position. Further (or any) loss of bladder control and protective sensation can compound the risk of decubiti in patients with incomplete SCI.

Traditionally, the entire thoracolumbar spine is fused from T1 or T2 to the sacrum/pelvis. This allows for complete control of the thoracolumbar spine as well as stabilization and correction of pelvic obliquity, which plays a significant role in sitting balance. Recent trends in instrumentation have shifted from "unit rods" and sublaminar wires/hooks to segmental pedicle screws and iliac wing fixation with large screws. Pedicle screw instrumentation provides purchase into all three columns of the vertebra, providing a powerful corrective and stabilizing force[24] (▶ Fig. 9.1c, d). Obtaining a DEXA (dual-energy X-ray absorptiometry) scan preoperatively to assess a patient's bone mineral density can be considered. This may impact the number and type (pedicle screws, hooks, wires, hybrid combination, etc.) of anchors necessary to achieve a stable spinal fusion construct.[25] Larger diameter pedicle screws or pedicle screws with both cortical and cancellous threads can be a good adjunct when bone density is low.

Intraoperatively, the authors have found the use of a "T square" as described by Vernon Tolo useful for confirming the proper correction of pelvic obliquity.[26] Two rods are attached in a perpendicular fashion to form a "T," with the horizontal rod overlying the acetabulum bilaterally parallel to the pelvis and the vertical rod over the center sacral vertical line, with positioning of both confirmed by fluoroscopy. If the spine and pelvis are properly balanced, the vertical rod will intersect the center of T1. If this is not the case, further correction in the form of compression, distraction, or rod contouring may be indicated (▶ Fig. 9.2a–e).

The surgeon must also be aware of hip instability in patients with SCI potentially resulting in hip subluxation or dislocation. McCarthy et al[27] reported hip instability in 100% of patients injured before the age of 5 years and in 93% of patients injured before the age of 10 years. The authors typically recommend treatment of the scoliosis prior to treatment of significant hip instability, if pelvic osteotomies would be required, as the orientation and alignment of the pelvis may change following spinal fusion. Hip contractures can often occur after spinal fusion in patients with SCI and may require soft-tissue releases if medication and stretching are ineffective.[28] Pelvic fixation screws placed near the acetabulum may interfere with subsequent pelvic osteotomies, of which both the hip and spine surgeons should be aware.

Postoperative Care

Postoperatively, there are significant forces placed on the fixation of the spinal implants into the bone, especially with rotation and bending of the trunk. These forces and a lack of sensation at times will lead to the development of a nonunion. For this reason, it is important to minimize these forces by restricting independent transfers and requesting use of a power wheelchair for 6 months. Patients may be prescribed a brace (TLSO) postoperatively to minimize motion across the fused segments and reduce stress within the implants. If a brace is recommended, a material should be considered that is not too rigid so the risk to insensate skin is minimized.

Since many of these patients are not continent of urine or stool, we strictly enforce covering the inferior one-third of the wound with a Bioclusive dressing at all times for the first 2 to 4 weeks after surgery. The authors recommend initiating DVT prophylaxis with the use of sequential compressive devices on the day of surgery until approximately 1 week postoperatively. At this point, pharmacologic DVT prophylaxis is suggested for a total of 6 weeks. Given the high risk of developing a DVT, the authors suggest a postoperative Doppler ultrasound of all four extremities at 1 to 2 weeks postoperatively.

9.4 Outcomes

The goals for spinal alignment include recreating a comfortable, functional, and cosmetically pleasing sitting position for the patient with balanced shoulders and a spine as well aligned in space as possible. Another important consideration is proper weight distribution and prevention of pressure sores. Preoperative skin pressure mapping assessment is possible to determine areas of concern for future skin breakdown. If the pressure distribution preoperatively is acceptable, then reproducing the patient's sagittal alignment should maintain a similar pressure distribution postoperatively. In a study by Drummond et al,[29] weight distributions in normal sitting should be 21% in each posterior thigh, 18% over each ischial tuberosity, and 5% over the sacrum. It is valuable to perform pressure mapping after spinal fusion when the patient first sits up to assure there are no abnormally high skin pressure areas. It is critical to proactively prevent pressure sores postoperatively not only for the patient's overall well-being, but also specifically to prevent development of decubiti that may also lead to a spinal wound infection.

9.5 Complications

The risks of major perioperative complications in the patient with neuromuscular scoliosis and SCI are certainly higher than in the able-bodied patient with idiopathic scoliosis. A recent study by Samdani et al[30] of 127 patients with cerebral palsy (CP) reported a 39% incidence of major perioperative complications following spinal fusion. Surgery for patients with SCI with spasticity is very similar to surgery for patients with CP and therefore shares similar risk factors. The magnitude of the spinal deformity was also identified as a risk factor for major complications in a second study of 45 patients with SCI who underwent posterior spinal fusion.[11] There was a significantly higher rate of major complications in patients with curves 70 degrees or greater (36%) versus curves less than 70 degrees (21%). The treatment for postoperative spinal fusion infection typically involves formal operative debridement(s). The need for complete removal of the implants has been shown to be reduced in neuromuscular scoliosis with the use of negative pressure wound dressings after debridement.[31] Given the risk of pseudarthrosis in this population, all attempts should be made to maintain the spinal instrumentation (or replace it) following a postoperative wound infection.[32]

9.5.1 Pseudarthrosis

A pseudarthrosis, or nonunion of the spinal fusion, has been reported in 2 to 29% of pediatric patients with SCI.[33] This may be identified by pain, progression of the deformity, and/or implant breakage. Treatment of the pseudarthrosis often

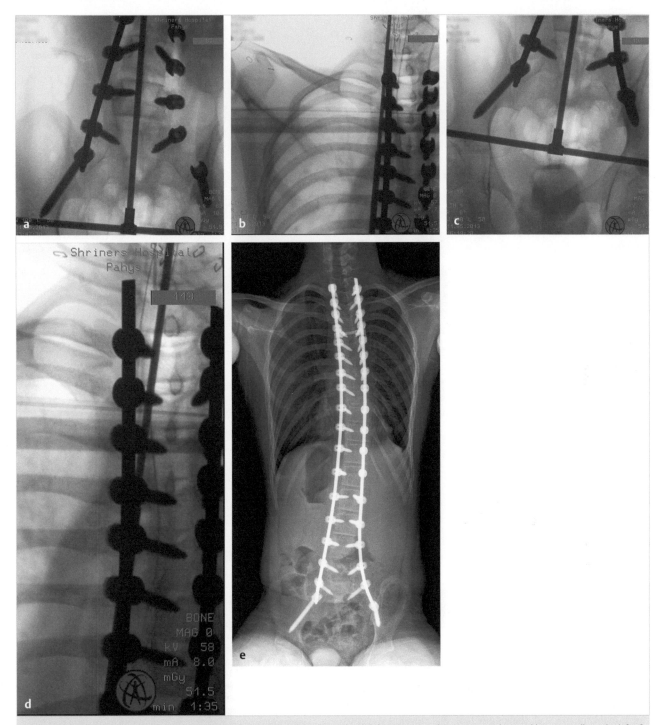

Fig. 9.2 Example of the use of an intraoperative T bar placed parallel to the pelvis (a) demonstrates the center sacral vertical line is initially to the left of T1 (b). Additional correction and placement of a second rod subsequently centers the T bar over T1 (c,d). This correlates with postoperative images that demonstrate proper coronal balance (e).

requires revision instrumentation and fusion. Bone morphogenetic protein (BMP) has been used in recent years to help obtain an early fusion or as an adjunct for pseudarthrosis treatment. The use of BMP may be acceptable for use in patients with SCI who are several years out from their initial injury. However, research has suggested that the use of BMP with a recent SCI may trigger detrimental changes and adversely affect functional recovery.[34] The importance of this is likely more related to the

use of BMP in the acute trauma setting, but further studies with chronic injuries are needed.

Untreated pseudarthrosis may lead to Charcot arthropathy of the spine. This phenomenon, unique to patients with SCI, arises from loss of joint sensation and proprioception. Delay in diagnosis of Charcot arthropathy in patients with SCI may lead to the development of neurologic changes including loss of previous spasticity. This complication can be devastating to a

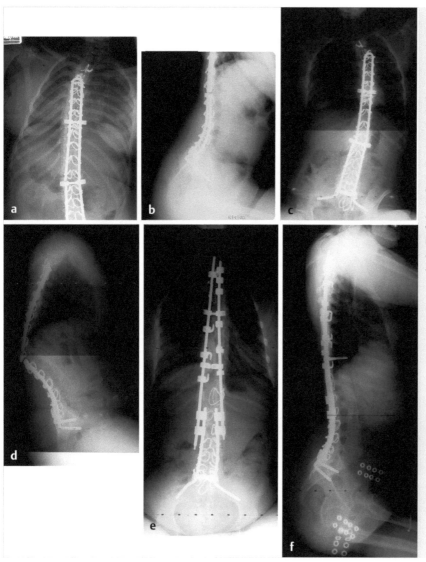

Fig. 9.3 Anteroposterior (**a**) and lateral (**b**) radiographs of a patient who had a fusion at 11 years of age. These radiographs reveal broken rods at T12–L1 that occurred 3½ years later, after a traumatic event. Anteroposterior (**c**) and lateral (**d**) radiographs of the same patient. While waiting for surgery (within 3 months of the traumatic event), she presented with a loss of spasticity, as well as severe instability and a kyphotic deformity. Anteroposterior (**e**) and lateral (**f**) postoperative radiographs after extensive surgery and multiple implants to repair the nonunion of the spine. In addition to the extensive posterior instrumentation, the patient had a vascularized rib graft placed anterolaterally across the spine to help healing. (Reproduced with permission from Vogel L, Zebracki K, Betz R, Mulcahey M, eds. Spinal Cord Injury in the Child and Young Adult. London: MacKeith Press; 2014:278.)

patient with SCI, as any loss of their already compromised neurologic function can significantly alter their independence and/or protective sensation[35] (▶ Fig. 9.3a–f).

9.6 Conclusion

The management of spinal deformity in patients with an SCI begins at the time of their initial treatment. The variety of both functional and medical challenges that will develop depends greatly on the level and completeness of the neurologic deficit as well as the age of onset. A collapsing spinal deformity may lead to deteriorating independence, increased risk of pressure-related skin breakdown, and loss of sitting height. The same concerns may also exist postoperatively for a poorly selected patient undergoing spinal instrumentation and fusion. Both the decision-making and technical execution require expertise in order to ideally manage a child with spinal deformity following an SCI. A team approach that engages the patient/family is required so that all of the risks, benefits, and expectations following a generally extensive posterior spinal fusion (T2–pelvis) can be understood.

References

[1] Mayfield JK, Erkkila JC, Winter RB. Spine deformity subsequent to acquired childhood spinal cord injury. J Bone Joint Surg Am. 1981; 63(9):1401–1411

[2] Lancourt JE, Dickson JH, Carter RE. Paralytic spinal deformity following traumatic spinal-cord injury in children and adolescents. J Bone Joint Surg Am. 1981; 63(1):47–53

[3] Dearolf WW, III, Betz RR, Vogel LC, Levin J, Clancy M, Steel HH. Scoliosis in pediatric spinal cord-injured patients. J Pediatr Orthop. 1990; 10(2):214–218

[4] Mulcahey MJ, Gaughan JP, Betz RR, Samdani AF, Barakat N, Hunter LN. Neuromuscular scoliosis in children with spinal cord injury. Top Spinal Cord Inj Rehabil. 2013; 19(2):96–103

[5] Mehta S, Betz RR, Mulcahey MJ, McDonald C, Vogel LC, Anderson C. Effect of bracing on paralytic scoliosis secondary to spinal cord injury. J Spinal Cord Med. 2004; 27 Suppl 1:S88–S92

[6] Miller DJ, Franzone JM, Matsumoto H, et al. Electronic monitoring improves brace-wearing compliance in patients with adolescent idiopathic scoliosis: a randomized clinical trial. Spine. 2012; 37(9):717–721

[7] Sison-Williamson M, Bagley A, Hongo A, et al. Effect of thoracolumbosacral orthoses on reachable workspace volumes in children with spinal cord injury. J Spinal Cord Med. 2007; 30 Suppl 1:S184–S191

[8] Kinali M, Main M, Eliahoo J, et al. Predictive factors for the development of scoliosis in Duchenne muscular dystrophy. Eur J Paediatr Neurol. 2007; 11 (3):160–166

[9] Smith AD, Koreska J, Moseley CF. Progression of scoliosis in Duchenne muscular dystrophy. J Bone Joint Surg Am. 1989; 71(7):1066–1074

[10] Müller EB, Nordwall A, von Wendt L. Influence of surgical treatment of scoliosis in children with spina bifida on ambulation and motoric skills. Acta Paediatr. 1992; 81(2):173–176

[11] Samdani AF, Cahill PJ, Hwang SW, et al. Larger curve magnitude is associated with markedly increased perioperative complications after scoliosis surgery in patients with spinal cord injury. 18th International Meeting on Advanced Spine Techniques July 13–16, 2011; Copenhagen, Denmark

[12] Samdani AF, Ranade A, Dolch HJ, et al. Bilateral use of the vertical expandable prosthetic titanium rib attached to the pelvis: a novel treatment for scoliosis in the growing spine. J Neurosurg Spine. 2009; 10(4):287–292

[13] Campbell RM, Jr, Smith MD, Mayes TC, et al. The effect of opening wedge thoracostomy on thoracic insufficiency syndrome associated with fused ribs and congenital scoliosis. J Bone Joint Surg Am. 2004; 86-A(8):1659–1674

[14] Sankar WN, Acevedo DC, Skaggs DL. Comparison of complications among growing spinal implants. Spine. 2010; 35(23):2091–2096

[15] Jones T, Ugalde V, Franks P, Zhou H, White RH. Venous thromboembolism after spinal cord injury: incidence, time course, and associated risk factors in 16,240 adults and children. Arch Phys Med Rehabil. 2005; 86(12):2240–2247

[16] Fayssoux RS, Samdani AF, Asghar J, Mulcahey MJ, McCarthy JJ, Betz RR. Sagittal profile of pediatric patients with spinal cord injury (SCI): a radiographic analysis. 14th International Meeting on Advanced Spine Techniques; July 11–14, 2007; Nassau, Bahamas

[17] Krassioukov A, Claydon VE. The clinical problems in cardiovascular control following spinal cord injury: an overview. Prog Brain Res. 2006; 152 (14):223–229

[18] Nash CL, Jr, Haller R, Brown RH. Succinylcholine, paraplegia, and intraoperative cardiac arrest. A case report. J Bone Joint Surg Am. 1981; 63(6):1010–1012

[19] Cahill PJ, Warnick DE, Lee MJ, et al. Infection after spinal fusion for pediatric spinal deformity: thirty years of experience at a single institution. Spine. 2010; 35(12):1211–1217

[20] Borkhuu B, Borowski A, Shah SA, Littleton AG, Dabney KW, Miller F. Antibiotic-loaded allograft decreases the rate of acute deep wound infection after spinal fusion in cerebral palsy. Spine. 2008; 33(21):2300–2304

[21] Sweet FA, Roh M, Sliva C. Intrawound application of vancomycin for prophylaxis in instrumented thoracolumbar fusions: efficacy, drug levels, and patient outcomes. Spine. 2011; 36(24):2084–2088

[22] Ashkenaze D, Mudiyam R, Boachie-Adjei O, Gilbert C. Efficacy of spinal cord monitoring in neuromuscular scoliosis. Spine. 1993; 18(12):1627–1633

[23] Schwartz DM, Sestokas AK, Dormans JP, et al. Transcranial electric motor evoked potential monitoring during spine surgery: is it safe? Spine. 2011; 36 (13):1046–1049

[24] Clements DH, Betz RR, Newton PO, Rohmiller M, Marks MC, Bastrom T. Correlation of scoliosis curve correction with the number and type of fixation anchors. Spine. 2009; 34(20):2147–2150

[25] Paxinos O, Tsitsopoulos PP, Zindrick MR, et al. Evaluation of pullout strength and failure mechanism of posterior instrumentation in normal and osteopenic thoracic vertebrae. J Neurosurg Spine. 2010; 13(4):469–476

[26] Andras L, Yamaguchi KT, Jr, Skaggs DL, Tolo VT. Surgical technique for balancing posterior spinal fusions to the pelvis using the T square of Tolo. J Pediatr Orthop. 2012; 32(8):e63–e66

[27] McCarthy JJ, Betz RR. Hip disorders in children who have spinal cord injury. Orthop Clin North Am. 2006; 37(2):197–202

[28] Betz RR, Murray HH. Orthopaedic complications. In: Vogel LC, Zebracki K, Betz RR, Mulcahey MJ, eds. Spinal Cord Injury in the Child and Young Adult. London: MacKeith Press; 2015:259–268

[29] Drummond DS, Narechania RG, Rosenthal AN, Breed AL, Lange TA, Drummond DK. A study of pressure distributions measured during balanced and unbalanced sitting. J Bone Joint Surg Am. 1982; 64(7):1034–1039

[30] Samdani AF, Belin EJ, Miyanji F, et al. Major perioperative complications after surgery for cerebral palsy: assessment of risk factors. 47th Scoliosis Research Society annual meeting; September 5–8, 2012; Chicago, IL

[31] Canavese F, Gupta S, Krajbich JI, Emara KM. Vacuum-assisted closure for deep infection after spinal instrumentation for scoliosis. J Bone Joint Surg Br. 2008; 90(3):377–381

[32] Muschik M, Lück W, Schlenzka D. Implant removal for late-developing infection after instrumented posterior spinal fusion for scoliosis: reinstrumentation reduces loss of correction. A retrospective analysis of 45 cases. Eur Spine J. 2004; 13(7):645–651

[33] Tsirikos AI, Markham P, McMaster MJ. Surgical correction of spinal deformities following spinal cord injury occurring in childhood. J Surg Orthop Adv. 2007; 16(4):174–186

[34] Dmitriev AE, Castner S, Lehman RA, Jr, Ling GS, Symes AJ. Alterations in recovery from spinal cord injury in rats treated with recombinant human bone morphogenetic protein-2 for posterolateral arthrodesis. J Bone Joint Surg Am. 2011; 93(16):1488–1499

[35] Brown CW, Jones B, Donaldson DH, Akmakjian J, Brugman JL. Neuropathic (Charcot) arthropathy of the spine after traumatic spinal paraplegia. Spine. 1992; 17(6) Suppl:S103–S108

10 The Spine in Duchenne Muscular Dystrophy

Benjamin Alman

Abstract

Duchenne muscular dystrophy (DMD) is a recessive X-linked disorder resulting in progressive muscle weakness. Untreated boys develop a relentlessly progressive scoliosis, resulting in historic recommendations for surgery once a curve progresses. There is no evidence that bracing alters the natural history. Glucocorticoid treatment results in a substantial modulation in the progressive decline in muscle strength and results in a decrease in the incidence of scoliosis and need for surgery. Boys should be offered this therapy when diagnosed. If surgery is required, instrumentation and fusion from the upper thoracic spine to the sacrum is recommended. There is no evidence that one instrumentation technique (e.g., sublaminar wiring vs. pedicle screws) is superior over others. While some have suggested shorter instrumentation and fusion levels, there is no evidence that longer levels are associated with complications, and given the progressive decline in muscle function over time, such approaches should be used with caution. When needed, spinal surgery should be undertaken before the progressive muscle weakness leads to a higher chance of perioperative pulmonary and cardiac complications. New drug therapies are under development, and these may further reduce the need for surgical intervention in boys with DMD.

Keywords: Duchenne muscular dystrophy, fusion levels, glucocorticoid, muscle weakness

10.1 Introduction

Duchenne muscular dystrophy (DMD) is a recessive X-linked disorder resulting from mutations in the gene encoding for dystrophin. Dystrophin is an intracytoplasmic protein that functions as a component of a large glycoprotein complex whose function is to stabilize the sarcolemma. When dystrophin is nonfunctional, the glycoprotein complex is compromised and the resulting membrane instability and increased mechanical stress results in myofiber necrosis, which triggers a state of muscle inflammation. A chronic state of mononuclear cell infiltration precedes the onset of weakness in the DMD muscle,[1] and this inflammatory state affects state affects the skeleton and spine.

DMD is the most prevalent form of muscular dystrophy in children, affecting approximately 1 in 4,700 males.[2] While there is variability in the phenotype of boys with DMD, the clinical manifestations in untreated children follow a predictable course. This progressive disorder is characterized by muscle fiber degeneration causing gradual worsening of muscle weakness. The onset of weakness usually occurs between 2 and 3 years of age, and is subtle at first. Weakness begins in the proximal musculature, and the Gower's sign, in which children use their arms to "climb up their body" when standing from the floor, can be used to suggest this diagnosis in young children. The weakness is progressive, and walking ability slowly declines. This decline in ambulatory capability is associated with hypertrophy of the musculature and the development of contractures. An infiltration of fatty-fibrous tissue into the muscles causes hypertrophy and contributes to contracture development. By the teen years, patients become full-time wheelchair users. The progressive muscle weakness affects respiratory function and eventually cardiac function. There is a roughly 2% per year decline in predicted pulmonary function tests. Ultimately, patients succumb to the disease in their third decade of life from respiratory decline and/or cardiomyopathy.

10.2 Natural History of Scoliosis

Almost all untreated boys with this disorder develop progressive scoliosis. While muscle weakness is the principle cause, some authors believe there may be other contributing factors.[3] For instance, kyphosis associated with full-time wheelchair use may unlock the facet joints allowing for more lateral motion[4]; others have suggested that the chronic inflammatory state causes contracture of the paraspinal musculature that in turn could act as a tether.[3,5] Spinal deformity starts after boys become full-time wheelchair users.[6,7] The one exception is boys with a hyperextended spine. However, this is a rare occurrence, and since studies evaluating the natural history were undertaken before genetic testing was in widespread use, it is not clear if these boys did indeed have a mutation in the DMD gene. There is relentless progression once a scoliotic curve reaches 20 degrees in a nonambulatory child, although the pace of progression varies from patient to patient.[8] A subpopulation of boys develop very large curves that make seating difficult, resulting in pain and a rather poor overall quality of life.[7] There is also a progressive decline in pulmonary function, although it is not clear if the scoliosis progression is directly related to the pulmonary decline.[9,10]

10.3 Glucocorticoid Treatment in Duchenne Muscular Dystrophy

Over the past decade, glucocorticoids, such as prednisone and deflazacort, have come into widespread use in DMD. These agents were initially utilized for short time periods in boys transitioning to full-time wheelchair use. They were found to slow the decline in strength, but concerns about side effects and the finding that once the agents were stopped strength returned to the same level as in boys who did not use the drugs limited their use. However, starting in the late 1990s, long-term glucocorticoid treatment was attempted in patients to determine if the benefits would outweigh possible side effects. The initial cohort of boys treated with long-term deflazacort now has been followed for 20 years. Treatment with deflazacort results in a significant slowing of the progressive decline in muscle strength and function, pulmonary function, and cardiac function. This results in continuation of mobility, a decreased incidence of skeletal deformity, and improved survival.[11,12,13] Side effects of therapy, however, do exist, such as cataracts and osteoporosis, resulting in long bone and vertebral compression fractures.[11,12,13] These side effects can be managed with appropriate ophthalmologic and medical management. Interestingly, however, a recent population study[14] found that steroid use did not increase fracture incidence, raising the possibility that long-term suppression of the inflammation associated with the disease by glucocorticoids may also improve bone health. While there have been discussions about the relative efficacy of different glucocorticoids, there is no comparative data showing the superiority of one drug over another.

10.4 Nonoperative Management of Scoliosis

Although there have been attempts to control scoliosis progression with bracing in DMD, spinal orthosis use has not been shown to alter the natural history of curve progression.[4] Extremity surgery and bracing to keep boys standing longer was at one time thought to slow scoliosis progression, by keeping the lumbar spine lordotic and "locking" the facets, but this too has not been shown to alter the natural history of relentless curve progression.[15]

Long-term use of glucocorticoids results in a substantial attenuation in the natural history of scoliosis development. Early analysis of a cohort of boys treated with glucocorticoids showed an 80% decline in the chance of developing scoliosis by age 20 years.[16] Long-term follow-up of this cohort showed that this reduced rate of developing scoliosis persists into adulthood (▶ Fig. 10.1).[17] In addition, data from acquired paralysis suggest that if the spine remains relatively straight after skeletal maturity, it is unlikely to progress in later life.[18,19] Data from more recent studies confirm a substantially reduced rate of development of scoliosis in other cohorts of boys treated with glucocorticoids.[12,20,21] Not all these studies found as dramatic a reduction in the development of scoliosis as in the early reported cohort. However, taken together, these studies suggest a dose response effect in the prevention of scoliosis and slowing its progression rate from over 90% to less than 30%. There is still much to be learned about the impact of this treatment on scoliosis, including the duration of treatment needed and long-term risks. Compliance is likely also an issue, and boys using the drug intermittently are less likely to show an effect.

10.5 Surgical Management

Because of the relentless progression, surgery is recommended for boys with progressive curves. Rationale for this is an improvement in quality of life and the belief that surgery will slow the decline in pulmonary function. However, the lack of clinical trials has led to a Cochrane collaborative report[22] on scoliosis surgery in DMD concluding that there is no evidence on which to recommend surgery. Furthermore, the effect of surgery on pulmonary function is controversial, with some studies showing a protective effect of surgery and others showing no effect.[10,23,24] Due to the inherent problems identifying an appropriate control group for pulmonary function studies, it is likely that the studies showing little or no positive effect on pulmonary function are accurate. In contrast, multiple studies show a positive impact on physical function, sitting balance and tolerance, pain, and quality of life.[25,26,27,28] Since curves progress after 20 degrees, spinal instrumentation and fusion are recommended in nonambulatory patients who have a spinal curve greater than this magnitude, primarily to prevent further curve progression and improve/maintain sitting balance. Early surgery is preferable, as the worsening of pulmonary and cardiac function over time increases the medical and anesthetic complications associated with surgery. While initial recommendations were for surgery to be performed in boys with pulmonary function tests above 30% predictive values, using more modern anesthetic approaches, surgery can be safely performed once values fall below this range.[29]

This relatively low Cobb angle threshold for surgery is selected since the curves are relentlessly progressive.[8,30] Patients taking corticosteroids may still develop a scoliosis, but the progression is less predictable, so waiting until there is evidence of clear progression is a reasonable approach. There are little data on which to base treatment recommendations in boys treated with corticosteroids, and as such there are no universally accepted treatment recommendations. A conservative approach is to instrument and fuse the spine once the curve progresses beyond 20 degrees. However, not all these curves

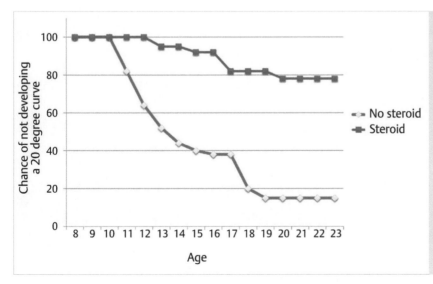

Fig. 10.1 Chance of developing a curve of greater than 20 degrees in a cohort of patients taking corticosteroids compared to a control group by age. There is a substantial reduction in the development of scoliosis in the group taking corticosteroids.

will progress, and since pulmonary and cardiac function does not deteriorate as quickly when taking steroids, one can reasonably monitor the boys' spines as long as they have pulmonary function testing above 30% predicted values. Surgery is recommended using the same criteria as for other etiologies of spinal deformity, primarily based on symptoms, seating difficulty, and progression. These boys may also develop a collapsing kyphosis after they become full-time wheelchair users. In a minority of boys, this may become severe and symptomatic, but this is usually due to associated vertebral compression fractures. Appropriate treatment to optimize bone health/density may help.

Surgical instrumentation should include the upper thoracic spine and extend into the pelvis in patients with a pelvic obliquity of greater than 15 degrees.[31,32,33,34] In those without pelvic obliquity, fusion to the lower lumbar vertebra is sufficient. It is important to balance the head over the pelvis, with the goal of surgical intervention to prevent further progression and improve sitting tolerance, as this can correlate with quality of life.[25,35] While there are a number of studies analyzing different instrumentation techniques,[30,33,36,37,38,39,40] there is no evidence that there is an advantage of any particular approach. Importantly, none of the comparative studies have the power or long enough follow-up to conclusively recommend one approach over another. Screws, wires, or hooks to achieve segmental instrumentation of the spine all can be successfully utilized, as long as the head can be centered over the pelvis (▶ Fig. 10.2). However, it makes practical sense that screws provide superior fixation in the lumbar spine and should be considered if instrumentation will stop in the lumbar region rather than extending distally, and this is supported by data from a comparative series.[36] Allograft is probably a better source of bone graft than autologous iliac crest, especially if instrumentation into the

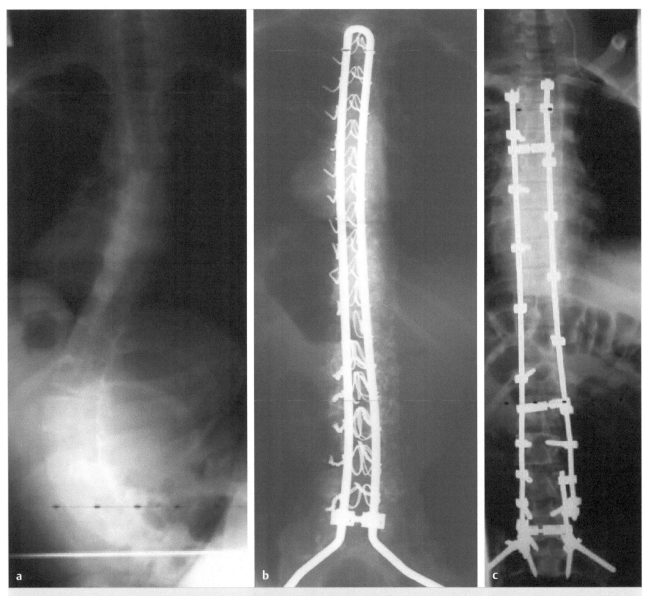

Fig. 10.2 Instrumentation and fusion of the spine in Duchenne muscular dystrophy to balance the head over the pelvis using different approaches. **(a)** A preoperative sitting radiograph. **(b)** A postoperative radiograph showing a balanced spine treated using a unit rod and sublaminar wires. **(c)** A postoperative radiograph from a similar case, using pedicle screws and hooks.

pelvis is used for stabilization to the sacrum.[41] The complication rate in DMD is not significantly different than that of other neuromuscular conditions, although hepatic failure has also been reported.[42,43] Anesthetic techniques can be optimized by undergoing careful preoperative assessment and avoiding inhalational agents that can have deleterious effects[44,45,46,47] so that patients ideally can be extubated in the operating room, and even patients with poor pulmonary function can safely undergo surgery.[27,48] Invasive ventilation with a tracheostomy can prolong survival required in more severely affected boys,[49] but end-of-life and palliative care discussions should be held when making decisions around this treatment approach.[50]

10.6 Conclusion

The management of the spine in DMD has changed dramatically in the past 20 years. The more widespread use of corticosteroids has substantially reduced the need for scoliosis surgery, and advances in anesthetic technique and instrumentation have resulted in substantially improved surgical outcomes. Current research into improved pharmacologic approaches to DMD will likely result in even fewer patients progressing to the need for scoliosis surgery and in improved overall survival rate and quality of life.

References

[1] Feener CA, Koenig M, Kunkel LM. Alternative splicing of human dystrophin mRNA generates isoforms at the carboxy terminus. Nature. 1989; 338 (6215):509–511

[2] Dooley J, Gordon KE, Dodds L, MacSween J. Duchenne muscular dystrophy: a 30-year population-based incidence study. Clin Pediatr (Phila). 2010; 49 (2):177–179

[3] Duval-Beaupère G, Lespargot A, Grossiord A. Scoliosis and trunk muscles. J Pediatr Orthop. 1984; 4(2):195–200

[4] Colbert AP, Craig C. Scoliosis management in Duchenne muscular dystrophy: prospective study of modified Jewett hyperextension brace. Arch Phys Med Rehabil. 1987; 68(5, Pt 1):302–304

[5] Dubowitz V. Recent advances in neuromuscular disorders. Rheumatol Phys Med. 1971; 11(3):126–130

[6] Shapiro F, Zurakowski D, Bui T, Darras BT. Progression of spinal deformity in wheelchair-dependent patients with Duchenne muscular dystrophy who are not treated with steroids: coronal plane (scoliosis) and sagittal plane (kyphosis, lordosis) deformity. Bone Joint J. 2014; 96-B(1):100–105

[7] Smith AD, Koreska J, Moseley CF. Progression of scoliosis in Duchenne muscular dystrophy. J Bone Joint Surg Am. 1989; 71(7):1066–1074

[8] Sussman MD. Advantage of early spinal stabilization and fusion in patients with Duchenne muscular dystrophy. J Pediatr Orthop. 1984; 4(5):532–537

[9] Chua K, Tan CY, Chen Z, et al. Long-term follow-up of pulmonary function and scoliosis in patients with Duchenne's muscular dystrophy and spinal muscular atrophy. J Pediatr Orthop. 2016; 36(1):63–69

[10] Roberto R, Fritz A, Hagar Y, et al. The natural history of cardiac and pulmonary function decline in patients with Duchenne muscular dystrophy. Spine. 2011; 36(15):E1009–E1017

[11] Biggar WD, Gingras M, Fehlings DL, Harris VA, Steele CA. Deflazacort treatment of Duchenne muscular dystrophy. J Pediatr. 2001; 138(1):45–50

[12] Biggar WD, Politano L, Harris VA, et al. Deflazacort in Duchenne muscular dystrophy: a comparison of two different protocols. Neuromuscul Disord. 2004; 14(8–9):476–482

[13] Houde S, Filiatrault M, Fournier A, et al. Deflazacort use in Duchenne muscular dystrophy: an 8-year follow-up. Pediatr Neurol. 2008; 38(3):200–206

[14] James KA, Cunniff C, Apkon SD, et al. Risk factors for first fractures among males with Duchenne or Becker muscular dystrophy. J Pediatr Orthop. 2015; 35(6):640–644

[15] Gardner-Medwin D. Controversies about Duchenne muscular dystrophy. (2) Bracing for ambulation. Dev Med Child Neurol. 1979; 21(5):659–662

[16] Alman BA, Raza SN, Biggar WD. Steroid treatment and the development of scoliosis in males with Duchenne muscular dystrophy. J Bone Joint Surg Am. 2004; 86-A(3):519–524

[17] Lebel DE, Corston JA, McAdam LC, Biggar WD, Alman BA. Glucocorticoid treatment for the prevention of scoliosis in children with Duchenne muscular dystrophy: long-term follow-up. J Bone Joint Surg Am. 2013; 95(12):1057–1061

[18] Mayfield JK, Erkkila JC, Winter RB. Spine deformity subsequent to acquired childhood spinal cord injury. J Bone Joint Surg Am. 1981; 63(9):1401–1411

[19] Lancourt JE, Dickson JH, Carter RE. Paralytic spinal deformity following traumatic spinal-cord injury in children and adolescents. J Bone Joint Surg Am. 1981; 63(1):47–53

[20] King WM, Ruttencutter R, Nagaraja HN, et al. Orthopedic outcomes of long-term daily corticosteroid treatment in Duchenne muscular dystrophy. Neurology. 2007; 68(19):1607–1613

[21] Balaban B, Matthews DJ, Clayton GH, Carry T. Corticosteroid treatment and functional improvement in Duchenne muscular dystrophy: long-term effect. Am J Phys Med Rehabil. 2005; 84(11):843–850

[22] Cheuk DK, Wong V, Wraige E, Baxter P, Cole A. Surgery for scoliosis in Duchenne muscular dystrophy. Cochrane Database Syst Rev. 2015; 10(10): CD005375

[23] Alexander WM, Smith M, Freeman BJ, Sutherland LM, Kennedy JD, Cundy PJ. The effect of posterior spinal fusion on respiratory function in Duchenne muscular dystrophy. Eur Spine J. 2013; 22(2):411–416

[24] Velasco MV, Colin AA, Zurakowski D, Darras BT, Shapiro F. Posterior spinal fusion for scoliosis in Duchenne muscular dystrophy diminishes the rate of respiratory decline. Spine. 2007; 32(4):459–465

[25] Suk KS, Baek JH, Park JO, et al. Postoperative quality of life in patients with progressive neuromuscular scoliosis and their parents. Spine J. 2015; 15 (3):446–453

[26] Van Opstal N, Verlinden C, Myncke J, Goemans N, Moens P. The effect of Luque-Galveston fusion on curve, respiratory function and quality of life in Duchenne muscular dystrophy. Acta Orthop Belg. 2011; 77(5):659–665

[27] Takaso M, Nakazawa T, Imura T, et al. Surgical management of severe scoliosis with high risk pulmonary dysfunction in Duchenne muscular dystrophy: patient function, quality of life and satisfaction. Int Orthop. 2010; 34(5):695–702

[28] Mercado E, Alman B, Wright JG. Does spinal fusion influence quality of life in neuromuscular scoliosis? Spine. 2007; 32(19) Suppl:S120–S125

[29] Takaso M, Nakazawa T, Imura T, et al. Surgical management of severe scoliosis with high-risk pulmonary dysfunction in Duchenne muscular dystrophy. Int Orthop. 2010; 34(3):401–406

[30] Cervellati S, Bettini N, Moscato M, Gusella A, Dema E, Maresi R. Surgical treatment of spinal deformities in Duchenne muscular dystrophy: a long term follow-up study. Eur Spine J. 2004; 13(5):441–448

[31] Alman BA, Kim HK. Pelvic obliquity after fusion of the spine in Duchenne muscular dystrophy. J Bone Joint Surg Br. 1999; 81(5):821–824

[32] Modi HN, Suh SW, Song HR, Yang JH, Jajodia N. Evaluation of pelvic fixation in neuromuscular scoliosis: a retrospective study in 55 patients. Int Orthop. 2010; 34(1):89–96

[33] Mubarak SJ, Morin WD, Leach J. Spinal fusion in Duchenne muscular dystrophy—fixation and fusion to the sacropelvis? J Pediatr Orthop. 1993; 13 (6):752–757

[34] Takaso M, Nakazawa T, Imura T, et al. Can the caudal extent of fusion in the surgical treatment of scoliosis in Duchenne muscular dystrophy be stopped at lumbar 5? Eur Spine J. 2010; 19(5):787–796

[35] Bowen RE, Abel MF, Arlet V, et al. Outcome assessment in neuromuscular spinal deformity. J Pediatr Orthop. 2012; 32(8):792–798

[36] Debnath UK, Mehdian SM, Webb JK. Spinal deformity correction in Duchenne Muscular Dystrophy (DMD): comparing the outcome of two instrumentation techniques. Asian Spine J. 2011; 5(1):43–50

[37] Takaso M, Nakazawa T, Imura T, et al. Two-year results for scoliosis secondary to Duchenne muscular dystrophy fused to lumbar 5 with segmental pedicle screw instrumentation. J Orthop Sci. 2010; 15(2):171–177

[38] Arun R, Srinivas S, Mehdian SM. Scoliosis in Duchenne's muscular dystrophy: a changing trend in surgical management: a historical surgical outcome study comparing sublaminar, hybrid and pedicle screw instrumentation systems. Eur Spine J. 2010; 19(3):376–383

[39] Mehta SS, Modi HN, Srinivasalu S, et al. Pedicle screw-only constructs with lumbar or pelvic fixation for spinal stabilization in patients with Duchenne muscular dystrophy. J Spinal Disord Tech. 2009; 22(6):428–433

[40] Modi HN, Suh SW, Yang JH, et al. Surgical complications in neuromuscular scoliosis operated with posterior- only approach using pedicle screw fixation. Scoliosis. 2009; 4:11

[41] Nakazawa T, Takaso M, Imura T, et al. Autogenous iliac crest bone graft versus banked allograft bone in scoliosis surgery in patients with Duchenne muscular dystrophy. Int Orthop. 2010; 34(6):855–861

[42] Ramirez N, Richards BS, Warren PD, Williams GR. Complications after posterior spinal fusion in Duchenne's muscular dystrophy. J Pediatr Orthop. 1997; 17(1):109–114

[43] Duckworth AD, Mitchell MJ, Tsirikos AI. Incidence and risk factors for postoperative complications after scoliosis surgery in patients with Duchenne muscular dystrophy : a comparison with other neuromuscular conditions. Bone Joint J. 2014; 96-B(7):943–949

[44] Segura LG, Lorenz JD, Weingarten TN, et al. Anesthesia and Duchenne or Becker muscular dystrophy: review of 117 anesthetic exposures. Paediatr Anaesth. 2013; 23(9):855–864

[45] Cripe LH, Tobias JD. Cardiac considerations in the operative management of the patient with Duchenne or Becker muscular dystrophy. Paediatr Anaesth. 2013; 23(9):777–784

[46] Hayes J, Veyckemans F, Bissonnette B. Duchenne muscular dystrophy: an old anesthesia problem revisited. Paediatr Anaesth. 2008; 18(2):100–106

[47] Girshin M, Mukherjee J, Clowney R, Singer LP, Wasnick J. The postoperative cardiovascular arrest of a 5-year-old male: an initial presentation of Duchenne's muscular dystrophy. Paediatr Anaesth. 2006; 16(2):170–173

[48] Almenrader N, Patel D. Spinal fusion surgery in children with non-idiopathic scoliosis: is there a need for routine postoperative ventilation? Br J Anaesth. 2006; 97(6):851–857

[49] Boussaïd G, Lofaso F, Santos DB, et al. Impact of invasive ventilation on survival when non-invasive ventilation is ineffective in patients with Duchenne muscular dystrophy: a prospective cohort. Respir Med. 2016; 115:26–32

[50] Birnkrant DJ, Noritz GH. Is there a role for palliative care in progressive pediatric neuromuscular diseases? The answer is "Yes! J Palliat Care. 2008; 24(4):265–269

11 Spinal Muscular Atrophy

Benjamin D. Roye and Michael G. Vitale

Abstract

The incidence of scoliosis in children with spinal muscular atrophy syndrome types I–III is 60 to 95%, with severity correlating directly with disease severity. Surgical management of progressive spinal (especially greater than 50 degrees) and truncal deformity in these patients is generally recommended to help preserve respiratory and gastrointestinal function as well as to facilitate positioning. Complications are not uncommon (averaging one complication per patient in some studies) and include surgical site infection, pneumonia, and implant fixation failure. These patients' myriad medical comorbidities necessitate focused attention and multidisciplinary management to minimize risks of surgery. Surgical options include insertion of growth-friendly implants, such as externally controlled magnetic growing rods, in the younger patients and spinal fusion in more mature patients. Surgical treatment of scoliosis has been shown to improve radiographic parameters, including Cobb angle, trunk height, space available for lung, and pelvic obliquity. Data regarding the effect of surgery on pulmonary parameters are less clear, with some studies showing slowed but not reversed deterioration of pulmonary function tests and moderate improvements in self-reported pulmonary function. With the advent of effective pharmacological treatments requiring intrathecal administration, it is paramount that when fusion is performed, at least two lumbar levels are skipped ("skip constructs") to allow continued intrathecal access.

Keywords: growing rods, intrathecal drug treatment, spinal muscular atrophy

11.1 Etiology and Pathogenesis of Spinal Muscular Atrophy

11.1.1 Introduction and Epidemiology

Spinal muscular atrophy (SMA) is one of a diverse group of neuromuscular disorders that presents variably from the newborn period to much later in life, even as late as the third or fourth decade.[1] The disease usually manifests itself as hypotonia and weakness.[1] This autosomal recessive neurodegenerative disorder occurs in as many as 1 of every 10,000 live births, with a reported carrier frequency between 1.7 and 2.5% of the general population.[1] Currently, there are no preventative therapies, and the mainstay of treatment after diagnosis is supportive therapy aimed at addressing specific symptoms.[2] Currently, an investigational gene therapy that acts to replace the defective gene through intrathecal injections holds promise.[3]

11.1.2 Etiology and Genetics

SMA is caused by the degeneration of the alpha motor neurons of the anterior horn cells of the spinal cord as well as the motor nuclei of the brainstem.[4] In approximately 99% of patients, the etiology of this degeneration is thought to be a homozygous deletion in the survival motor neuron 1 gene (SMN1),[5,6] found on chromosome 5q13.2. The most often reported mutation within the SMN1 gene is a deletion of exon 7, with approximately 94% of patients with SMA having a homozygous deletion of exon 7.[7] The SMN1 gene codes for a protein which, when produced correctly, inhibits neuronal apoptosis.[8] In patients with SMA, it is this loss-of-function mutation that results in the neurodegenerative aspects of the disease process.[8]

Disease severity seems to be closely related to the levels of SMN1 protein deficiency, although the ability to predict SMA severity from genotype alone is limited and not recommended in clinical practice.[6,9] There is also evidence that survival motor neuron 2 (SMN2), a gene differing only in the nucleotide change from C to T in exon 7, affects phenotypical expression of disease.[4,9,10] SMN2 codes for the production of survival motor neurons, albeit in smaller numbers than SMN1, and there is evidence that increased levels of SMN2 correlate with less severe forms of SMA[11]

There are currently two theories as to how the deletion within SMN1 causes SMA. The first theory asserts that this deletion impairs the assembly of small ribonucleoprotein (RNP) subunits of the spliceosome, resulting in disruption of motor neuron circuitry.[6,12] A second theory postulates that the SMN1 deletion inhibits mRNA transport within neurons.[6,13]

11.1.3 Initial Presentation, Diagnosis, and Genetic Screening

A diagnosis of SMA should be entertained in any child presenting with delayed milestones, symmetric proximal muscle weakness (ranging from mild to flaccid paralysis [greater in the lower limbs]), or diminished or absent deep tendon reflexes, with or without fasciculations.[14] A weak cry, poor suck and swallow reflex resulting in excess secretions, and aspiration may also be indicative of SMA, and should prompt further investigation.[14]

Once clinical suspicion is established, genetic testing for a homozygous deletion in exons 7 and 8 of the SMN1 gene can confirm the diagnosis.[13] In most cases, genetic testing alone can make a diagnosis, but if an SMN1 deletion is not found, a diagnosis can be confirmed through the use of electromyography, muscle biopsy, and nerve conduction studies.[7,13] In those with a family history of SMA, a prenatal diagnosis can be made, although population-wide genetic screening is not currently recommended.[1,15]

11.1.4 Classification Types and Pathogenesis

Once a diagnosis is made, it is important to determine the subtype of disease. There are currently four subtypes of SMA, which are defined by age on onset and functional disability.[6] SMA type I, or Werdnig–Hoffmann disease, is the most severe form of this disorder and presents within the neonatal period, typically before 6 months of age, although some signs may be evident in utero, such as decreased fetal movement.[13] Neonates with SMA often present with poor swallowing, loss of deep tendon reflexes, poor head control, tongue atrophy, and fasciculations, as well as intercostal muscle weakness.[6] They never develop the ability to sit independently. In the past, this disease has led to very early death, often within the first year of life.[16] However, advances in treatment, including aggressive respiratory support that often includes tracheostomy and ventilator support, has dramatically increased the life expectancy of these children.[13]

SMA type II (intermediate) presents between 7 and 18 months. These patients present with delayed milestones, although most develop the ability to sit independently, with the defining characteristic of this subtype being the ability to maintain a sitting position unsupported.[13] Some patients with SMA type II are ultimately able to stand with the support of a standing frame or leg braces, although they lack the ability to walk.[13] Children with SMA type II also typically suffer from swallowing difficulty due to bulbar weakness and may have trouble gaining weight.[13] They also have weak intercostal muscles, resulting in difficulty clearing tracheal secretions.[13] Patients also suffer from joint contractures, scoliosis, and pulmonary comorbidities that contribute to a decreased life expectancy.[6,13]

SMA type III (Kugelberg–Welander disease) presents after 18 months of age.[6,13] Patients within this subtype achieve independent ambulation, although this may deteriorate throughout life.[13] Difficulty with mucociliary clearance and swallowing, while less common than in SMA type II, is also present in patients with SMA type III.[13] These patients often have less severe pulmonary manifestations of their disease, and in those who continue to ambulate, life expectancy may often approach that of the general population.[17] These patients suffer from musculoskeletal overuse syndromes, scoliosis, hip abductor weakness (which causes a Trendelenburg lurch), and increased lumbar lordosis.[6]

SMA type IV (adult onset), the least severe subtype of this condition, presents within the second or third decade of life and results in similar, albeit less severe, symptomatology as SMA type III.[16] Patients are able to ambulate without assistance and may experience mild motor impairment but do not typically suffer from respiratory or gastrointestinal manifestations of disease.[13]

11.1.5 Relevance to Orthopaedics

In all subtypes of SMA, there are significant comorbidities, including pulmonary, gastrointestinal, and orthopaedic complications. Scoliosis, in particular, has been reported in between 60 and 95% of patients with SMA types I–III, with the severity of scoliosis and degree of progression directly related to SMA subtype and age of onset.[6,18] The prevalence of scoliosis is also highly influenced by the ambulatory status of the patient.[18] Nearly all patients with SMA types I and II will develop scoliosis, while the incidence is as low as 50% in those with SMA type III.[7,18] Pelvic obliquity and kyphosis are also associated with SMA, further complicating the clinical picture.[6] Hip dislocations are ubiquitous in more involved patients, although, as these patients are not ambulatory, surgical treatment is rarely indicated. Given the extent of orthopaedic complications in SMA, all patients with SMA should be seen regularly by an orthopaedic surgeon with experience treating patients with neuromuscular disease.

11.2 Disease-Specific Deformity Characteristics and Comorbidities

11.2.1 Patterns of Deformity

The orthopaedic manifestations of SMA include hip dislocations, joint contractures of the upper and lower extremities, and, perhaps most significantly, scoliosis. While the patterns of deformity are generally similar to those seen in other neuromuscular diseases, there are without question distinct characteristics that are specific to SMA that need to be understood to properly care for this challenging population. These include early age of onset, rapid rate of progression, and the unique severe chest wall deformities.

Spinal Deformity

Scoliosis is nearly ubiquitous in children with SMA types I and II. Not surprisingly, the pattern of deformity does vary with disease involvement. For example, while most cases of scoliosis in this population are long **C**-shaped thoracolumbar curves (▶ Fig. 11.1),[19] as commonly seen in a variety of neuromuscular diseases,[6] double major curve patterns are more common in children who are less severely affected. The incidence of double major curves is approximately 33% in children who can sit (type II) and only 12% in those who are unable to sit (type I).[19] The laterality of the curves varies significantly and is approximately 2:1 left:right for curves in patients with type II, while it is closer to 1:1 in patients with type III.[19] In addition to the frontal plane deformity, sagittal plane deformities are common as in other paralytic disorders such as Duchenne muscular dystrophy.[20]

The age of onset of scoliosis for these patients is almost always early in life (4.5 years for type II).[21] Pelvic obliquity is common, which affects sitting balance, and is typically proportional to the magnitude of scoliosis.[22] For children with SMA capable of ambulation (type III), the incidence of scoliosis is lower, with the

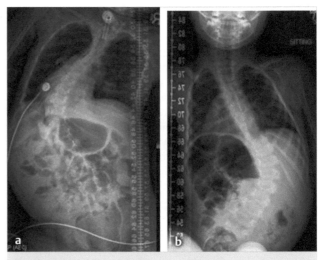

Fig. 11.1 (a,b) Typical **C**-shaped deformities with pelvic obliquity.

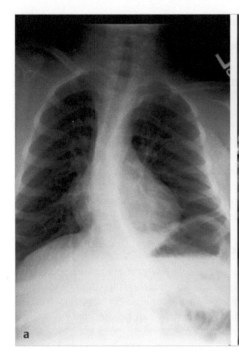
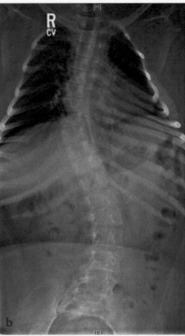

Fig. 11.2 **(a)** Chest radiograph of 4-year-old boy with type I SMA. Scoliosis is clearly present, but his ribs look to be in good position. **(b)** Several years later, there is clear drooping, or "parasoling" of the ribs, especially on the left. The ribs are much more drooped despite minimal changes in the scoliosis.

timing of onset typically related to the age at which SMA becomes manifest. Overall, for children with all types of SMA type III, the age of onset of deformity is approximately 10 years.[21]

Chest Wall Deformity

Dr. Robert Campbell helped us recognize that in many cases of early-onset scoliosis, it was not the spine deformity per se that causes problems, but rather the resultant deformities of the chest wall that can be the major source of morbidity.[23] In some cases, there can be chest wall deformities that are secondary to spinal deformities, while in other cases the primary issue can be the rib cage such as in cases of rib fusions and some syndromes including Jeune's syndrome.[24] The effect of the thoracic wall deformity is diminished effective lung capacity because of decreasing space available for the lung and often chest wall compliance as well.[25] In SMA, there is typically a chest wall deformity, known as a parasol deformity, that develops independently of any underlying spinal deformity (▶ Fig. 11.2). This is seen in other paralytic neuromuscular disorders, such as Duchenne muscular dystrophy, and has a negative effect on lung function that is amplified by any underlying scoliosis.[26]

11.2.2 Comorbidities

Children with SMA, especially those with types I and II, are among the most fragile orthopaedic patients. There are multiple issues that need to be tightly managed to minimize complications in the perioperative period. Many of these factors were recently delineated in a consensus statement from a group of medical experts specializing in SMA.[13]

Respiratory Issues

Pulmonary problems are probably the most significant challenge in managing patients with SMA. Their profound weakness impairs coughing, making it difficult to clear secretions.[13] The weakness also results in hypoventilation when sleeping. These two factors lead to frequent, recurrent infections, both from aspiration and from more typical airborne pathogens, and the recurrent infections themselves can exacerbate muscle weakness.[13]

Gastrointestinal and Nutritional Issues

Gastrointestinal dysfunction results from both bulbar dysfunction and gastroesophageal dysmotility.[6] They thus have difficulties swallowing and protecting their airway, as well as with digestion once the food has passed the oropharynx. This results in a high rate of aspiration pneumonia, which can be deadly in these patients. The other result of these difficulties is malnutrition. This leads to poor growth, which, combined with their scant subcutaneous fat, makes prominence of most spinal implants a potential problem. These issues are most noticeable in patients with SMA types I and II, and are less of an issue with less involved type II and type III patients, where excessive weight can occur.[13]

11.2.3 Disorder-Specific Techniques

Perioperative Considerations

Surgical management of spinal deformity in children with SMA begins well before entering the operating room. As discussed previously, these patients are fragile, and complication rates are significant. It is critical to optimize these patients prior to surgery to ensure the best possible outcomes. Preoperative evaluation by their pulmonary and gastrointestinal (GI) specialists to optimize their preoperative status and to obtain guidance on postoperative management is mandatory. It is important not to overlook the nutritional status and to consider delaying cases where nutrition is suboptimal for a given patient.

When obtaining consent from these families for surgery, one must make sure the family is aware of the risks involved, including possible need for prolonged ventilatory support and the risk of infection and instrumentation-related problems. There is much literature on the risks of surgery in these fragile and complex patients, and the number of complications *per patient* in many studies exceeds 1 with growth-sparing techniques.

Infection control is of particular concern as infection rates in this population can exceed 10 to 15%. Certainly, proper management of the patient's nutritional status is important in minimizing infection risk, but also having and following a stringent protocol that includes pre-, intra-, and postoperative interventions is critical.[27]

Postsurgical medical management is critical. There are several established protocols with recommendations for this period. In general, most patients with SMA undergoing spinal surgery should be extubated to BiPAP (bilevel positive airway pressure) in the pediatric intensive care unit, and this should be followed by an aggressive program of pulmonary toilet to include cough assist and chest physiotherapy.[28,29,30]

Nutritionally, it is important to avoid prolonged fasting after surgery—many patients may require prolonged intubation or may be unable to otherwise take enteral feedings. Additionally, any patient undergoing major surgery suffers a period of relative stasis of their GI tract, and this is especially true for patients with underlying dysmotility issues. For this reason, the use of peripheral parenteral nutrition should be strongly considered to reduce the likelihood of the patient becoming catabolic and developing metabolic decompensation.[13]

Surgical Management

Surgery is almost always indicated for progressive scoliosis in this population. Orthotic treatment with spine bracing is used frequently on the hope that it will slow progression of the curve,[31] although there is no evidence for this. The authors rarely use bracing, except for soft jackets to assist with positioning, because of the detrimental effect on respiratory capacity.[32]

Surgical Indications

Although it sounds obvious, the first consideration in surgical management is the surgical indication. There are multiple factors at play here, including the age and size of the patient, his/her medical fragility, the magnitude of the deformity, the rate of change of the deformity (i.e., how quickly has it progressed), and the impact of the deformity on the patient's health and quality of life. Clearly, in such a complex setting, there is no one formulaic approach that works for every patient.

Another factor to consider is what type of surgery to perform—while growth-sparing surgeries are widely used in this population, there are those who make the argument that waiting until the child is mature enough for a definitive fusion makes sense, even if that means accepting a relative large deformity in the interim. There is no published evidence for this in the SMA population, but this approach does obviate the significant problems with stiffness and difficulty getting additional correction in fusion procedures done in the growth-friendly surgical "graduate."[33]

Growth-Sparing Techniques

Soft-Tissue Considerations

As most patients with SMA develop scoliosis early in life, the initial management of spinal deformity usually utilizes growth-sparing techniques. These patients are often very small without much subcutaneous fat or lean muscle mass. This makes meticulous handling of the soft tissues critical. Any skin flaps that are needed during exposure must be full thickness, and, if possible, incisions in fascia should not be directly over the anchor points to help protect the suture line from breakdown. There is some evidence to suggest that use of plastic surgeons to assist with opening and closing some difficult wounds may reduce the rate of infection in patients with neuromuscular disorders.[34]

Implant Considerations

It behooves the surgeon to use low-profile implants, preferably one of the few systems designed for this indication. There are several options for anchor points. For cephalad fixation, there are hooks and cradles that can be used for rib fixation (► Fig. 11.3) as well as more standard pedicle screws. Other options include sublaminar fixation with bands, wires, or even hooks, although the authors prefer other points of fixation due to the particularly tenuous nature of laminar bone in these patients. In general, the authors prefer multiple points of rib fixation with broad up-going hooks (► Fig. 11.4a–c), and pedicle screws are reserved as a backup when rib fixation fails (► Fig. 11.4c). We have found that using at least three points of fixation per side has reduced our cephalad fixation failure rate, and there is recent published evidence to support this as well.[35] Additionally, we try to achieve some of our rib fixation laterally to support the rib cage and protect against parasoling of the rib cage (► Fig. 11.5). Although a recent study showed no difference in rib cage morphology between spine-based and rib-based fixation,[26] the study did not seem to utilize lateral attachment of the rib fixation, which creates a longer lever arm to push up on the rib.

For caudal fixation, the options are pelvic hooks that sit on the iliac crest or screws in the lumbosacral spine. Both work well, but prominence and pain seem to be more common with pelvic hooks, so we currently tend to utilize screws. In keeping with our philosophy of three fixation points, we us L5, S1, and S2 alar-iliac screws when possible. These provide a solid base

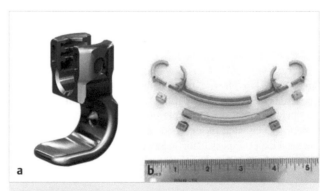

Fig. 11.3 Images of hooks (a) and cradles (b) frequently used for rib fixation in growing constructs.

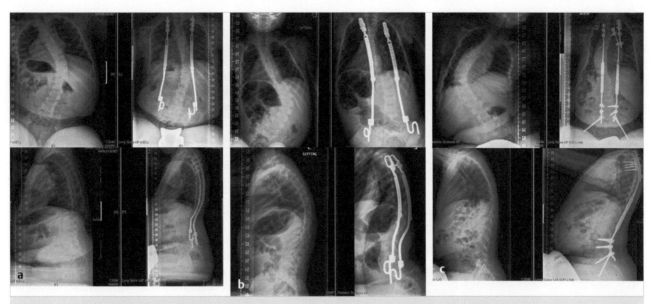

Fig. 11.4 Typical growing constructs with **(a)** rib hook to pelvic hook fixation, **(b)** rib cradle to pelvic hook, and **(c)** proximal rib hooks and screws to pelvic/sacral screw fixation.

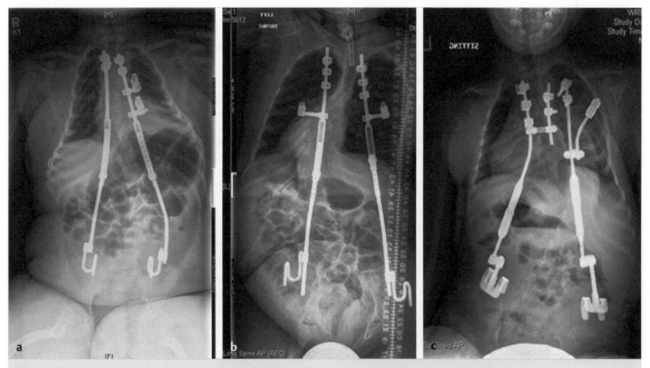

Fig. 11.5 (a-c) Growing constructs with outriggers designed to support the rib cage laterally to help control drooping of the rib cage.

and the screws can be used at the time of definitive fusion in the future.

Definitive Fusion Techniques

While fusing the spine of a child with SMA is similar to the procedure done in children with other neuromuscular disease, there is one specific technical aspect to consider. With the advent of intrathecal medications that have been shown to reverse the effects of SMA syndrome in many patients,[36] access to the intrathecal space must be maintained when fusing these spines. That means skipping one to two levels in the fusion by neither exposing nor instrumenting levels in the mid-to-lower lumbar spine (e.g., L2–L3, L3–L4). This "skip construct" (▶ Fig. 11.6) preserves the interlaminar space to permit future medication administration. There are even some patients who had their fusions done prior to the advent of this treatment who are requesting surgery to create access with a laminotomy.

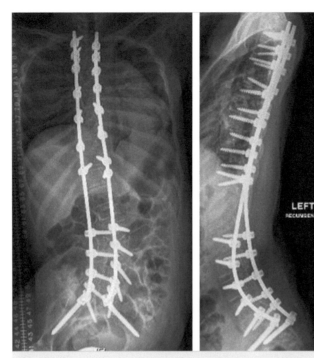

Fig. 11.6 "Skip construct" used when doing long fusion in patients with spinal muscular atrophy.

The same pre- and postoperative medical considerations certainly still apply, however, and the need for parenteral nutrition is highlighted to a greater degree as these surgeries take a major toll and children are likely to be intubated for a longer period of time.

For the population of children with SMA syndrome who undergo growing instrumentation, transitioning them from their growth-friendly implant as they approach maturity is a challenging problem with more than one answer. One factor to consider is that the spines of children who have had growing instrumentation for any period of time become incredibly stiff. Therefore, if planning to achieve any significant change in the curve magnitude or balance, then it is usually necessary to plan on doing osteotomies. This certainly increases the magnitude and risk of the surgery. The best way to avoid this is to achieve and maintain good balance with the growing system the child lives with prior to fusion.

A second consideration would be to not perform a definitive fusion on a child who has been treated with growing instrumentation. These are obviously low-demand patients and, as we have seen, their spines become to a large degree autofused over time with growing instrumentation. While there is little literature to guide us on the ideal way to handle the so-called "growing instrumentation graduate" leaving the implants in place may be an option for some patients.

11.3 Evidence-Based Outcomes

There are few outcomes studies evaluating spine surgery specifically in children with SMA. To be sure, there are many published articles assaying outcomes in children with neuromuscular scoliosis, but even in the studies that selectively look at flaccid forms of scoliosis, SMA makes up a small percentage of these patient populations.[20,37,38,39] This makes it difficult to draw meaningful conclusions from these studies. Additionally, the vast majority of the studies here are only level 4 evidence. In this section, we focus on studies specifically describing outcomes in patients with SMA.

11.3.1 Outcomes of Growing Instrumentation

Complications

As mentioned earlier, the majority of scoliosis in this population begins early in life and requires growth-sparing implants. Many studies have demonstrated the high rate of complications with this surgery. A preliminary short-term study showed a 20% complication rate with minimum follow-up of 24 months.[40] A separate study conducted from a database review had a minimum follow-up of 54 months and demonstrated that complications after surgery occur at double the rate when compared to idiopathic infantile or juvenile scoliosis treated similarly with growing instrumentation (1.1 complication per patient vs. 0.5 complications per patient).[41] Complications include infection and implant fixation failure, as well as respiratory problems.

Radiographic and Physiologic Outcomes

There seems to be agreement in multiple studies that good radiographic outcomes are achievable. Improvements in Cobb angle ranged from 40 to 60% with little loss at last follow-up.[40,41] Improvements in pelvic obliquity (65%), space available for lung ratio (9%), and trunk height (8.7 cm) have also been demonstrated.[41,42] On the other hand, rib collapse (parasoling) was shown not to improve in two separate studies.[26,41] Finally, while absolute forced vital capacity (FVC) has been shown to improve, there is evidence that predicted FVC diminishes over time in children with type II SMA.[42]

11.3.2 Outcomes of Spinal Fusion

There are less data on the results of fusion in this population. A study out of Singapore demonstrated 65% improvement in Cobb angle and, even more importantly, demonstrated a slowing in the rate of decline in respiratory function as defined by FVC. In this study of children with type II and III SMA, with most surgeries occurring in the 1980s, FVC declined at 7.7% per year before surgery and at 3.8% postoperatively (44-month follow-up).[43] A second study of fusion in immature patients with SMA (open triradiate cartilage) also demonstrated an initial correction in Cobb angle of 61% and pelvic obliquity improvement of 53%.[44] There was loss of correction, and at last follow-up (minimum 5 years), Cobb correction had fallen to 44%. They found that fusing to the pelvis was protective as all patients who were not fused to the pelvis had significant progression of their fused major curve. Two other recent articles, both out of Asia, showed not only good radiographic results, but also stabilization, and in some cases improvement, of respiratory function in long-term follow-up.[45,46]

References

[1] ACOG Committee on Genetics. ACOG committee opinion No. 432: spinal muscular atrophy. Obstet Gynecol. 2009; 113(5):1194–1196

[2] Darras BT. Spinal muscular atrophies. Pediatr Clin North Am. 2015; 62 (3):743–766

[3] Passini MA, Bu J, Richards AM, et al. Translational fidelity of intrathecal delivery of self-complementary AAV9-survival motor neuron 1 for spinal muscular atrophy. Hum Gene Ther. 2014; 12:1–12

[4] Lorson CL, Rindt H, Shababi M. Spinal muscular atrophy: mechanisms and therapeutic strategies. Hum Mol Genet. 2010; 19 R1:R111–R118

[5] Lefebvre S, Bürglen L, Reboullet S, et al. Identification and characterization of a spinal muscular atrophy-determining gene. Cell. 1995; 80(1):155–165

[6] Mesfin A, Sponseller PD, Leet AI. Spinal muscular atrophy: manifestations and management. J Am Acad Orthop Surg. 2012; 20(6):393–401

[7] Ogino S, Wilson RB. Genetic testing and risk assessment for spinal muscular atrophy (SMA). Hum Genet. 2002; 111(6):477–500

[8] Roy N, Mahadevan MS, McLean M, et al. The gene for neuronal apoptosis inhibitory protein is partially deleted in individuals with spinal muscular atrophy. Cell. 1995; 80(1):167–178

[9] Lefebvre S, Burlet P, Liu Q, et al. Correlation between severity and SMN protein level in spinal muscular atrophy. Nat Genet. 1997; 16(3):265–269

[10] Burghes AHM, Beattie CE. Spinal muscular atrophy: why do low levels of survival motor neuron protein make motor neurons sick? Nat Rev Neurosci. 2009; 10(8):597–609

[11] Feldkötter M, Schwarzer V, Wirth R, Wienker TF, Wirth B. Quantitative analyses of SMN1 and SMN2 based on real-time lightCycler PCR: fast and highly reliable carrier testing and prediction of severity of spinal muscular atrophy. Am J Hum Genet. 2002; 70(2):358–368

[12] Eggert C, Chari A, Laggerbauer B, Fischer U. Spinal muscular atrophy: the RNP connection. Trends Mol Med. 2006; 12(3):113–121

[13] Wang CH, Finkel RS, Bertini ES, et al. Participants of the International Conference on SMA Standard of Care. Consensus statement for standard of care in spinal muscular atrophy. J Child Neurol. 2007; 22(8):1027–1049

[14] Arnold WD, Kassar D, Kissel JT. Spinal muscular atrophy: diagnosis and management in a new therapeutic era. Muscle Nerve. 2015; 51(2):157–167

[15] Prior TW. Spinal muscular atrophy: a time for screening. Curr Opin Pediatr. 2010; 22(6):696–702

[16] Thomas NH, Dubowitz V. The natural history of type I (severe) spinal muscular atrophy. Neuromuscul Disord. 1994; 4(5–6):497–502

[17] Zerres K, Rudnik-Schöneborn S, Forrest E, Lusakowska A, Borkowska J, Hausmanowa-Petrusewicz I. A collaborative study on the natural history of childhood and juvenile onset proximal spinal muscular atrophy (type II and III SMA): 569 patients. J Neurol Sci. 1997; 146(1):67–72

[18] Sucato DJ. Spine deformity in spinal muscular atrophy. J Bone Joint Surg Am. 2007; 89 Suppl 1:148–154

[19] Fujak A, Raab W, Schuh A, Richter S, Forst R, Forst J. Natural course of scoliosis in proximal spinal muscular atrophy type II and IIIa: descriptive clinical study with retrospective data collection of 126 patients. BMC Musculoskelet Disord. 2013; 14:283

[20] Chong HS, Moon ES, Park JO, et al. Value of preoperative pulmonary function test in flaccid neuromuscular scoliosis surgery. Spine. 2011; 36(21):E1391–E1394

[21] Granata C, Merlini L, Magni E, Marini ML, Stagni SB. Spinal muscular atrophy: natural history and orthopaedic treatment of scoliosis. Spine. 1989; 14 (7):760–762

[22] Patel J, Shapiro F. Simultaneous progression patterns of scoliosis, pelvic obliquity, and hip subluxation/dislocation in non-ambulatory neuromuscular patients: an approach to deformity documentation. J Child Orthop. 2015; 9 (5):345–356

[23] Campbell RM, Jr, Smith MD, Mayes TC, et al. The characteristics of thoracic insufficiency syndrome associated with fused ribs and congenital scoliosis. J Bone Joint Surg Am. 2003; 85-A(3):399–408

[24] Lacher M, Dietz H-G. VEPTR (Vertical Expandable Prosthetic Titanium Rib) treatment for Jeune syndrome. Eur J Pediatr Surg. 2011; 21(2):138–139

[25] Lissoni A, Aliverti A, Tzeng AC, Bach JR. Kinematic analysis of patients with spinal muscular atrophy during spontaneous breathing and mechanical ventilation. Am J Phys Med Rehabil. 1998; 77(3):188–192

[26] Livingston K, Zurakowski D, Snyder B, Growing Spine Study Group, Children's Spine Study Group. Parasol rib deformity in hypotonic neuromuscular scoliosis: a new radiographical definition and a comparison of short-term treatment outcomes with VEPTR and growing rods. Spine. 2015; 40(13):E780–E786

[27] Vitale MG, Riedel MD, Glotzbecker MP, et al. Building consensus: development of a Best Practice Guideline (BPG) for surgical site infection (SSI) prevention in high-risk pediatric spine surgery. J Pediatr Orthop. 2013; 33 (5):471–478

[28] Mills B, Bach JR, Zhao C, Saporito L, Sabharwal S. Posterior spinal fusion in children with flaccid neuromuscular scoliosis: the role of noninvasive positive pressure ventilatory support. J Pediatr Orthop. 2013; 33(5):488–493

[29] Khirani S, Bersanini C, Aubertin G, Bachy M, Vialle R, Fauroux B. Non-invasive positive pressure ventilation to facilitate the post-operative respiratory outcome of spine surgery in neuromuscular children. Eur Spine J. 2014; 23 Suppl 4:S406–S411

[30] Bach JR, Sabharwal S. High pulmonary risk scoliosis surgery: role of noninvasive ventilation and related techniques. J Spinal Disord Tech. 2005; 18 (6):527–530

[31] Fujak A, Kopschina C, Forst R, Mueller LA, Forst J. Use of orthoses and orthopaedic technical devices in proximal spinal muscular atrophy. Results of survey in 194 SMA patients. Disabil Rehabil Assist Technol. 2011; 6(4):305–311

[32] Tangsrud SE, Carlsen KC, Lund-Petersen I, Carlsen KH. Lung function measurements in young children with spinal muscle atrophy; a cross sectional survey on the effect of position and bracing. Arch Dis Child. 2001; 84(6):521–524

[33] Cahill PJ, Marvil S, Cuddihy L, et al. Autofusion in the immature spine treated with growing rods. Spine. 2010; 35(22):E1199–E1203

[34] Ward JP, Feldman DS, Paul J, et al. Wound closure in nonidiopathic scoliosis: does closure matter? J Pediatr Orthop. 2017; 37(3):166–170

[35] Vitale M, Sullivan M, Trupia E, et al. Prospective study comparing the effects of proximal rib anchors versus proximal spine anchors: examining complications, curve correction, and quality of life [abstract]. In: Proceedings of the 8th International Congress on Early Onset Scoliosis and Growing Spine (ICEOS); November 20–21, 2014; Warsaw, Poland

[36] Finkel RS, Chiriboga CA, Vajsar J, et al. Treatment of infantile-onset spinal muscular atrophy with nusinersen: a phase 2, open-label, dose-escalation study. Lancet. 2016; 388(10063):3017–3026

[37] Modi HN, Suh S-W, Hong J-Y, Park Y-H, Yang J-H. Surgical correction of paralytic neuromuscular scoliosis with poor pulmonary functions. J Spinal Disord Tech. 2011; 24(5):325–333

[38] Chang D-G, Suk S-I, Kim J-H, Ha K-Y, Na K-H, Lee J-H. Surgical outcomes by age at the time of surgery in the treatment of congenital scoliosis in children under age 10 years. Spine J. 2015; 15(8):1783–1795

[39] Modi HN, Suh S-W, Hong J-Y, Cho J-W, Park J-H, Yang J-H. Treatment and complications in flaccid neuromuscular scoliosis (Duchenne's muscular dystrophy and spinal muscular atrophy) with posterior-only pedicle screw instrumentation. Eur Spine J. 2010; 19(3):384–393

[40] Chandran S, McCarthy J, Noonan K, Mann D, Nemeth B, Guiliani T. Early treatment of scoliosis with growing rods in children with severe spinal muscular atrophy: a preliminary report. J Pediatr Orthop. 2017; 26(6):1721–1726

[41] McElroy MJ, Shaner AC, Crawford TO, et al. Growing rods for scoliosis in spinal muscular atrophy: structural effects, complications, and hospital stays. Spine. 2011; 36(16):1305–1311

[42] Lenhart RL, Youlo S, Schroth MK, et al. Radiographic and respiratory effects of growing rods in children with spinal muscular atrophy. J Pediatr Orthop. 7-7-17

[43] Chng SY, Wong YQ, Hui JH, Wong HK, Ong HT, Goh DY. Pulmonary function and scoliosis in children with spinal muscular atrophy types II and III. J Paediatr Child Health. 2003; 39(9):673–676

[44] Zebala LP, Bridwell KH, Baldus C, et al. Minimum 5-year radiographic results of long scoliosis fusion in juvenile spinal muscular atrophy patients: major curve progression after instrumented fusion. J Pediatr Orthop. 2011; 31 (5):480–488

[45] Chua K, Tan CY, Chen Z, et al. Long-term follow-up of pulmonary function and scoliosis in patients with duchenne's muscular dystrophy and spinal muscular atrophy. J Pediatr Orthop. 2016; 36(1):63–69

[46] Chou SH, Lin GT, Shen PC, et al. The effect of scoliosis surgery on pulmonary function in spinal muscular atrophy type II patients. Eur Spine J. 2016

12 Other Neuromuscular Conditions: Rett Syndrome, Charcot–Marie–Tooth Disease, and Friedreich's Ataxia

Keith R. Bachman and Vidyadhar V. Upasani

Abstract

Rett syndrome, Charcot–Marie–Tooth disease, and Friedreich's ataxia are unique neuromuscular conditions which require special attention. As our understanding of the underlying etiology for these diseases continues to expand, our treatment approaches need to be refined to improve patient outcomes. Ultimately, genetic and medical advances may improve the musculoskeletal impact of these diseases and lead to improved quality of life for these patients and their families.

Keywords: Charcot–marie–tooth disease, Friedreich's ataxia, Rett syndrome

12.1 Rett Syndrome

12.1.1 Etiology and Pathogenesis

Rett syndrome is a progressive neurodevelopmental disorder. It was first described by Dr. Andreas Rett[1] in 1966 and given the eponym by Hagberg et al in 1983.[2] This condition is thought to affect approximately 1 in 10,000 females and is often due to a sporadic mutation of the methyl-CpG-binding protein 2 gene (MECP2) on the X-chromosome.[3,4,5] This gene mutation has been shown to affect cells in the locus coeruleus, which is responsible for noradrenergic innervation to the cerebral cortex and hippocampus.[6] In fewer than 10% of cases, mutations in other genes including CDKL5 or FOXG1 have also been identified in these patients.[7] The predominance of females with Rett syndrome is due to the sex-linked mutation, and males with MECP2 gene mutations either do not survive to term or die before the age of 2 years due to a severe encephalopathy.

Children with Rett syndrome typically undergo normal development in the early stages of growth and then regress in motor and language function. Four stages of this syndrome have been described.[8,9] During the antenatal period, the child develops normally for the first 6 to 10 months of life. Between 1.5 to 3 years of age, there is regression of volitional hand movements and speech, as well as social withdrawal. This is followed by a plateau phase during which the symptoms stabilize for several years, until eventually there is late regression of motor function resulting in progressive scoliosis, dystonia, and spasticity. Due to this characteristic progression of symptoms, the diagnosis of Rett syndrome is often based on clinical assessment and is then verified by genetic testing.[10]

Females with Rett syndrome can often live up to 40 years or more. A recent publication from the Australian Rett Syndrome Database reported a likelihood of survival of 77.6% at 20 years and 59.8% at 37 years.[11] In their cohort of 396 adult female patients with Rett syndrome, over 50% were ambulating (most with assistive devices), and two-thirds (64%) were taking antiepileptic medications. Scoliosis was the most common orthopaedic condition in these patients, affecting 86% of the cohort, with 40% of those having undergone corrective surgery. Bassett and Tolo reported on 258 patients from the International Rett Syndrome Association and identified a 46% incidence of scoliosis in that cohort.[12] They reported that bracing was largely unsuccessful to control curve progression during adolescence, and surgical correction and fusion was required in the majority of patients.

12.1.2 Disease-Specific Deformity Characteristics and Comorbidities

Patients with Rett syndrome typically present with a long C-shaped thoracolumbar curve in the coronal plane and increased global sagittal kyphosis similar to the deformity observed in other neuromuscular conditions. Most patients also develop a pelvic obliquity with concomitant hip instability. The deformity can be rapidly progressive during adolescence due to vertebral growth as well as progressive neuromuscular imbalance and spasticity as described previously in the fourth stage of this disease. Some studies have reported deformity progression of 14 to 21 degrees per year,[13,14] with continued progression after skeletal maturity.[15] While the spinal deformity remains flexible during childhood, the curve often becomes structural and rigid early in adolescence (▶ Fig. 12.1). Brace treatment can be used as a temporizing measure in patients with a flexible deformity or in patients with significant medical comorbidities and contraindications to surgical treatment.

Patients with Rett syndrome are especially medically labile and have numerous medical comorbidities that need to be managed by a multidisciplinary team. Epilepsy is present in up to 80% of affected individuals.[16] Although about 50% of seizures can be controlled by medications, intractable epilepsy is more common in girls with decelerated head growth and can be triggered in the perioperative period due to physiologic stresses of surgery. Irregular breathing and nonepileptic vacant spells can also occur in these patients due to their immature brainstems, leading to sudden death.[17] Additionally, a defective control mechanism of carbon dioxide exhalation leads to respiratory alkalosis or acidosis requiring prolonged ventilator support and intensive care management.[18] Some patients also experience sudden violent screaming that can last for hours or even days. This behavior may signal extreme pain, although on examination there does not seem to be any somatic abnormality.[19] This phenomenon has been described as "brain-pain-crying" and may lead to overmedication and sedation, further depressing the respiratory drive in these patients.

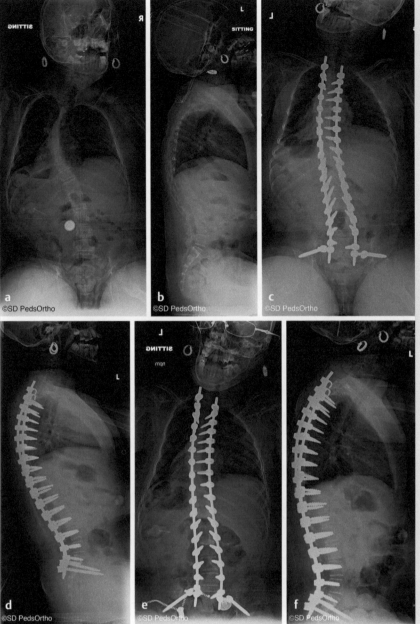

Fig. 12.1 Preoperative sitting posteroanterior (PA) **(a)** and lateral **(b)** radiographs of a 10-year-old girl with Rett syndrome and a progressive scoliotic deformity. Four-week postoperative PA **(c)** and lateral **(d)** radiographs after a posterior T2 to pelvis segmental instrumentation and fusion with iliac bolts. Four-year postoperative PA **(e)** and lateral **(f)** radiographs demonstrating maintenance of deformity correction and sitting balance.

12.1.3 Disorder-Specific Techniques

In 2009, a modified Delphi technique was used to integrate available published evidence, parental input, and expert opinion to arrive at a general consensus for managing scoliosis in patients with Rett syndrome.[20] This study concluded that surgery should be considered when the deformity magnitude was approximately 40 to 50 degrees. The primary indications for surgery were progressive deformity, pain, loss of sitting balance, deteriorating ambulatory status, and progressive restrictive lung disease.[20,21] Surgery should also only be considered after all medical comorbidities are optimized and with close involvement of specialized anesthesia and intensive care teams

to minimize perioperative complications. Despite these measures, the incidence of complications after scoliosis surgery in this patient population remains high, ranging from 50 to 100%.[22,23,24] The most common complications were due to pulmonary (ventilator-acquired pneumonia, pneumothorax, pulmonary effusion) or gastrointestinal compromise (pancreatitis, gastric ulceration, superior mesenteric artery syndrome, acute abdominal distension).

Surgical considerations specific to this patient population should aim to minimize blood loss, minimize infections, monitor neurologic changes, and optimize fixation in osteoporotic bone. Lessons learned from other neuromuscular conditions can be applied to this patient population. Tranexamic acid or

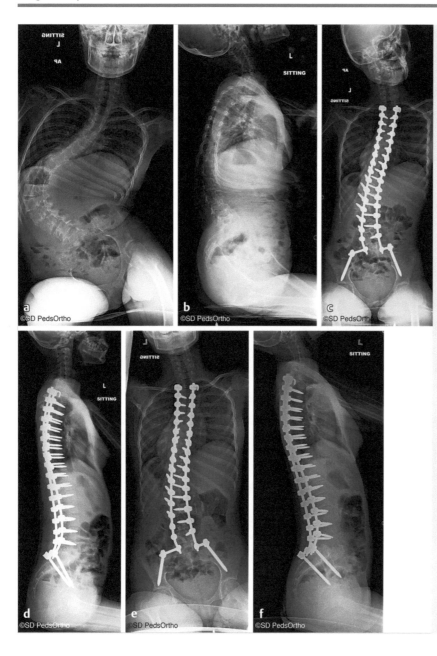

Fig. 12.2 Preoperative sitting PA (**a**) and lateral (**b**) radiographs of an 11-year-old girl with Rett syndrome and a 110-degree thoracolumbar scoliotic deformity with significant pelvic obliquity. Four-week postoperative PA (**c**) and lateral (**d**) radiographs after a posterior T2 to pelvis segmental instrumentation and fusion with iliac bolts. Five-year postoperative PA (**e**) and lateral (**f**) radiographs demonstrating maintenance of deformity correction and sitting balance.

other antifibrinolytic agents should be considered to decrease blood loss and transfusion requirements.[25] Established operating room teams with consistent anesthesiologists, surgical technicians, and two experienced surgeons can be used to decrease surgical time. Preoperative skin preparation, prophylaxis with gram-positive and gram-negative coverage, and vancomycin powder in the surgical wound may decrease infection rates.[26] Neuromonitoring with somatosensory and motor evoked potentials is often possible in this population and should be used to prevent spinal cord injury during surgical correction.[27]

The spinal deformity in Rett syndrome often requires instrumentation and fusion of the entire thoracolumbar spine. The majority of the patients will require extension to the pelvis if there is a substantial pelvic obliquity present. We recommend the pelvic obliquity be corrected with pelvic instrumentation (iliac bolts or sacroiliac screws) as in the cerebral palsy population (see Chapter 16). With the seizure activity, the most rigid spinal instrumentation should be used (▶ Fig. 12.2). Our preference is to use segmental fixation to the spine with pedicle screws and sublaminar wires/bands as needed to stabilize osteoporotic bone. Intraoperative traction may be used to facilitate deformity correction and instrumentation. Anterior spinal release/instrumentation and fusion may be rarely required in very immature patients or with rigid spinal deformities. However, the underlying cardiopulmonary compromise should alert the surgeon in exercising caution if considering anterior thoracic spine surgery.

12.1.4 Evidence-Based Outcomes

Outcome studies of scoliosis surgery in patients with Rett syndrome are primarily case series. They report approximately 50 to 60% correction of the main spinal deformity with a well-balanced sagittal profile and improved pelvic obliquity. Hammett et al[28] published their results in 2014 on 11 patients with Rett syndrome and average 5-year postoperative follow-up (range: 2–8 years). The mean preoperative spinal deformity measured 71 degrees (range: 44–105 degrees) and was corrected to an average of 27 degrees (range: 10–46 degrees). Patients were treated with posterior segmental instrumentation and fusion to the pelvis with either hybrid (sublaminar wires, hook, and screws) instrumentation or an all–pedicle screw construct. Eight patients (73%) had significant complications, primarily respiratory and wound infections. Similarly, in 2012, Gabos et al[22] reported on 16 patients with mean 4.7-year follow-up. All patients were instrumented from T1 to the pelvis using unit rod instrumentation. The coronal deformity improved on average from 68 degrees (range: 38–100 degrees) preoperatively to 16 degrees (range: 5–40 degrees) at final follow-up. No patients in this series experienced deterioration in ambulatory status over the follow-up period despite fusion to the pelvis.

Larsson et al[29] reported on postoperative function, seating position, and self-reported quality of care measures in 23 girls with Rett syndrome and neuromuscular scoliosis. All patients were treated with posterior segmental instrumentation and fusion with hybrid constructs (sublaminar wires, hooks, and screws), with a majority of patients (83%) being fused to the pelvis. Seven patients had concomitant anterior instrumentation and fusion with the Zielke apparatus ($n = 3$) or Aaro instrumentation ($n = 4$). Ten patients (44%) experienced postoperative complications in the short term, requiring pulmonary support and antibiotics for superficial wound infections, while three patients experienced deformity progression in the midterm with extension of the fusion into the cervical spine ($n = 1$) or to the pelvis ($n = 2$). Preoperative median deformity magnitude was 66 degrees (range q1–q3: 51–83 degrees) and at average 74-month follow-up (range: 49–99 months) was 17 degrees (range q1–q3: 8–33 degrees). The caregivers reported improvement in seating position, daily activities, time used for rest, and cosmetic appearance. The authors concluded that surgical intervention was successful in improving posture, which would decrease the risk for pressure sores, improve pulmonary function, and improve the general health of the child.

12.2 Charcot–Marie–Tooth Disease

12.2.1 Etiology and Pathogenesis

Charcot–Marie–Tooth disease (CMT) is one of the most common hereditary motor and sensory neuropathies with an estimated prevalence of 0.5 to 1 per 2,500.[30,31] This condition was described by French (Charcot and Marie) and British (Tooth) neurologists in 1886 as a peroneal muscle atrophy.[32] In 1968,

Dyck and Lambert identified the electrophysiologic characteristics of these inherited neuropathies and used them to develop the first classification system.[33,34] The type I neuropathies are associated with slow nerve conduction velocities with histologic findings of hypertrophic demyelination, while the type II neuropathies have normal or mildly reduced nerve conduction velocities with pathologic evidence of axonopathy. More recently, genetic testing has been used to classify these neuropathies and more than 80 genes have been identified.[35] CMT type I represents about 70% of all inherited neuropathies. It has an autosomal dominant inheritance and is due to duplication of the peripheral myelin protein 22 gene (PMP22) on chromosome 17.[36] Overexpression of PMP22 results in a toxic aggregation of this protein, resulting in demyelination of the nerves and prolonged conduction velocities.

CMT neuropathy is length dependent, affecting the longest nerves first and most significantly. Distal limb weakness and muscle atrophy are the first clinical features of this disease, and the lower extremities are often affected earlier than the upper extremities. This diagnosis should be included in the differential when examining toddlers with delayed motor development, toe walking, or frequent tripping and falling. Patients also often present with complaints of foot abnormalities including flat feet or high arches. CMT is less likely if these findings are unilateral, and the child should be evaluated for a mononeuropathy or another spinal cord disease. Sensory deficits in CMT are less severe than motor nerve dysfunction and typically result in decreased vibration or joint position sense instead of changes in pin-prick or temperature sensation.[37]

12.2.2 Disease-Specific Deformity Characteristics and Comorbidities

Previous studies have reported a 10 to 40% prevalence of scoliosis in patients with CMT[38,39,40]; however, certain genetic subtypes have been associated with a higher prevalence.[41,42] Unlike idiopathic scoliosis, there seems to be a predominance of male CMT patients with scoliosis. In the series by Karol and Elerson,[39] 60% of the patients with scoliosis were male. The most common spinal deformity pattern is also different from the right thoracic hypokyphotic deformity observed in most patients with idiopathic scoliosis. In the series by Karol and Elerson,[39] there was a 33% prevalence of left thoracic curves, and nearly 50% of the curves were hyperkyphotic. They also report that spinal deformity progression in patients with CMT may be dependent on the extent of neurologic disease and the magnitude of hyperkyphosis. Nonambulatory patients all had significant curve progression requiring surgical treatment.

Comorbidities in this patient population often involve the musculoskeletal system. Foot and ankle abnormalities are common, often resulting in pes cavus and claw feet; however, occasionally these patients can also present with pes plano valgus.[43] Gait abnormalities are often due to foot and ankle weakness and contractures resulting in functional compensation as seen with excessive hip abduction or steppage gait pattern. Upper extremity involvement initially presents with hypothenar atrophy and can progress to finger flexion contractures and interosseous muscle wasting. Decreased vibration and altered proprioception may be more difficult to identify.

12.2.3 Disorder-Specific Techniques

Hensinger and MacEwen believed that spinal deformity in patients with CMT could be managed using the treatment principles for adolescent idiopathic scoliosis. They reported on the effective use of a Milwaukee brace in 50% of the patients in their series.[40] Similar success rates with brace treatment were reported by Daher et al[44] and Walker et al.[38] On the other hand, Karol and Elerson[39] reported a lower success rate with brace treatment. Only 3 of the 16 patients with CMT who were braced

(19%) did not progress more than 5 degrees, and a majority (69%) required surgical stabilization for a progressive deformity. Brace compliance was not evaluated in any of these previous publications and may likely affect the nonoperative success rates in this patient population.

Surgical techniques in this patient population are not significantly different from those used for managing idiopathic scoliosis. Posterior spinal instrumentation and fusion is most commonly used to address the deformities. Often, only the structural curves need to be addressed; however, minimal data exist regarding spontaneous lumbar curve correction in this population. Instrumentation and fusion to the pelvis is rarely required, and these patients often do not develop significant pelvic obliquity (▶ Fig. 12.3). The sagittal plane abnormalities,

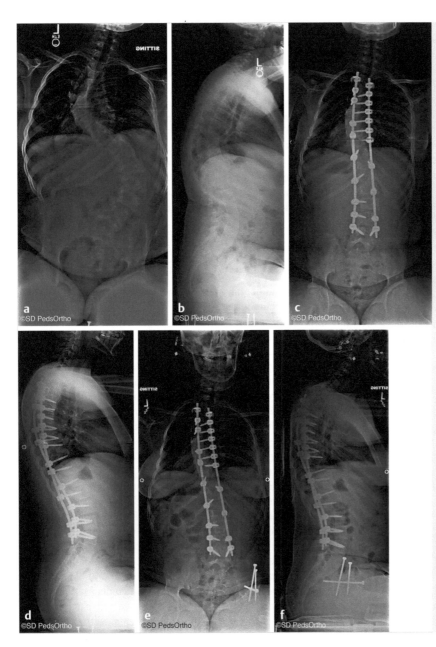

Fig. 12.3 Preoperative sitting PA (a) and lateral (b) radiographs of a 12-year-old girl with Charcot–Marie–Tooth disease and a progressive double major scoliotic deformity. Six-week postoperative PA (c) and lateral (d) radiographs after a posterior T3–L4 segmental instrumentation and fusion. Motor evoked potentials and somatosensory monitoring was not possible during the surgical procedure, and a Stagnara wake-up test was performed. The patient tolerated the procedure with no postoperative complications. Three-year postoperative PA (e) and lateral (f) radiographs demonstrating maintenance of deformity correction and sitting balance.

especially thoracic hyperkyphosis, must be addressed when selecting fusion levels to prevent proximal or distal junctional kyphosis. Krishna et al[45] reported on the difficulties of conventional somatosensory evoked potential monitoring in these patients due to their demyelinating polyneuropathy. Although intraoperative monitoring should be attempted in these cases, the anesthesia team should be prepared to conduct an intraoperative wake-up test.

12.2.4 Evidence-Based Outcomes

Surgical outcomes in patients with CMT have been reported in a number of small case series. In the series by Daher et al,[44] two out of four surgically treated patients developed pseudarthrosis, and one developed a superior mesenteric artery syndrome. In a series by Walker et al,[38] 2 of 37 patients with CMT and scoliosis required surgical treatment, and no peri- or postoperative complications were reported. Karol and Elerson[39] reported on 14 surgically treated patients with CMT and also found no postoperative complications. Recently, a pediatric multidimensional neuropathy scoring system has been developed and validated for use in pediatric patients with CMT (http://cmtpeds.org).[46,47] This tool is now being used to study the natural history of this progressive neuropathy as well as the changes to the natural history with medical and surgical intervention.

12.3 Friedreich's Ataxia

12.3.1 Etiology and Pathogenesis

Friedreich's ataxia is a multisystem autosomal recessive condition first described in 1863 by Friedreich, a German neurologist. It is the most common inheritable ataxia with an incidence of approximately 1:20,000 to 1:125,000.[48] It is more likely in Caucasians with a carrier frequency of 1:60 to 1:110.[49,50,51] Friedreich's ataxia is due to a mutation in the gene FXN (frataxin) on chromosome 9q13. This results in a reduction in frataxin, which is a protein involved in iron storage and transport. Around 1 to 3% of cases represent a compound heterozygous mutation with a point mutation or deletion of the frataxin gene.[52,53,54] Although the exact role of frataxin in this disease is unknown, it is thought to result in increased levels of total iron, which results in degeneration of nerve tissue in the spinal cord.

Patients with Friedreich's ataxia typically present with symptoms around puberty or slightly before with a mean age at onset ranging from 10.5 to 15.5 years.[49,55,56] Patients most commonly present with gait ataxia and general clumsiness.[49,55,56,57] Some patients may present with a late-onset scoliosis and neurologic signs, but the orthopaedic surgeon needs to include early-onset cerebellar ataxia, neuropathy, spasticity, and CMT disease in the differential diagnosis.[58,59]

12.3.2 Disease-Specific Deformity Characteristics and Comorbidities

The incidence of scoliosis in Friedreich's ataxia has been noted to be 100%[60] when using the clinical criteria of Geoffroy et al[61]

and 63 to 78% when genetic testing was used for diagnosis.[57,62] The curve in Friedreich's ataxia demonstrates several neuromuscular scoliosis characteristics: increased kyphosis, more common thoracolumbar curve apex, and left-sided curves.[62] It does not tend to be a large sweeping collapsing C-shaped curve; instead, the curve is more similar to idiopathic. Digitized radiographic measurements have demonstrated that the amount of vertebral axial rotation for the amount of vertebral lateral deviation in this population was more similar to idiopathic curves than to cerebral palsy curves.[63] Cady and Bobechko[64] reported 3 out of 38 C-shaped curves; Tsirikos and Smith[65] noted 2 out of 31 in their study. Labelle et al[60] noted sweeping C-shaped curves in 14% and demonstrated that not all curves were relentlessly progressive. They felt that curve onset before age 10 years was a large determinant of that trend toward progression. Milbrandt et al[62] advocated for considering the curves to be neuromuscular and incorporating all curves in a fusion, as attempting selective fusion may have a higher rate of decompensation and need for revision.

Foot deformity with pes cavus or talipes equinovarus is the other common skeletal abnormality in genetically proven cases of Friedreich's ataxia (74%).[57] Abnormality of eye movements is a common early sign,[66,67,68] as are dysarthria and mild dysphagia.[55,56,68,69] Hearing difficulties are common,[49,56,61,68] and some investigators feel this is more common than reported,[70] with disordered neural conduction in the central auditory pathways resulting in impaired speech and understanding, especially where background noise is present. This impaired hearing may have been part of what led early investigators to include diminished IQ as part of the phenotype,[61] but later investigators felt it was more a sign of slowed information processing and impairments in motor, speech, and auditory function.[71] Diabetes is present in about a third of cases,[72] and cardiomyopathy is present in around 66%.[57] Death has been found to occur in the fourth decade of life, with cardiac complications accounting for the majority.[55,73,74]

12.3.3 Disorder-Specific Techniques

Labelle et al[60] advocated for two groups in Friedreich's ataxia, onset of scoliosis before 10 and after 10, thinking that the earlier onset leads to higher rates of progression, while the later onset may be able to be observed without significant progression. Tsirikos and Smith presented a series of 31 patients with scoliosis and Friedreich's ataxia.[65] Seventeen patients had progressive deformity and underwent posterior instrumented spinal fusion (▶ Fig. 12.4). Similarly, Daher et al[75] reported on 19 patients with Friedreich's ataxia and scoliosis, of which 12 required surgical treatment for a progressive deformity (▶ Fig. 12.5).

Bracing is widely considered unsuccessful in Friedreich's ataxia. Out of six patients braced in the Daher et al[75] series, only two (33%) were successfully braced through maturity. They postulated that brace failure occurs at a higher rate because of brace intolerance due to difficulties with balance and coordination in the brace. Tsirikos and Smith[65] reported bracing nine patients, with only one successfully braced to maturity. Milbrandt et al[62] reported failure of bracing in 8 out of 10 patients but still recommend a trial.

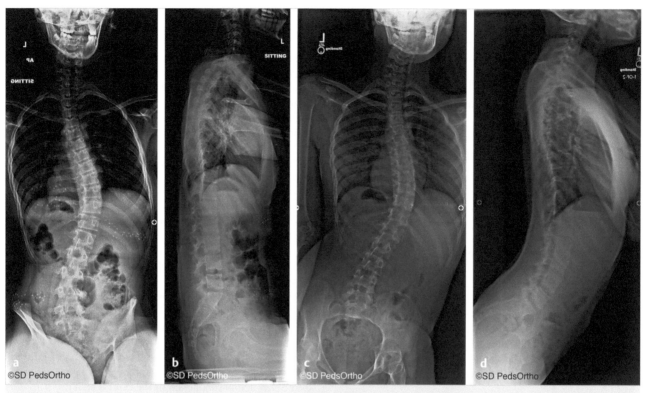

Fig. 12.4 Seated PA (a) and lateral (b) radiographs of a 13-year-old girl with Friedreich's ataxia and a 40-degree scoliosis. One-year follow-up standing PA (c) and lateral (d) radiographs reveal relatively stable scoliosis with a Cobb angle of 42 degrees. The issues with balance can be appreciated and this patient will be followed with seated radiographs as she progresses into a wheelchair.

Surgical techniques involve incorporating all curves as in most cases of neuromuscular scoliosis.[62] Since patients with Friedreich's ataxia can maintain ambulation for an average of 15 years after diagnosis,[49] fusion levels attempt to avoid fixation to the pelvis. Cady and Bobechko[64] fused 1 out of 25 patients to the sacrum, Daher et al[75] 1 out of 12, and Tsirikos and Smith[65] 1 out of 17. While the authors above did not frequently fuse to the pelvis, they all commented on extending fusions below L2, thereby incorporating all curves. Others have reported on fusing to the pelvis; however, these reports are primarily general technique reviews in neuromuscular scoliosis of a heterogenic population of which patients with Friedreich's ataxia were few in number.[76,77,78,79,80]

Variability in spinal cord monitoring has also been highlighted by a number of authors in this patient population.[81] Pelosi et al[82] included motor evoked potentials with somatosensory evoked potentials and could not record a signal in either channel in two out of two patients with Friedreich's ataxia. Milbrandt et al[62] recommended planning for a wake-up test if needed.

12.3.4 Evidence-Based Outcomes

Case series make up the surgical outcomes literature for patients with Friedreich's ataxia and scoliosis. Cady and Bobechko[64] reported on 11 surgical patients with average correction of 41% with an average starting curve of 56 degrees.

They had one death at 6 weeks due to congestive heart failure. Daher et al[75] evaluated 12 cases with Harrington or Luque instrumentation: estimated blood loss was 1,440 mL, and 10 of 12 patients were immobilized in a cast or brace for an average of 9 months with curve correction from mean 49 degrees pre-op to 26 degrees post-op. Tsirikos and Smith[65] reported on 17 patients with instrumentation ranging from Harrington rods to all–pedicle screw constructs. They had one death early in the series due to cardiorespiratory compromise, one patient had rod breakage at the thoracolumbar junction, and four patients fused to T4 experienced proximal junctional kyphosis that was asymptomatic and left untreated.

Milbrandt et al[62] reported on all patients with Friedreich's ataxia at two institutions. Of 49 patients, 16 with scoliosis underwent surgery with an average of 13.25 levels fused. Estimated blood loss was 1,268 mL, and operative time averaged 5.6 hours. They reported one patient with neuromonitoring signals, but in all other patients the monitoring was ineffective and they performed a wake-up test in four patients. Initial postoperative correction was 49%, but this decreased to 39% over a mean follow-up of 3.7 years. They had one patient each with multiple complications of infection, junctional kyphosis, adding on, and instrumentation failure.

There has been interest recently in attempting to chart the progression of Friedreich's ataxia with development of several rating scales. These rating scales are replacing simpler measures such as time to wheelchair dependence.[83,84,85,86,87]

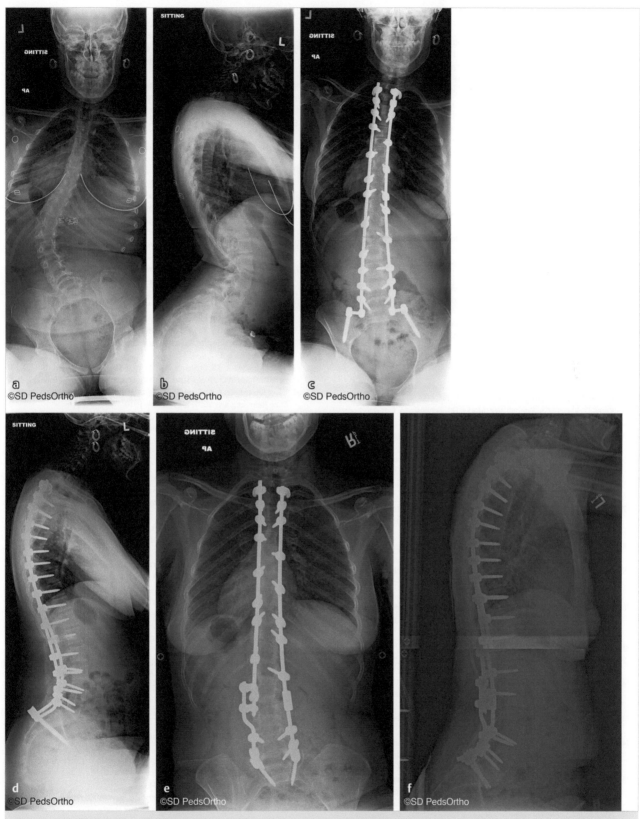

Fig. 12.5 Preoperative sitting PA (**a**) and lateral (**b**) radiographs of a 13-year-old girl with Friedreich's ataxia and a collapsing **C**-shaped curve with pelvic obliquity. Four-week postoperative PA (**c**) and lateral (**d**) radiographs after a posterior T2 to pelvis segmental instrumentation and fusion with iliac bolts. She developed pain with transfers and household ambulation and underwent revision with fixation to the sacrum. Three-year postoperative PA (**e**) and lateral (**f**) radiographs after the revision demonstrating maintenance of deformity correction and sitting balance.

References

[1] Rett A. On a unusual brain atrophy syndrome in hyperammonemia in childhood [in German]. Wien Med Wochenschr. 1966; 116(37):723–726

[2] Hagberg B, Aicardi J, Dias K, Ramos O. A progressive syndrome of autism, dementia, ataxia, and loss of purposeful hand use in girls: Rett's syndrome: report of 35 cases. Ann Neurol. 1983; 14(4):471–479

[3] Fehr S, Bebbington A, Nassar N, et al. Trends in the diagnosis of Rett syndrome in Australia. Pediatr Res. 2011; 70(3):313–319

[4] Amir RE, Zoghbi HY. Rett syndrome: methyl-CpG-binding protein 2 mutations and phenotype-genotype correlations. Am J Med Genet. 2000; 97 (2):147–152

[5] Wan M, Lee SS, Zhang X, et al. Rett syndrome and beyond: recurrent spontaneous and familial MECP2 mutations at CpG hotspots. Am J Hum Genet. 1999; 65(6):1520–1529

[6] Berridge CW, Waterhouse BD. The locus coeruleus-noradrenergic system: modulation of behavioral state and state-dependent cognitive processes. Brain Res Brain Res Rev. 2003; 42(1):33–84

[7] Weaving LS, Ellaway CJ, Gécz J, Christodoulou J. Rett syndrome: clinical review and genetic update. J Med Genet. 2005; 42(1):1–7

[8] Hagberg B. Clinical manifestations and stages of Rett syndrome. Ment Retard Dev Disabil Res Rev. 2002; 8(2):61–65

[9] Hagberg B, Witt-Engerström I. Early stages of the Rett syndrome and infantile neuronal ceroid lipofuscinosis–a difficult differential diagnosis. Brain Dev. 1990; 12(1):20–22

[10] The Rett Syndrome Diagnostic Criteria Work Group. Diagnostic criteria for Rett syndrome. Ann Neurol. 1988; 23(4):425–428

[11] Anderson A, Wong K, Jacoby P, Downs J, Leonard H. Twenty years of surveillance in Rett syndrome: what does this tell us? Orphanet J Rare Dis. 2014; 9:87

[12] Bassett GS, Tolo VT. The incidence and natural history of scoliosis in Rett syndrome. Dev Med Child Neurol. 1990; 32(11):963–966

[13] Keret D, Bassett GS, Bunnell WP, Marks HG. Scoliosis in Rett syndrome. J Pediatr Orthop. 1988; 8(2):138–142

[14] Harrison DJ, Webb PJ. Scoliosis in the Rett syndrome: natural history and treatment. Brain Dev. 1990; 12(1):154–156

[15] Lidström J, Stokland E, Hagberg B. Scoliosis in Rett syndrome. Clinical and biological aspects. Spine. 1994; 19(14):1632–1635

[16] Steffenburg U, Hagberg G, Hagberg B. Epilepsy in a representative series of Rett syndrome. Acta Paediatr. 2001; 90(1):34–39

[17] Smeets EEJ, Julu POO, van Waardenburg D, et al. Management of a severe forceful breather with Rett syndrome using carbogen. Brain Dev. 2006; 28 (10):625–632

[18] Julu PO, Engerström IW, Hansen S, et al. Cardiorespiratory challenges in Rett's syndrome. Lancet. 2008; 371(9629):1981–1983

[19] Smeets E, Schollen E, Moog U, et al. Rett syndrome in adolescent and adult females: clinical and molecular genetic findings. Am J Med Genet A. 2003; 122A(3):227–233

[20] Downs J, Bergman A, Carter P, et al. Guidelines for management of scoliosis in Rett syndrome patients based on expert consensus and clinical evidence. Spine. 2009; 34(17):E607–E617

[21] Berven S, Bradford DS. Neuromuscular scoliosis: causes of deformity and principles for evaluation and management. Semin Neurol. 2002; 22(2):167–178

[22] Gabos PG, Inan M, Thacker M, Borkhu B. Spinal fusion for scoliosis in Rett syndrome with an emphasis on early postoperative complications. Spine. 2012; 37(2):E90–E94

[23] Kerr AM, Webb P, Prescott RJ, Milne Y. Results of surgery for scoliosis in Rett syndrome. J Child Neurol. 2003; 18(10):703–708

[24] Karmaniolou I, Krishnan R, Galtrey E, Cleland S, Vijayaraghavan R. Perioperative management and outcome of patients with Rett syndrome undergoing scoliosis surgery: a retrospective review. J Anesth. 2015; 29(4):492–498

[25] Verma K, Errico TJ, Vaz KM, Lonner BS. A prospective, randomized, double-blinded single-site control study comparing blood loss prevention of tranexamic acid (TXA) to epsilon aminocaproic acid (EACA) for corrective spinal surgery. BMC Surg. 2010; 10:13

[26] Vitale MG, Riedel MD, Glotzbecker MP, et al. Building consensus: development of a Best Practice Guideline (BPG) for surgical site infection (SSI) prevention in high-risk pediatric spine surgery. J Pediatr Orthop. 2013; 33 (5):471–478

[27] Pastorelli F, Di Silvestre M, Plasmati R, et al. The prevention of neural complications in the surgical treatment of scoliosis: the role of the neurophysiological intraoperative monitoring. Eur Spine J. 2011; 20 Suppl 1:S105–S114

[28] Hammett T, Harris A, Boreham B, Mehdian SMH. Surgical correction of scoliosis in Rett syndrome: cord monitoring and complications. Eur Spine J. 2014; 23 Suppl 1:S72–S75

[29] Larsson E-L, Aaro S, Ahlinder P, Normelli H, Tropp H, Oberg B. Long-term follow-up of functioning after spinal surgery in patients with Rett syndrome. Eur Spine J. 2009; 18(4):506–511

[30] Skre H. Genetic and clinical aspects of Charcot-Marie-Tooth's disease. Clin Genet. 1974; 6(2):98–118

[31] Martyn CN, Hughes RA. Epidemiology of peripheral neuropathy. J Neurol Neurosurg Psychiatry. 1997; 62(4):310–318

[32] Jani-Acsadi A, Ounpuu S, Pierz K, Acsadi G. Pediatric Charcot-Marie-Tooth disease. Pediatr Clin North Am. 2015; 62(3):767–786

[33] Dyck PJ, Lambert EH. Lower motor and primary sensory neuron diseases with peroneal muscular atrophy. II. Neurologic, genetic, and electrophysiologic findings in various neuronal degenerations. Arch Neurol. 1968; 18(6):619–625

[34] Dyck PJ, Lambert EH. Lower motor and primary sensory neuron diseases with peroneal muscular atrophy. I. Neurologic, genetic, and electrophysiologic findings in hereditary polyneuropathies. Arch Neurol. 1968; 18(6):603–618

[35] Timmerman V, Strickland AV, Züchner S. Genetics of Charcot-Marie-Tooth (CMT) disease within the frame of the human genome project success. Genes (Basel). 2014; 5(1):13–32

[36] Raeymaekers P, Timmerman V, Nelis E, et al. The HMSN Collaborative Research Group. Duplication in chromosome 17p11.2 in Charcot-Marie-Tooth neuropathy type 1a (CMT 1a). Neuromuscul Disord. 1991; 1(2):93–97

[37] Thomas PK. Overview of Charcot-Marie-Tooth disease type 1A. Ann NY Acad Sci. 1999; 883:1–5

[38] Walker JL, Nelson KR, Stevens DB, Lubicky JP, Ogden JA, VandenBrink KD. Spinal deformity in Charcot-Marie-Tooth disease. Spine. 1994; 19(9):1044–1047

[39] Karol LA, Elerson E. Scoliosis in patients with Charcot-Marie-Tooth disease. J Bone Joint Surg Am. 2007; 89(7):1504–1510

[40] Hensinger RN, MacEwen GD. Spinal deformity associated with heritable neurological conditions: spinal muscular atrophy, Friedreich's ataxia, familial dysautonomia, and Charcot-Marie-Tooth disease. J Bone Joint Surg Am. 1976; 58(1):13–24

[41] Azzedine H, Ravisé N, Verny C, et al. Spine deformities in Charcot-Marie-Tooth 4C caused by SH3TC2 gene mutations. Neurology. 2006; 67(4):602–606

[42] Mikesová E, Hühne K, Rautenstrauss B, et al. Novel EGR2 mutation R359Q is associated with CMT type 1 and progressive scoliosis. Neuromuscul Disord. 2005; 15(11):764–767

[43] Hoellwarth JS, Mahan ST, Spencer SA. Painful pes planovalgus: an uncommon pediatric orthopedic presentation of Charcot-Marie-Tooth disease. J Pediatr Orthop B. 2012; 21(5):428–433

[44] Daher YH, Lonstein JE, Winter RB, Bradford DS. Spinal deformities in patients with Charcot-Marie-tooth disease. A review of 12 patients. Clin Orthop Relat Res. 1986(202):219–222

[45] Krishna M, Taylor JF, Brown MC, et al. Failure of somatosensory-evoked-potential monitoring in sensorimotor neuropathy. Spine. 1991; 16(4):479

[46] Burns J, Ouvrier R, Estilow T, et al. Validation of the Charcot-Marie-Tooth disease pediatric scale as an outcome measure of disability. Ann Neurol. 2012; 71(5):642–652

[47] Burns J, Raymond J, Ouvrier R. Feasibility of foot and ankle strength training in childhood Charcot-Marie-Tooth disease. Neuromuscul Disord. 2009; 19 (12):818–821

[48] Filla A, De Michele G, Marconi R, et al. Prevalence of hereditary ataxias and spastic paraplegias in Molise, a region of Italy. J Neurol. 1992; 239(6):351–353

[49] Harding AE, Zilkha KJ. 'Pseudo-dominant' inheritance in Friedreich's ataxia. J Med Genet. 1981; 18(4):285–287

[50] Cossée M, Schmitt M, Campuzano V, et al. Evolution of the Friedreich's ataxia trinucleotide repeat expansion: founder effect and premutations. Proc Natl Acad Sci U S A. 1997; 94(14):7452–7457

[51] Epplen C, Epplen JT, Frank G, Miterski B, Santos EJ, Schöls L. Differential stability of the (GAA)n tract in the Friedreich ataxia (STM7) gene. Hum Genet. 1997; 99(6):834–836

[52] Campuzano V, Montermini L, Moltò MD, et al. autosomal recessive disease caused by an intronic GAA triplet repeat expansion. Science. 1996; 271 (5254):1423–1427

[53] Cossée M, Dürr A, Schmitt M, et al. Friedreich's ataxia: point mutations and clinical presentation of compound heterozygotes. Ann Neurol. 1999; 45 (2):200–206

[54] Gellera C, Castellotti B, Mariotti C, et al. Frataxin gene point mutations in Italian Friedreich ataxia patients. Neurogenetics. 2007; 8(4):289–299

[55] Filla A, DeMichele G, Caruso G, Marconi R, Campanella G. Genetic data and natural history of Friedreich's disease: a study of 80 Italian patients. J Neurol. 1990; 237(6):345–351

[56] Dürr A, Cossee M, Agid Y, et al. Clinical and genetic abnormalities in patients with Friedreich's ataxia. N Engl J Med. 1996; 335(16):1169–1175

[57] Delatycki MB, Paris DB, Gardner RJ, et al. Clinical and genetic study of Friedreich ataxia in an Australian population. Am J Med Genet. 1999; 87(2):168–174

[58] Schulz JB, Boesch S, Bürk K, et al. Diagnosis and treatment of Friedreich ataxia: a European perspective. Nat Rev Neurol. 2009; 5(4):222–234

[59] Delatycki MB, Corben LA. Clinical features of Friedreich ataxia. J Child Neurol. 2012; 27(9):1133–1137

[60] Labelle H, Tohmé S, Duhaime M, Allard P. Natural history of scoliosis in Friedreich's ataxia. J Bone Joint Surg Am. 1986; 68(4):564–572

[61] Geoffroy G, Barbeau A, Breton G, et al. Clinical description and roentgenologic evaluation of patients with Friedreich's ataxia. Can J Neurol Sci. 1976; 3 (4):279–286

[62] Milbrandt TA, Kunes JR, Karol LA. Friedreich's ataxia and scoliosis: the experience at two institutions. J Pediatr Orthop. 2008; 28(2):234–238

[63] Aronsson DD, Stokes IA, Ronchetti PJ, Labelle HB. Comparison of curve shape between children with cerebral palsy, Friedreich's ataxia, and adolescent idiopathic scoliosis. Dev Med Child Neurol. 1994; 36(5):412–418

[64] Cady RB, Bobechko WP. Incidence, natural history, and treatment of scoliosis in Friedreich's ataxia. J Pediatr Orthop. 1984; 4(6):673–676

[65] Tsirikos AI, Smith G. Scoliosis in patients with Friedreich's ataxia. J Bone Joint Surg Br. 2012; 94(5):684–689

[66] Furman JM, Perlman S, Baloh RW. Eye movements in Friedreich's ataxia. Arch Neurol. 1983; 40(6):343–346

[67] Fahey MC, Cremer PD, Aw ST, et al. Vestibular, saccadic and fixation abnormalities in genetically confirmed Friedreich ataxia. Brain. 2008; 131(Pt 4):1035–1045

[68] Schöls L, Amoiridis G, Przuntek H, Frank G, Epplen JT, Epplen C. Friedreich's ataxia. Revision of the phenotype according to molecular genetics. Brain. 1997; 120(Pt 12):2131–2140

[69] Folker J, Murdoch B, Cahill L, Delatycki M, Corben L, Vogel A. Dysarthria in Friedreich's ataxia: a perceptual analysis. Folia Phoniatr Logop. 2010; 62 (3):97–103

[70] Rance G, Corben LA, Du Bourg E, King A, Delatycki MB. Successful treatment of auditory perceptual disorder in individuals with Friedreich ataxia. Neuroscience. 2010; 171(2):552–555

[71] Corben LA, Georgiou-Karistianis N, Fahey MC, et al. Towards an understanding of cognitive function in Friedreich ataxia. Brain Res Bull. 2006; 70(3):197–202

[72] Hewer RL, Robinson N. Diabetes mellitus in Friedreich's ataxia. J Neurol Neurosurg Psychiatry. 1968; 31(3):226–231

[73] Andermann E, Remillard GM, Goyer C, Blitzer L, Andermann F, Barbeau A. Genetic and family studies in Friedreich's ataxia. Can J Neurol Sci. 1976; 3 (4):287–301

[74] Tsou AY, Paulsen EK, Lagedrost SJ, et al. Mortality in Friedreich ataxia. J Neurol Sci. 2011; 307(1–2):46–49

[75] Daher YH, Lonstein JE, Winter RB, Bradford DS. Spinal deformities in patients with Friedreich ataxia: a review of 19 patients. J Pediatr Orthop. 1985; 5 (5):553–557

[76] Piazzolla A, Solarino G, De Giorgi S, Mori CM, Moretti L, De Giorgi G. Cotrel-Dubousset instrumentation in neuromuscular scoliosis. Eur Spine J. 2011; 20 Suppl 1:S75–S84

[77] La Rosa G, Giglio G, Oggiano L. Surgical treatment of neurological scoliosis using hybrid construct (lumbar transpedicular screws plus thoracic sublaminar acrylic loops). Eur Spine J. 2011; 20 Suppl 1:S90–S94

[78] Bell DF, Moseley CF, Koreska J. Unit rod segmental spinal instrumentation in the management of patients with progressive neuromuscular spinal deformity. Spine. 1989; 14(12):1301–1307

[79] Bui T, Shapiro F. Posterior spinal fusion to sacrum in non-ambulatory hypotonic neuromuscular patients: sacral rod/bone graft onlay method. J Child Orthop. 2014; 8(3):229–236

[80] Stricker U, Moser H, Aebi M. Predominantly posterior instrumentation and fusion in neuromuscular and neurogenic scoliosis in children and adolescents. Eur Spine J. 1996; 5(2):101–106

[81] Lubicky JP, Spadaro JA, Yuan HA, Fredrickson BE, Henderson N. Variability of somatosensory cortical evoked potential monitoring during spinal surgery. Spine. 1989; 14(8):790–798

[82] Pelosi L, Lamb J, Grevitt M, Mehdian SMH, Webb JK, Blumhardt LD. Combined monitoring of motor and somatosensory evoked potentials in orthopaedic spinal surgery. Clin Neurophysiol. 2002; 113(7):1082–1091

[83] Fahey MC, Corben L, Collins V, Churchyard AJ, Delatycki MB. How is disease progress in Friedreich's ataxia best measured? A study of four rating scales. J Neurol Neurosurg Psychiatry. 2007; 78(4):411–413

[84] Bürk K, Mälzig U, Wolf S, et al. Comparison of three clinical rating scales in Friedreich ataxia (FRDA). Mov Disord. 2009; 24(12):1779–1784

[85] Friedman LS, Farmer JM, Perlman S, et al. Measuring the rate of progression in Friedreich ataxia: implications for clinical trial design. Mov Disord. 2010; 25(4):426–432

[86] Regner SR, Wilcox NS, Friedman LS, et al. Friedreich ataxia clinical outcome measures: natural history evaluation in 410 participants. J Child Neurol. 2012; 27(9):1152–1158

[87] Metz G, Coppard N, Cooper JM, et al. Rating disease progression of Friedreich's ataxia by the International Cooperative Ataxia Rating Scale: analysis of a 603-patient database. Brain. 2013; 136(Pt 1):259–268

13 Neurosurgical Causes of Scoliosis

Marie Roguski, Steven W. Hwang, and Amer F. Samdani

Abstract

The most common cause of scoliosis is idiopathic. However, in infantile and juvenile scoliosis, up to 20% of patients may harbor an underlying neurologic cause.[1,2,3,4] Recognition of a potentially reversible underlying neurologic process is vital in order to prevent progressive and irreversible neurologic injury. Several clinical conditions may predispose to the development and progression of scoliosis. Neurological signs and symptoms, such as pain, weakness, sensory changes, gait abnormalities, and bowel and bladder changes, as well as the presence of orthopaedic and cutaneous anomalies, are important indicators that a neurologic condition may exist.[5] Early age of onset, presence of a left curvature, increased kyphosis, and rapid progression are additional clinical indicators that should prompt the acquisition of a magnetic resonance image (MRI) of the spine.[6] Once a neurologic cause is identified, treatment is focused toward correcting the underlying pathology, and deformity correction is reserved for large or progressive curves following treatment. This chapter will focus on the etiology and pathogenesis, disease-specific deformity, comorbidities, techniques, and evidence-based outcomes of three specific causes of neurogenic scoliosis: Chiari I malformation, tethered cord, and split cord malformation.

Keywords: Chiari I malformation, neurogenic scoliosis, spinal dysraphism, split cord malformation, tethered spinal cord syndrome

13.1 Chiari I Malformation and Syringomyelia

13.1.1 Etiology and Pathogenesis

Although there are four recognized varieties of Chiari I malformations, they are vastly different pathophysiologic processes, and patients with both type I and II Chiari's malformations may develop scoliosis. Chiari I malformations are generally defined as cerebellar tonsillar ectopia with descent of the tonsils greater than 5 mm below the foramen magnum.[7,8,9] In contrast, Chiari II malformations involve the herniation of the inferior cerebellar vermis and are associated with myelomeningocele and frequently hydrocephalus.[10,11,12] Although scoliosis is frequently encountered among patients with spina bifida and Chiari II malformations, scoliosis is unlikely to be the primary presenting sign, and, thus, this chapter will focus largely on Chiari I malformations. Among patients presenting with pediatric scoliosis, Chiari I malformations are the most common neural axis abnormality detected.[2,3,4]

Marin-Padilla and Marin-Padilla suggested that a hypoplastic posterior fossa during fetal development may limit the expansion of the rhombencephalon, resulting in the herniation of the cerebellar tonsils through the foramen magnum.[13] Morphometric studies demonstrating a small posterior fossa provide further support for this theory.[9,14] Scoliosis may coexist with a Chiari I malformation in up to 42% of patients,[9] and an association exists between those with progressive scoliosis and the presence of a syrinx.[15,16,17] The association of syringomyelia with progressive scoliosis among patients with Chiari I malformation has been theorized to result from paresis of the axial musculature, congenital vertebral structural changes, and interference of postural tonic reflexes.[18]

Several theories have been hypothesized to explain the development of syringomyelia in the setting of Chiari malformation. Gardner's hydrodynamic theory suggests that cerebrospinal fluid (CSF) pulsations from the choroid plexus normally play a role in neural tube expansion during fetal development; unbalanced CSF pulsations between supratentorial and infratentorial compartments result in a small posterior fossa, tonsillar ectopia, and forced diversion of CSF into the central canal of the spinal cord due to obstruction of the fourth ventricular outflow tracts at the foramen magnum.[19] Williams postulated that transient intracranial pressure elevations due to Valsalva's maneuvers resulted in bulk flow of CSF caudally; CSF outflow obstruction resists flow caudally and creates a differential pressure between the cranial and spinal compartments that contributes to worsening syringomyelia.[20] Although these theories offer insight into the etiology of syringomyelia in the setting of Chiari I malformation, they provide an incomplete explanation for the pathogenesis of syringomyelia because syringomyelia is often acquired and the syrinx does not always directly communicate with the fourth ventricle. Oldfield et al attempted to address these inconsistencies by postulating that the movement of the cerebellar tonsils during systole creates a systolic pressure wave in the spinal CSF that results in the movement of fluid into the spinal cord via perivascular and interstitial spaces rather than through the central canal at the obex.[21]

13.1.2 Disease-Specific Deformity and Comorbidities

Chiari I malformations are defined by tonsillar ectopia of greater than 5 mm on magnetic resonance images (MRI). However, the degree of tonsillar descent does not always correlate with symptom severity, and Elster and Chen demonstrated that nearly 30% of patients with 5 to 10 mm of tonsillar herniation may be asymptomatic.[8] Patients with Chiari I malformations present with a myriad of symptoms and signs, but they most commonly present with occipital or cervical headache that is worsened with exertion or Valsalva. Weakness, paresthesia, numbness, nystagmus, gait imbalance, ataxia, dysphagia, dysarthria, and drop attacks are other symptoms that may result from Chiari I malformation.[5] Children may not portray typical symptoms and, instead, may present with irritability, opisthoclonus, or failure to thrive.

In addition to tonsillar ectopia, associated vertebral column or neural abnormalities are present in between 24 and 50% of patients with Chiari I malformation, and include Klippel–Feil deformity and atlantoaxial assimilation.[22] Syringomyelia occurs in between 50 and 75% of patients, is most commonly located in the cervical spine, and is associated with progressive scoliosis.[9,15,16,17,22,23] Overall, scoliosis is present in nearly 42% of patients.[9]

13.1.3 Disorder-Specific Techniques

Treatment of Chiari I malformation–associated scoliosis is surgical and aims to relieve cervicomedullary compression at the foramen magnum in order to halt progression of scoliosis. Posterior fossa decompression is most commonly performed with a suboccipital craniectomy. There remains significant controversy regarding whether duraplasty is necessary and whether coagulation of the cerebellar tonsils should be performed in order to achieve adequate decompression.[24]

13.1.4 Evidence-Based Outcomes

Arnautovic et al performed a meta-analysis and systematic review of 145 publications (8,605 patients) studying the role of decompressive surgery for Chiari I malformations.[25] The vast majority of included series involved suboccipital craniectomy with duraplasty. Neurological improvement or resolution occurred in 72%. Nearly 65% of patients harbored a spinal cord syrinx, and postoperative improvement in syringomyelia was noted in 78% of patients. Other series report that nearly 85% of patients note improvement in headache and neck pain.[22,26] These good outcomes, however, must be balanced by a reported median complication rate of 3.5%. Complications include pseudomeningocele, aseptic meningitis, CSF leak, meningitis, and neurologic injury. Only 11% of the series included by Arnautovic et al mentioned death as an observed complication of surgery; among these, the overall mortality rate was estimated at 3%.[25] In addition, although syringomyelia commonly improves after surgery, incomplete resolution or residual paresthesias may be present in over 50% of patients.[27]

Several series have demonstrated that suboccipital decompression may halt or improve the progression of scoliosis.[15,16,28,29] A recent systematic review estimated that curve magnitude improved in 37% and progressed in 45% of patients with Chiari I malformations following surgical intervention.[30] Brockmeyer et al further demonstrated that curves improved or remained stable in nearly 91% of children younger than 10 years suboccipital decompression and duraplasty.[31] Other authors have linked older age, curves of greater than 40 degrees, double scoliosis patterns, kyphosis, and curve rotations with progression despite foramen magnum decompression.[17,31,32,33] The association of smaller curves with improvement or stabilization of curve magnitude highlights the importance of early detection and treatment in patients with Chiari I malformation and scoliosis (▶ Fig. 13.1, ▶ Fig. 13.2).

13.2 Tethered Cord Syndrome and Spinal Dysraphism

13.2.1 Etiology and Pathogenesis

Tethered cord syndrome (TCS) results from a number of congenital conditions and causes progressive neurological decline due to tension on the spinal cord. The filum terminale is a fibroelastic structure that extends from the conus to the sacrum and is theorized to stabilize the conus medullaris during spinal column movement. Pathological stretch applied to the spinal cord is associated with metabolic derangements resembling those seen with ischemia.[34] These metabolic changes may be related to reduction in blood flow to the spinal cord during flexion movements, impairment of oxidative metabolism, or physical neuronal damage related to tethering. Given that the spinal canal length changes by as much as 7% during flexion and stretch applied to neural tissue results in metabolic derangements, some authors have hypothesized that the signs and symptoms of TCS are due to failure of the filum terminale to alleviate spinal cord stretch during flexion-related changes in spinal canal length.[35] Although tethering by a tight filum terminale may be the causative problem in many patients with TCS, any pathology that limits spinal cord movement, including spinal dysraphism, may result in pathologic stretch and associated signs and symptoms. Mild or moderate damage may sometimes be reversible with alleviation of the pathological spinal cord stretch via detethering procedures; however, damage due to severe stretch may be irreversible, highlighting the need for early recognition and treatment.[35,36]

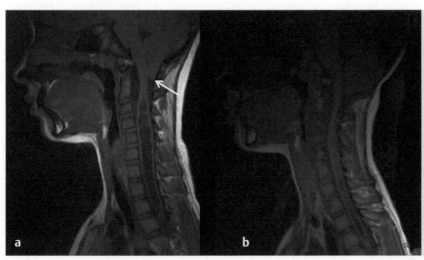

Fig. 13.1 An 11-year-old girl with Chiari I malformation and scoliosis. **(a)** Preoperative sagittal T1-weighted MRI showing tonsillar descent and a syrinx. **(b)** Postoperative sagittal MRI showing decompression of the posterior fossa and decrease in the syrinx size.

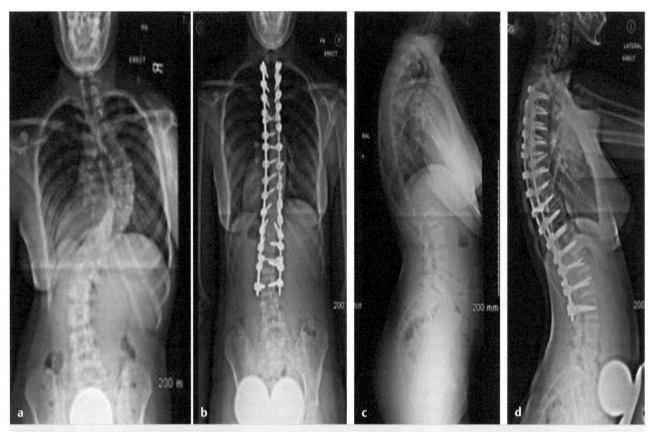

Fig. 13.2 (a) Preoperative posteroanterior (PA) radiograph showing a progressive thoracic curve. (b) Postoperative PA X-ray. (c) Preoperative lateral radiograph showing increased kyphosis. (d) Postoperative lateral X-ray.

Spinal dysraphism refers to a number of congenital anomalies of the spine that result from malformation of midline dorsal neural, mesenchymal, and cutaneous ectodermal structures during early embryogenesis.[37] Development of the spinal cord occurs via neurulation, canalization of the tail bud, and regression of the caudal cell mass (CCM). The process begins at gestational day 18 when differential proliferation of the neuroectoderm is induced by the underlying notochord, resulting in folding of the flat neural plate into a neural tube (neurulation). The neuroectoderm and ectoderm then separate and form a neural tube that is covered by cutaneous ectoderm (dysjunction). This process begins in the upper cervical region and extends rostrally and caudally toward L1/L2. This process results in the formation of the cephalic portion of the spinal cord. Caudal portions, including the conus medullaris and filum terminale, develop through canalization of the tail bud and regression of the CCM. The tail bud or CCM is formed by neuroectodermal cells that are located caudal to the neural tube; vacuoles form and coalesce within the tail bud to form a central canal beginning at day 28, continuing through day 48. The central canal then connects with the rostral neural tube and forms the embryologic basis of the lower lumbar, sacral, and coccygeal spine. Lastly, regression of the caudal portion of the CCM forms the filum terminale and terminal ventricle, which eventually forms the conus medullaris.[38] Errors in neurulation, dysjunction, canalization, and regression result in congenital malformations, including myelomeningocele, meningocele, lipomyelomeningocele, dermal sinus tract, dermoid and epidermoid tumors, and

fatty filum, all of which may result in tethering and caudal traction on the spinal cord (▶ Fig. 13.3).

TCS is often associated with syringomyelia. Thus, progression of neurological symptoms may be due to both metabolic changes within the spinal cord related to stretch and cystic dilation of the spinal cord itself. The syrinx in patients with TCS is often located in the terminal spinal cord, suggesting that the traditional pathogenic theories noted previously may not be relevant to the development of dysraphism- or TCS- associated syringes.[39] The association of TCS with scoliosis was first demonstrated by McLone et al.[40] By demonstrating stabilization or improvement in scoliosis following detethering in patients who had previously undergone myelomeningocele repair, they postulated that tethering may cause scoliosis via ischemic spinal cord injury at the site of tethering, dysfunction of sensory tracts, and asymmetric paravertebral muscle tone.[5]

13.2.2 Disease-Specific Deformity and Comorbidities

Patients with TCS present with progressive neurological deterioration, musculoskeletal abnormalities (such as scoliosis and limb anomalies), cutaneous stigmata, and dysraphic posterior spinal elements.[41,42,43] Neurological symptoms in children with TCS include gait abnormalities, regression of gait training, urological symptoms (including recurrent urinary tract infections and enuresis), or numbness; pain tends to be less prominent than in adult patients with TCS.[44] Cutaneous findings include

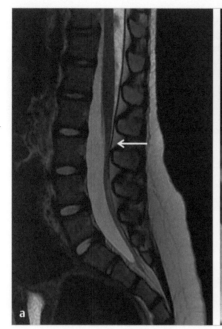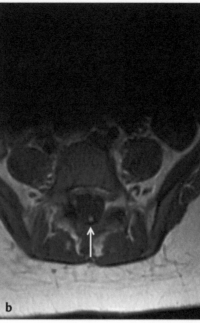

Fig. 13.3 (a) Sagittal T2-weighted MRI showing a low-lying conus and a thickened filum in a symptomatic 3-year-old girl. (b) Axial T1-weighted MRI showing a fatty filum (white arrow).

hypertrichosis, pigmented nevi, subcutaneous lipomas, dermal dimples, and dermal sinuses. Musculoskeletal abnormalities include vertebral body anomalies, scoliosis, accentuated lumbosacral lordosis, and leg deformities, including hammertoes, talipes cavus, pes equinus high arched feet, and different leg lengths.[42,45] Up to 29% of patients may present with scoliosis or kyphosis.[46]

Radiographic diagnosis is made when the conus medullaris lies below the level of the second lumbar vertebrae. However, among patients with myelomeningocele who have previously undergone myelomeningocele repair, the diagnosis must be made clinically as there is universally radiographic evidence of tethering.

13.2.3 Disorder-Specific Techniques

Because patients present with progressive neurological deficits due to caudal traction from tethering, many neurosurgeons advocate operative detethering to prevent further progression of neurological signs.[47] The primary goal of surgery is to completely untether the spinal cord. Procedures to achieve this goal range from transection of the filum terminale to more extensive procedures for complex malformations.[48] Laser microsurgery has been used to aid in the resection of spinal lipomas.[49]

Prevention of recurrent tethering is critical during TCS surgery as recurrent tethering occurs in 5 to 50% of patients.[50,51,52] Meticulous hemostasis is needed in order to prevent arachnoiditis. In addition, the use of a duraplasty graft rather than a primary dural closure is advocated by some in order to enlarge the subarachnoid space.[53,54,55,56] Repeated detethering procedures have multiple shortcomings related to increased difficulty due to arachnoid adhesions and scarring. Patients often relapse and develop progressive neurological deterioration following a short period of improvement.[57] Given the difficulty, increased morbidity, and poor outcomes associated with multiple repeated detethering procedures, Grande et al proposed vertebral column subtraction osteotomy (VCSO) or spinal shortening

as a possible alternative treatment for patients with progressive TCS in whom multiple retethering operations have failed.[58]

13.2.4 Evidence-Based Outcomes

Surgical detethering in TCS is associated with improvements in neurologic and urologic function in 90% and 50% of patients, respectively.[59] Complications include spinal fluid leak, wound infection, meningitis, and neurologic injury, and the risk of the procedure varies according to the complexity of the underlying pathology. Younger children tend to fare better than older children or adults.[5,60]

Several authors have demonstrated a correlation between tethering and scoliosis. McLone et al demonstrated stabilization or improvement in progressive scoliosis after detethering in patients with myelomeningocele and recurrent tethering.[40] By observing that only one child among six with a curve greater than 50 degrees improved following detethering, this study identified degree of deformity as an important predictor of progression following spinal cord release. In contrast, of 24 children with curves less than 50 degrees, nearly all patients had stable or improved curves at 1 year, and 63% remained stable or improved at a later follow-up (2–7 years).[40] Other authors have also demonstrated a plateau or improvement in curve progression following tethered spinal cord release.[61,62,63]

13.3 Split Cord Malformation

13.3.1 Etiology and Pathogenesis

Split cord malformations (SCMs) are rare congenital malformations in which the spinal cord is comprised of two hemicords. Pang and Wilberger proposed a unified theory of embryogenesis postulating that the formation of adhesions between ectoderm and endoderm leads to the formation of an accessary neuroenteric canal. An endomesenchymal tract condenses around the accessary canal and bisects the developing

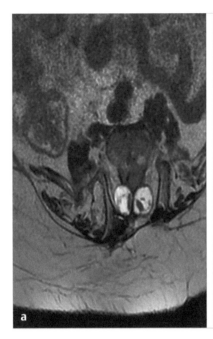
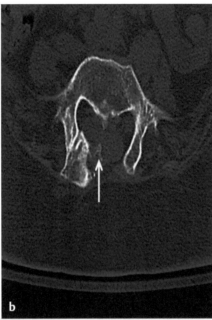

Fig. 13.4 **(a)** Axial T2-weighted MRI showing a split cord malformation with two dural sheaths (type 1). **(b)** Axial CT showing associated calcification across neuroenteric band.

notochord, leading to the development of two hemicords (▶ Fig. 13.4).[64] This alteration results in variable configuration and orientation of the hemicords, and median septum and is associated with vascular, lipomatous, neural, and fibrous anomalies.

In offering a pathogenic theory, Pang and Wilberger also classified SCMs into two types based on the orientation of the two hemicords. In type I SCM, each hemicord is contained in a separate dural tube and is separated by a rigid osseocartilaginous septum. In type II SCM the two hemicords are contained within the same dural tube separated by a fibrous median septum.[64]

13.3.2 Disease-Specific Deformity and Comorbidities

SCMs present with a constellation of cutaneous, musculoskeletal, and neurological signs. Nearly 80% of 254 patients with SCM presented with sensorimotor and autonomic disturbances in a series reported by Mahapatra and Gupta.[65] Symptoms included motor deficits, atrophy, gait disturbance, dysesthetic pain, trophic ulcers, and bowel and bladder disturbances. Furthermore, orthopaedic lower limb deformities and scoliosis were present in 43 and 52% of patients, respectively. Cutaneous findings were present in 59% of patients and included hypertrichosis, dimple, dermal sinus, hyperpigmented patch, capillary hemangiomas, and subcutaneous lipoma. The septum of the SCM is most commonly located in the lumbar spine, and the anomaly often coexists with another abnormality that may also cause spinal cord tethering.[5,65]

13.3.3 Disorder-Specific Techniques

The technique of detethering is similarly described above. However, once the fibrous band is removed, a caudal laminectomy should be performed to transect the filum. Classically, patients were recommended for detethering prior to correction of spinal deformity to theoretically minimize the risk of spinal cord injury. However, recently a series of 247 patients with diastematomyelia without neurological symptoms or signs of TCS clinically underwent deformity correction without prior detethering. Approximately 4% had nerve root complications, but none developed complications from spinal cord injury.[66]

13.3.4 Evidence-Based Outcomes

The risk of progressive neurological decline in the setting of an SCM and spinal cord tethering has been estimated to be greater than 50%.[67] As such, surgical release of the tethered hemicords by resection of bone spurs, fibrous septa, or fibrous bands (meningocele manqué) is recommended by many authors prior to development of neurological signs and symptoms.[5,65,68] With regard to neurological status, Pang reported that 89% of patients with SCM improved or stabilized following surgery for SCM.[67] Transient deterioration in neurological status is common (7%) postoperatively.[65] Although no study exists examining the effect of detethering of SCM on associated spinal deformities, it is possible that detethering of SCM may have a similar effect on stabilization or improvement of progressive scoliosis as detethering in other pathologic entities.

13.4 Conclusion

Recognition of a potentially reversible underlying neurologic process is vital in order to prevent progressive and irreversible neurologic injury. A low index of suspicion to obtain an MRI when atypical features are present can be very helpful to identify these neurological etiologies causing scoliosis, such as Chiari malformations, syringomyelia, spinal dysraphisms, TCS, congenital abnormalities, and spinal cord tumors. Once identified radiographically, neurosurgical consultation can help determine the optimal treatment for these patients, as their care can be tailored to balance our understanding of the natural history, surgical complications, and the clinical picture.

References

[1] McMaster MJ. Occult intraspinal anomalies and congenital scoliosis. J Bone Joint Surg Am. 1984; 66(4):588–601

[2] Dobbs MB, Lenke LG, Szymanski DA, et al. Prevalence of neural axis abnormalities in patients with infantile idiopathic scoliosis. J Bone Joint Surg Am. 2002; 84-A(12):2230–2234

[3] Evans SC, Edgar MA, Hall-Craggs MA, Powell MP, Taylor BA, Noordeen HH. MRI of 'idiopathic' juvenile scoliosis. A prospective study. J Bone Joint Surg Br. 1996; 78(2):314–317

[4] Gupta P, Lenke LG, Bridwell KH. Incidence of neural axis abnormalities in infantile and juvenile patients with spinal deformity. Is a magnetic resonance image screening necessary? Spine. 1998; 23(2):206–210

[5] Cardoso M, Keating RF. Neurosurgical management of spinal dysraphism and neurogenic scoliosis. Spine. 2009; 34(17):1775–1782

[6] Schwend RM, Hennrikus W, Hall JE, Emans JB. Childhood scoliosis: clinical indications for magnetic resonance imaging. J Bone Joint Surg Am. 1995; 77(1):46–53

[7] Dyste GN, Menezes AH, VanGilder JC. Symptomatic Chiari malformations. An analysis of presentation, management, and long-term outcome. J Neurosurg. 1989; 71(2):159–168

[8] Elster AD, Chen MY. Chiari I malformations: clinical and radiologic reappraisal. Radiology. 1992; 183(2):347–353

[9] Milhorat TH, Chou MW, Trinidad EM, et al. Chiari I malformation redefined: clinical and radiographic findings for 364 symptomatic patients. Neurosurgery. 1999; 44(5):1005–1017

[10] Chiari H. Uber Veranderungen des Kleinhiens, des pons und der medulla oblongata. Folge voncongenitaler hydrocephalie des grossherns. Deskschr Akad Wiss Wien. 1895; 63:71–116

[11] Peach B. The Arnold-Chiari malformation; morphogenesis. Arch Neurol. 1965; 12:527–535

[12] Gilbert JN, Jones KL, Rorke LB, Chernoff GF, James HE. Central nervous system anomalies associated with meningomyelocele, hydrocephalus, and the Arnold-Chiari malformation: reappraisal of theories regarding the pathogenesis of posterior neural tube closure defects. Neurosurgery. 1986; 18(5):559–564

[13] Marin-Padilla M, Marin-Padilla TM. Morphogenesis of experimentally induced Arnold–Chiari malformation. J Neurol Sci. 1981; 50(1):29–55

[14] Schady W, Metcalfe RA, Butler P. The incidence of craniocervical bony anomalies in the adult Chiari malformation. J Neurol Sci. 1987; 82(1–3):193–203

[15] Nohria V, Oakes WJ. Chiari I malformation: a review of 43 patients. Pediatr Neurosurg. 1990–1991; 16(4–5):222–227

[16] Muhonen MG, Menezes AH, Sawin PD, Weinstein SL. Scoliosis in pediatric Chiari malformations without myelodysplasia. J Neurosurg. 1992; 77(1):69–77

[17] Eule JM, Erickson MA, O'Brien MF, Handler M. Chiari I malformation associated with syringomyelia and scoliosis: a twenty-year review of surgical and nonsurgical treatment in a pediatric population. Spine. 2002; 27(13):1451–1455

[18] Robin GC. Scoliosis and neurological disease. Isr J Med Sci. 1973; 9(5):578–586

[19] Gardner WJ, Angel J. The cause of syringomyelia and its surgical treatment. Cleve Clin Q. 1958; 25(1):4–8

[20] Williams B. On the pathogenesis of syringomyelia: a review. J R Soc Med. 1980; 73(11):798–806

[21] Oldfield EH, Muraszko K, Shawker TH, Patronas NJ. Pathophysiology of syringomyelia associated with Chiari I malformation of the cerebellar tonsils. Implications for diagnosis and treatment. J Neurosurg. 1994; 80(1):3–15

[22] Menezes AH. Chiari I malformations and hydromyelia–complications. Pediatr Neurosurg. 1991–1992; 17(3):146–154

[23] Batzdorf U. Chiari I malformation with syringomyelia. Evaluation of surgical therapy by magnetic resonance imaging. J Neurosurg. 1988; 68(5):726–730

[24] Hankinson T, Tubbs RS, Wellons JC. Duraplasty or not? An evidence-based review of the pediatric Chiari I malformation. Childs Nerv Syst. 2011; 27(1):35–40

[25] Arnautovic A, Splavski B, Boop FA, Arnautovic KI. Pediatric and adult Chiari malformation Type I surgical series 1965–2013: a review of demographics, operative treatment, and outcomes. J Neurosurg Pediatr. 2015; 15(2):161–177

[26] Nagib MG. An approach to symptomatic children (ages 4–14 years) with Chiari type I malformation. Pediatr Neurosurg. 1994; 21(1):31–35

[27] Wetjen NM, Heiss JD, Oldfield EH. Time course of syringomyelia resolution following decompression of Chiari malformation Type I. J Neurosurg Pediatr. 2008; 1(2):118–123

[28] Sengupta DK, Dorgan J, Findlay GF. Can hindbrain decompression for syringomyelia lead to regression of scoliosis? Eur Spine J. 2000; 9(3):198–201

[29] Bertrand SL, Drvaric DM, Roberts JM. Scoliosis in syringomyelia. Orthopedics. 1989; 12(2):335–337

[30] Hwang SW, Samdani AF, Jea A, et al. Outcomes of Chiari I-associated scoliosis after intervention: a meta-analysis of the pediatric literature. Childs Nerv Syst. 2012; 28(8):1213–1219

[31] Brockmeyer D, Gollogly S, Smith JT. Scoliosis associated with Chiari 1 malformations: the effect of suboccipital decompression on scoliosis curve progression: a preliminary study. Spine. 2003; 28(22):2505–2509

[32] Flynn JM, Sodha S, Lou JE, et al. Predictors of progression of scoliosis after decompression of an Arnold Chiari I malformation. Spine. 2004; 29(3):286–292

[33] Attenello FJ, McGirt MJ, Atiba A, et al. Suboccipital decompression for Chiari malformation-associated scoliosis: risk factors and time course of deformity progression. J Neurosurg Pediatr. 2008; 1(6):456–460

[34] Yamada S, Won DJ, Pezeshkpour G, et al. Pathophysiology of tethered cord syndrome and similar complex disorders. Neurosurg Focus. 2007; 23(2):E6

[35] Yamada S, Iacono RP, Andrade T, Mandybur G, Yamada BS. Pathophysiology of tethered cord syndrome. Neurosurg Clin N Am. 1995; 6(2):311–323

[36] Schneider SJ, Rosenthal AD, Greenberg BM, Danto J. A preliminary report on the use of laser-Doppler flowmetry during tethered spinal cord release. Neurosurgery. 1993; 32(2):214–217, discussion 217–218

[37] Cochrane DD. Occult spinal dysraphism. In: Albright AL, Pollack IF, Adelson PD, eds. Principles and Practices of Pediatric Neurosurgery. 2nd ed. New York, NY: Thieme; 2008:367–393

[38] French BN. The embryology of spinal dysraphism. Clin Neurosurg. 1983; 30:295–340

[39] Iskandar BJ, Oakes WJ, McLaughlin C, Osumi AK, Tien RD. Terminal syringohydromyelia and occult spinal dysraphism. J Neurosurg. 1994; 81(4):513–519

[40] McLone DG, Herman JM, Gabrieli AP, Dias L. Tethered cord as a cause of scoliosis in children with a myelomeningocele. Pediatr Neurosurg. 1990–1991; 16(1):8–13

[41] Hertzler DA, II, DePowell JJ, Stevenson CB, Mangano FT. Tethered cord syndrome: a review of the literature from embryology to adult presentation. Neurosurg Focus. 2010; 29(1):E1

[42] Warder DE. Tethered cord syndrome and occult spinal dysraphism. Neurosurg Focus. 2001; 10(1):e1

[43] Anderson FM. Occult spinal dysraphism: a series of 73 cases. Pediatrics. 1975; 55(6):826–835

[44] Pang D, Wilberger JE, Jr. Tethered cord syndrome in adults. J Neurosurg. 1982; 57(1):32–47

[45] Tubbs RS, Bui CJ, Loukas M, Shoja MM, Oakes WJ. The horizontal sacrum as an indicator of the tethered spinal cord in spina bifida aperta and occulta. Neurosurg Focus. 2007; 23(2):E11

[46] Greenberg MS. Handbook of Neurosurgery. 7th ed. New York, NY: Thieme; 2010

[47] Tubbs RS, Pugh J, Wellons JC III. Tethered spinal cord: fatty filum terminale, meningocele manque, and dermal sinus tracts. In: Winn H, ed. Youmans Neurological Surgery. Philadelphia, PA: Elsevier Saunders; 2011:2227–2232

[48] Klekamp J. Tethered cord syndrome in adults. J Neurosurg Spine. 2011; 15(3):258–270

[49] McLone DG, Naidich TP. Laser resection of fifty spinal lipomas. Neurosurgery. 1986; 18(5):611–615

[50] Filler AG, Britton JA, Uttley D, Marsh HT. Adult postrepair myelomeningocoele and tethered cord syndrome: good surgical outcome after abrupt neurological decline. Br J Neurosurg. 1995; 9(5):659–666

[51] Hsieh PC, Ondra SL, Grande AW, et al. Posterior vertebral column subtraction osteotomy: a novel surgical approach for the treatment of multiple recurrences of tethered cord syndrome. J Neurosurg Spine. 2009; 10(4):278–286

[52] Herman JM, McLone DG, Storrs BB, Dauser RC. Analysis of 153 patients with myelomeningocele or spinal lipoma reoperated upon for a tethered cord. Presentation, management and outcome. Pediatr Neurosurg. 1993; 19(5):243–249

[53] Colak A, Pollack IF, Albright AL. Recurrent tethering: a common long-term problem after lipomyelomeningocele repair. Pediatr Neurosurg. 1998; 29(4):184–190

[54] Kang JK, Lee KS, Jeun SS, Lee IW, Kim MC. Role of surgery for maintaining urological function and prevention of retethering in the treatment of lipomeningomyelocele: experience recorded in 75 lipomeningomyelocele patients. Childs Nerv Syst. 2003; 19(1):23–29

[55] Samuels R, McGirt MJ, Attenello FJ, et al. Incidence of symptomatic retethering after surgical management of pediatric tethered cord syndrome with or without duraplasty. Childs Nerv Syst. 2009; 25(9):1085–1089

[56] Zide B, Constantini S, Epstein FJ. Prevention of recurrent tethered spinal cord. Pediatr Neurosurg. 1995; 22(2):111–114

[57] Lagae L, Verpoorten C, Casaer P, Vereecken R, Fabry G, Plets C. Conservative versus neurosurgical treatment of tethered cord patients. Z Kinderchir. 1990; 45 Suppl 1:16–17

[58] Grande AW, Maher PC, Morgan CJ, et al. Vertebral column subtraction osteotomy for recurrent tethered cord syndrome in adults: a cadaveric study. J Neurosurg Spine. 2006; 4(6):478–484

[59] Lee GY, Paradiso G, Tator CH, Gentili F, Massicotte EM, Fehlings MG. Surgical management of tethered cord syndrome in adults: indications, techniques, and long-term outcomes in 60 patients. J Neurosurg Spine. 2006; 4(2):123–131

[60] Keating MA, Rink RC, Bauer SB, et al. Neurourological implications of the changing approach in management of occult spinal lesions. J Urol. 1988; 140 (5, Pt 2):1299–1301

[61] Reigel DH, Tchernoukha K, Bazmi B, Kortyna R, Rotenstein D. Change in spinal curvature following release of tethered spinal cord associated with spina bifida. Pediatr Neurosurg. 1994; 20(1):30–42

[62] McGirt MJ, Mehta V, Garces-Ambrossi G, et al. Pediatric tethered cord syndrome: response of scoliosis to untethering procedures. Clinical article. J Neurosurg Pediatr. 2009; 4(3):270–274

[63] Pierz K, Banta J, Thomson J, Gahm N, Hartford J. The effect of tethered cord release on scoliosis in myelomeningocele. J Pediatr Orthop. 2000; 20(3):362–365

[64] Pang D, Dias MS, Ahab-Barmada M. Split cord malformation: Part I: A unified theory of embryogenesis for double spinal cord malformations. Neurosurgery. 1992; 31(3):451–480

[65] Mahapatra AK, Gupta DK. Split cord malformations: a clinical study of 254 patients and a proposal for a new clinical-imaging classification. J Neurosurg. 2005; 103(6) Suppl:531–536

[66] Shen JFF. Evaluation of surgical treatment of congenital scoliosis associated with split cord malformation. In: IMAST 22nd Annual Meeting; July 10, 2015; Kuala Lumpur, Malaysia

[67] Pang D. Split cord malformation: Part II: Clinical syndrome. Neurosurgery. 1992; 31(3):481–500

[68] Miller A, Guille JT, Bowen JR. Evaluation and treatment of diastematomyelia. J Bone Joint Surg Am. 1993; 75(9):1308–1317

14 Sagittal Plane Spinal Deformity in Patients with Neuromuscular Disease

Kirk W. Dabney

Abstract

Isolated sagittal plane spinal deformities (kyphosis and hyperlordosis) are uncommon in neuromuscular disease but can interfere with proper sitting and standing in this patient population. Scoliosis accompanied by sagittal plane deformity is common. Mild and some moderate deformity can be treated by wheelchair modifications and bracing. Symptomatic moderate and severe deformity may require surgical treatment. More flexible kyphosis and hyperlordosis can be corrected by posterior spinal fusion and segmental instrumentation alone, while more rigid deformity may require posterior osteotomies (for kyphosis) or anterior diskectomies (for hyperlordosis). Instrumentation and correction techniques vary from screw/rod constructs using distraction/compression correction to wire or screw/rod constructs using cantilever correction. Overall, outcomes literature focused on sagittal plane deformity in the patient with neuromuscular disease is limited and somewhat inconsistent; however, authors who do measure function report improvements in pain, sitting balance, head and neck control, breathing, and hand use. Patients with kyphosis undergoing spinal fusion with instrumentation are at risk for loss of proximal and/or distal fixation.

Keywords: hyperlordosis, kyphosis, neuromuscular disease, spinal deformity, spinal fusion

14.1 Introduction

Neuromuscular diseases are heterogeneous and are due to a vast number of pathologies involving the brain, spinal cord, peripheral nervous system, and muscle. The prevalence of spinal deformity is typically proportional to the severity of neurologic impairment. While scoliosis is the most commonly treated neuromuscular spinal deformity, sagittal plane deformities (excessive kyphosis or lordosis) can occur in combination with scoliosis or in isolation. Deterioration in pulmonary status is generally not an issue in isolated sagittal plane spinal deformities; however, they can cause difficulty with seating as well as pain, especially when the deformity is greater than 70 degrees.[1] In addition, some authors have identified hyperlordosis as a cause of superior mesenteric artery syndrome in a small number of patients.[1,2] Indications for corrective surgery include pain and difficulty with seating. Surgical methods for correcting sagittal plane spinal deformities require specific strategies, and it is also important to recognize the associated comorbidities in order to optimize the outcomes of treatment.

14.2 Etiology/Pathogenesis/ Natural History

Similar to neuromuscular scoliosis, neuromuscular sagittal plane deformities are a consequence of muscle imbalance and may occur in patients with a wide variety of neuromuscular diseases that includes: cerebral palsy; poliomyelitis; myelomeningocele; spinal muscle atrophy; muscular dystrophies; myopathies; and infectious, metabolic, and traumatic encephalopathy.

In cerebral palsy, there is felt to be a correlation between loss of lumbar lordosis or even frank lumbar kyphosis with hamstring contracture[3] that may cause a posteriorly tilted pelvis with a prominent vertically oriented sacrum. Alternatively, iliopsoas contracture can result in lumbar hyperlordosis, severe anterior pelvic tilting, and a horizontal sacrum. Lumbar hyperlordosis may result in a sacral pressure sore as the weight-bearing load during seating is shifted posterior onto the sacrum. Poor head control and truncal hypotonia may also result in a postural thoracic kyphosis that may gradually evolve into a more rigid deformity over time. Like scoliosis, the cause of sagittal plane deformity appears to be related to the severity of the neurological deficit. Understanding whether the neuromuscular disease is static or progressive is helpful in determining the rationale for treatment of spinal deformity, including sagittal plane deformity.

The natural history of specific neuromuscular diseases causing spinal deformity is critically important so that the surgeon can understand the impact that the sagittal plane deformity will have on the child's quality of life. In addition, the natural history of the disease impacts the associated comorbidities, surgical timing, and the subsequent risks associated with surgery. Sagittal plane kyphotic deformity was noted in 62% and lumbar hyperlordosis in 38% of patients with Duchenne muscular dystrophy not receiving steroid treatment.[4] Unlike scoliosis, however, little is known about the natural history of kyphosis and hyperlordosis within specific neuromuscular diseases.

14.3 Patient Assessment and Preoperative Considerations

With an informed decision by the family to proceed with surgery, an adequate preoperative evaluation must ensure that all associated comorbid conditions are medically optimized. All children with neuromuscular conditions should have a detailed preoperative assessment. Patients with neuromuscular disease often have associated medical comorbidities, which correlate strongly with postoperative complications and include cardiac disease, gastroesophageal reflux, reactive airway disease, restrictive lung disease, aspiration pneumonia and reactive airway disease, heart disease, poor nutrition, seizure disorders, and low bone mineral density.[5] These should be identified in the medical history preoperatively and comanaged medically.[5]

Physical examination should assess sitting and/or standing balance, coronal, sagittal, and any rotational deformity of the pelvis, and stiffness of the kyphosis (assessed on physical exam and bending films over a bolster). Curvatures that are stiff in both the coronal (scoliosis) and sagittal planes (severe hyperlordosis and hyperkyphosis) may require anterior release or preoperative traction.[6,7,8] Sagittal plane stiffness should be assessed by physical examination with an attempt to reduce the deformity in the supine position over a bolster. Additionally, one may observe the flexibility of a hyperlordotic deformity by hyperflexing both hips and the pelvis in the supine position. Supine sagittal bend radiographs can also be performed by using these same maneuvers while the radiograph is performed.

It is also important to assess and distinguish the coexistence of a hip flexion contracture and adduction contracture in high-tone neuromuscular conditions (e.g., cerebral palsy) with spinal deformity. This can be done by stabilizing the pelvis in a neutral position (flexing the opposite hip to level the pelvis to detect hip flexion contracture and assessing hip adduction contracture by the amount of abduction achieved with the pelvis in neutral obliquity). If these contractures are present, the parents should be warned that muscle releases may be necessary 4 to 6 months after spinal surgery. In addition, an assessment for hip subluxation should always be done in patients with spinal deformity.

The surgeon must also assess the need for fusing to the pelvis especially when the pelvis is included in the kyphosis. In the patient with cerebral palsy, this is almost always necessary to prevent distal extension of the deformity. Also, in patients with poor head control, the surgeon should consider instrumenting/fusing up to T1 or T2 to prevent a junctional kyphosis in routine cases and in those with more proximal kyphotic deformities even into the cervical spine. In addition, great care should be taken to preserve the posterior longitudinal ligament to prevent proximal falloff. Finally, the child should also have a detailed neurological examination that includes sensory and motor testing as well as reflexes including abdominal reflexes to establish baseline neurological function and the need to look for any undiagnosed intraspinal pathology such as tumor, tethered cord, and syringomyelia.

14.3.1 Nonoperative Treatment

Postural (flexible) kyphosis in neuromuscular disease may initially be managed utilizing wheelchair modifications such as a tilt-in-space wheelchair with an adequate chest harness to prevent the trunk from leaning forward (▶ Fig. 14.1a). In addition, a wheelchair tray table is also helpful in preventing forward lean, and a Hensinger or cervical soft collar may assist with trunk and head control (▶ Fig. 14.1b). As thoracic kyphosis becomes more rigid, bracing with a clam-shell orthosis that is high in the front of the trunk and lower in the back (usually below the scapulae) (▶ Fig. 14.1c) may provide some assistance with upright seating. Larger patients and/or those with stiff kyphotic deformities are generally not amenable to bracing but can be treated nonoperatively with a custom-molded seat-back if the kyphosis is not causing pain, recognizing that this only accommodates the kyphotic deformity. On the other hand, hyperlordosis is generally not amenable to bracing. Problems with bracing patients with neuromuscular disease may include discomfort, excessive sweating in warm weather, pressure sores, restriction of the child's breathing ability, and abdominal restriction when feeding the child. The latter can be alleviated by simply removing the orthosis during and for an hour after feeding.

14.4 Surgical Treatment

The principles of spinal deformity correction are to: (1) correct pelvic deformity (both coronal and sagittal) by leveling the pelvis with the sitting or standing surface and restoring anatomic sagittal alignment of the pelvis (average sacral slope of approximately 40 degrees, pelvic tilt of 13 degrees, and lumbar lordosis of 40–60 degrees); (2) restore trunk balance; (3) center the head over the trunk and pelvis; (4) restore sagittal balance (lumbar lordosis and thoracic kyphosis—including the correction of anterior and posterior pelvic tilt, respectively);

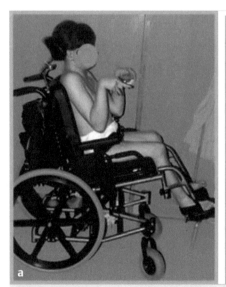
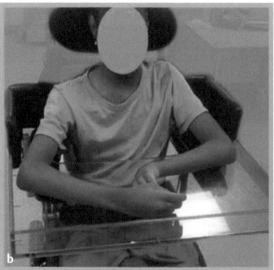
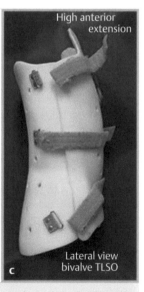

Fig. 14.1 Nonoperative methods for flexible kyphosis. **(a)** Tilt-in-space chair can be used to reduce a flexible neuromuscular kyphosis by tilting the chair back. **(b)** In children with flexible kyphosis, the tray table prevents the child from leaning too far forward. **(c)** Clam-shell brace used for kyphosis with high anterior extension.

(5) maximize segmental fixation in the face of what is often osteoporotic bone; and (6) minimize operative time in this patient population who often have multiple comorbidities and excessive bleeding, and who are at greater risk for wound infection.[9,10]

14.5 Preoperative Planning

Three main technical preoperative considerations deserve careful consideration: (1) Is fusion to the pelvis necessary? (2) Is there a significant rotational component to the spinal deformity that is contributing to difficulty in seating? (3) Is the rigidity of the deformity severe enough to warrant halo-femoral traction, posterior osteotomy, or total vertebral resection? In addition, strut graft can be added in severe/rigid kyphotic deformity.

The only treatment that has made a definitive impact on the correction of neuromuscular spinal deformity is instrumentation and fusion. The standard surgical procedure for neuromuscular sagittal plane deformity is a posterior spinal fusion with segmental instrumentation from T1 or T2 down to the sacrum if the pelvis is part of the deformity. In hyperlordosis, the pelvis and lumbar spine are almost always involved. Even if the pelvis is not involved in a severely involved nonambulatory patient or an ambulatory patient with poor balance, the surgeon should consider fusion to the pelvis to prevent the development of late pelvic deformity. The gold standard in the past for the correction of neuromuscular scoliosis[11,12,13] had been Luque rod instrumentation (with Galveston instrumentation to the pelvis), cross-linkage to prevent rod shift and rotation, and sublaminar wires; however, this approach has not been nearly as successful in managing hyperkyphosis.[14]

14.6 Author's Preferred Surgical Method of Treatment

14.6.1 Intraoperative Positioning

The patient is positioned prone on a Jackson table (a Relton-Hall frame can also be used) with the abdominal area free (▶ Fig. 14.2). We have adapted special radiolucent posts for the Jackson table that can be spaced at a narrower distance compared to the standard posts. In lumbar hyperlordosis, the hips and knees are bent and left to hang freely (reducing the excessive lordosis), which helps to optimize insertion in the case of unit rods. In addition, it helps to minimize the stress on the wire or screw/bone interface during the reduction of the hyperlordosis. All bony prominences should be well padded. Many children with cerebral palsy have significant contractures, making their extremities hard to position. Minimal tension should be placed on the joints. Urinary catheters should be free flowing, especially in children with neurogenic bladder with a vesicostomy or other bladder reconstruction.

Newer methods of instrumentation allow modularization of the unit rod concept and cantilever correction by combining wires and/or pelvic screws, precontoured rods, and a proximal connector (▶ Fig. 14.3a, b). Both the unit rod and the precontoured rods (in the modular construct) have prebent sagittal contour. With the modular system, precontoured rods are connected with a proximal connector, in addition to a pelvic screw

with diameter (7–10 mm) and length (65–100 mm) that can be selected according to pelvic size. Achieving proper sagittal balance is critical, particularly in those who are ambulatory. Precontoured rods typically place slightly more lumbar lordosis in order to shift weightbearing onto the posterior thigh musculature in wheelchair ambulatory patients, while ambulators should have a balanced thoracic kyphosis/lumbar lordosis contour. Dearolf et al[15] have described allowing greater thoracic kyphosis in patients with spinal cord injury in order to maintain activities of daily living. Many surgeons use pedicle screws instead of wires for segmental fixation, especially if there is a severe kyphotic component to the deformity, whereas sublaminar wires/tapes may be efficient at pulling a hyperlordotic lumbar spine into more normal alignment.[6] Caution should be taken to prevent pedicle screw pullout when the bone is

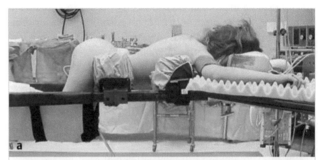
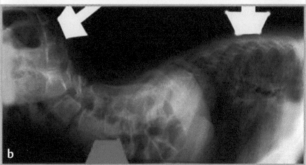

Fig. 14.2 (a,b) Positioning of the patient should allow the abdomen to be free, and in the case of hyperlordosis, the hips are flexed to 90 degrees with the trunk and the legs hanging freely to allow as much passive correction of the hyperlordosis as possible.

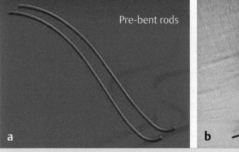
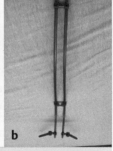

Pre-bent rods

Fig. 14.3 This modular system consists of **(a)** two rods with a sagittal contour which are **(b)** connected by a close connector proximally and a cross-link at the thoracolumbar junction. The pelvic screws are anchored into the pelvis separately, which allows easier pelvic placement than the unit rod.

severely osteopenic. If significant sagittal plane stiffness exists as assessed by the physical and radiographic examination with the inability to reduce the deformity, anterior diskectomy should be considered in hyperlordosis and halo-femoral traction or posterior osteotomy with or without anterior diskectomy considered in hyperkyphosis.

14.6.2 Medical/Anesthesia Considerations

In patients with neuromuscular disease, the general medical condition of the child should always be assessed prior to undertaking the surgical correction. Many children with neuromuscular conditions will have comorbidities such as pulmonary disease, cardiac disease, seizure disorder, gastrointestinal reflux, poor nutrition, osteoporosis, and so forth. Samdani et al[16] reported a major complication rate of 39.4% in a multicenter study of 127 patients with cerebral palsy. These major complications prolonged both the length of intensive care unit and hospital stays. Perioperative pulmonary complications were the most frequent. Risk factors of major perioperative complications included a greater preoperative kyphosis, staged procedures, lack of antifibrinolytic use, and greater intraoperative blood loss. Accordingly, all patients with complex preoperative medical conditions should undergo the appropriate preoperative medical workup.

The surgeon and anesthesiologist should plan for the possibility of large intraoperative blood loss.[17] Jain et al[9] reported higher intraoperative blood loss in patients undergoing spinal fusion with cerebral palsy and other neuromuscular diagnoses compared to idiopathic scoliosis and Scheuermann's kyphosis. In our own experience, this is especially true in hyperlordosis where the surgical dissection is often more difficult, especially exposing sublaminar spaces if sublaminar wires are being used. Type and cross-matched blood (up to twice the patient's blood volume), fresh-frozen plasma, and platelets should be available. In addition, the use of cell-saver blood should be considered. Currently, tranexamic acid is used to decrease fibrinolysis, decreasing overall blood loss.[18] Good vascular access is required, often through a central venous catheter, in patients with poor peripheral access. For good access and the purposes of possible postoperative hyperalimentation for nutrition, we place a central venous catheter in all patients with neuromuscular disease.

Another consideration in the treatment of neuromuscular spinal deformity is neurologic risk and the use of spinal cord monitoring. Rigid thoracic lordosis may cause the cord to displace more posteriorly, which places it more at risk while exposing sublaminar spaces for sublaminar wiring. Correction of a rigid thoracic kyphosis may result in stretching the anterior spine, resulting in an anterior cord syndrome. In cases where there is rigid deformity, multiple level diskectomies with anterior osteotomies, which shorten the spinal column, may help lessen the risk of spinal cord stretch. While somewhat unclear in patients with neuromuscular spinal deformity, most children with neuropathies, myopathies, and mild-to-moderate cerebral palsy (without severe motor cortex involvement) can be monitored using a combination of somatosensory and motor evoked potentials.[19] However, in one study, approximately 40% of children with severe quadriplegic cerebral palsy and poor motor function could not be monitored.[19] In addition, it is difficult to justify completely removing implant instrumentation if there are signal changes in the child with minimal motor function, since the risk of repeat operation to reimplant instrumentation is quite high in this population. As a general rule, somatosensory and motor evoked potential monitoring should be attempted for any child with ambulatory or functional standing (able to assist with standing transfers). There may also be some efficacy in monitoring neuromuscular patients with intact sensation and bowel and bladder control. Any child with neurogenic bladder should be carefully evaluated for urinary tract infection preoperatively and, if present, should be treated to clear the urine prior to surgery.

Bone density of the child undergoing spinal fusion should also be considered. The child who is nonambulatory, poorly nourished, and on seizure medication is at highest risk. Children with low bone density may be difficult to instrument owing to the possibility of sublaminar wires pulling through or pedicle screws pulling out of osteopenic bone. Any nonambulatory child with low-impact long bone fracture should be checked for low bone density using dual-energy X-ray absorptiometry scan. Children on seizure medication should have calcium, phosphorous, and vitamin D levels measured. Patients with bone density two or more Z-scores below the mean with frequent fracture should be considered for treatment using intravenous pamidronate.[20]

Another important preoperative and intraoperative consideration is the prevention of infection after spinal fusion. The range of infection has been shown to be from 4.2 to 20%.[21] Sponseller et al[22,23] reported on two multicenter analyses of infection risk factors and treatment in cerebral palsy. High preoperative white blood cell count, older age, higher preoperative curve magnitude, longer operative time, the presence of a gastrostomy or gastrojejunostomy tube, and the use of a unit rod were associated with deep wound infection. Final curve correction was lower for patients with infections. Several infected patients required intensive and prolonged irrigation/debridement and antibiotic therapy. At our institution, prophylactic intravenous antibiotics cover staph species with intravenous cefazolin. Consideration of prophylactic dosages of vancomycin or clindamycin should be given in patients with methicillin-resistant *Staphylococcus aureus* (MRSA)-positive nasal swabs (which should be considered in all institutionalized patients). We also give one preoperative dosage of gentamycin for gram-negative coverage to patients with stool incontinence, gastrostomy tubes, and a history of gram-negative urinary tract infections. In addition, we mix allograft bone graft with gentamycin and/or vancomycin.[24] Mohamed et al[21] showed that skin breakdown was one of the most significant predisposing factors to deep wound infection. Careful attention is placed on meticulous fascial closure to prevent leakage, covering the skin surface external to the subcuticular closure with a surgical glue barrier, and covering the wound dressing with a plastic stick-on barrier to prevent stool and urine from getting into the wound. Best practice guidelines for pediatric spine surgery have been recently proposed for high-risk pediatric spine surgery patients relevant for the majority of neuromuscular patients: (1) patients should have a chlorhexidine skin wash the night before surgery; (2) patients should have preoperative urine cultures obtained; (3) patients should receive a preoperative patient

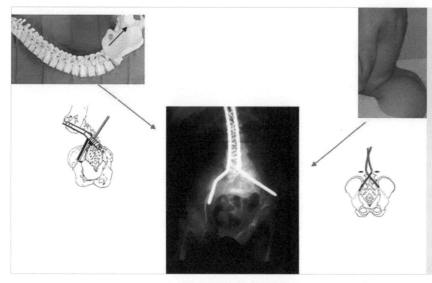

Fig. 14.4 Placement of the pelvic limbs of the unit rod is difficult in hyperlordosis due to the far anterior start point required for the pelvic limbs to enter the pelvis. The drill hole and rod limbs (the latter of which must be crossed in order to enter the pelvis properly) must aim just in front of the sciatic notch and aim distal and posterior. Failure to do so may cause the rod limb to penetrate the inner pelvic table as shown.

education sheet; (4) patients should have a preoperative nutritional assessment; (5) if removing hair, clipping is preferred to shaving; (6) patients should receive perioperative intravenous cefazolin; (7) patients should receive perioperative intravenous prophylaxis for gram-negative bacilli; (8) adherence to perioperative antimicrobial regimens should be monitored; (9) operating room access should be limited during scoliosis surgery (whenever practical); (10) UV lights need *not* be used in the operating room; (11) patients should have intraoperative wound irrigation; (12) vancomycin powder should be used in the bone graft and/or the surgical site; (13) impervious dressings are preferred postoperatively; and (14) postoperative dressing changes should be minimized before discharge to the extent possible.[25]

14.7 Specific Surgical Techniques

14.7.1 Pelvic Fixation

Fixation and fusion to the pelvis should be considered in every neuromuscular patient with a sagittal plane deformity that extends into the pelvis. Cantilever correction is a powerful method to correct both anterior and posterior pelvic tilt in the sagittal plane. It requires instrumentation that can firmly anchor into the pelvis and can then be used as a lever arm to bring the pelvis into a corrected position that is perpendicular to the longitudinal axis of the spine. Traditionally, the unit rod is ideal for pelvic fixation; however, it can be difficult to place the pelvic limbs of the rod in cases of severe lumbar lordosis because it must be placed into the pelvis in one unit (▶ Fig. 14.4). Cantilever correction using pelvic screws connected to dual precontoured rods connected to one another by a proximal connector (▶ Fig. 14.3) can also accomplish this and is easier to place than the unit rod. The pelvis is exposed by dissecting up over the sacroiliac joint onto the lumbar muscle attachment on the inner table of the pelvis. It is important not to dissect into the sacroiliac joint subperiosteally as one can encounter significant bleeding here. By dissecting over the joint itself, little bleeding is encountered. The muscle is then sharply and bluntly dissected up over the iliac crest apophysis. The

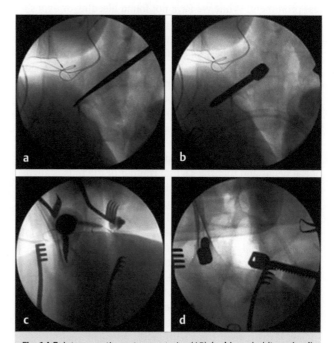

Fig. 14.5 Intraoperative anteroposterior (AP) (**a, b**), and oblique (**c, d**) views showing proper placement of pelvic screw. The AP view shows the trajectory of the pedicle probe from the posterior superior iliac spine (PSIS) to just superior and adjacent to the sciatic notch and the final screw position at least 1 cm lateral to the notch. The oblique view is taken parallel with the probe and shows the probe and the final screw position between the inner and outer cortex just superior to the sciatic notch, which appears as a "teardrop."

overlying fascia is then divided and the outer wing of the ilium is then subperiosteally exposed from the posterosuperior iliac spine (PSIS) forward along the posterior one-third of the pelvis and down to the sciatic notch. A guide which hooks into the sciatic notch is then utilized to aim a drill hole from the PSIS start point to just anterior and superior to the sciatic notch. If a guide is not available, the pedicle probe alone can be used and aimed just above the sciatic notch by direct palpation or by using intraoperative fluoroscopy (▶ Fig. 14.5a–d). This is the region where the pelvis is most dense for pelvic screw fixation.[26] Intra-operative anteroposterior and oblique fluoroscopic views are taken to confirm the placement of the drill or probe to make sure that there is no penetration through the inner or outer pelvic table, or into the sciatic notch. Pelvic screw fixation in the largest diameter possible (usually 7–10 mm) is placed in this trajectory and should be of sufficient length to pass the sciatic notch by at least 1 cm. The author prefers to use a closed poly-axial screw head to maximize the rigidity of the final rod–pelvic screw construct. Typically, pelvic screws alone are used; however, when additional fixation is needed to improve the rigidity of pelvic fixation, S1 screws can be added to the construct. I prefer this over sacral screw fixation alone, because pelvic screw fixation provides a better lever arm to correct both pelvic obliquity and sagittal plane pelvic deformity.

Alternatively, pelvic screws can be placed using the medial portal (S2-iliac approach) as described by Chang et al[27] and Sponseller et al.[28] Advocates for this method state that there is less exposure time and less bleeding and that the screw head is less prominent. While we have not found bleeding or exposure time to be less in our hands, the screw is less prominent using this approach and lines up more directly with the rods, obviating the need for lateral rod connectors. If the PSIS start point is used, notching the ilium at the entrance point with a rongeur and countersinking the screw prevents screw head prominence. A fixed lateral rodded connector (usually 10 or 20 mm) is used to connect each pelvic screw to a precontoured rod. Critical to the correction is to attach and secure each of the precontoured rods to the iliac screws with the fixed lateral connectors so that each of the rods is perfectly perpendicular to the horizontal axis of the pelvis and that the sagittal contour of the rods is aligned with the sacrum (▶ Fig. 14.6a, b). The sagittal bend should be identical on each rod and should also be aligned so that the contour matches from proximal to distal. If these steps are not meticulously adhered to, the pelvic obliquity will not be optimally corrected with the cantilever maneuver. Once this is done, the set screws on both the pelvic screws are tightened and torqued down onto the rod. A proximal connector is added at the top of the construct, which strengthens the proximal construct. A drop entry cross-connector can be added in the lumbar spine to augment the stability of the construct.

Only if the patient has a level pelvis, adequate sagittal pelvic position, and adequate balance should the surgeon consider ending fixation more proximal (e.g., at the L4 or L5 vertebral levels). If fixation to the pelvis is not done, pedicle screw fixation in the lumbar spine at a minimum of four levels is recommended. Cantilever correction and fixation to the remainder of the spine using pedicle screws or sublaminar wires can then be utilized.

14.8 Kyphosis

14.8.1 Lumbar/Thoracolumbar Kyphosis

Cantilever correction is very effective in correcting neuro-muscular kyphosis. Lumbar and thoracolumbar kyphosis is effectively corrected utilizing a distal-to-proximal cantilever correction beginning with fixation to the pelvis.[6] Once pelvic screws are placed, precontoured rods are anchored to the pelvic screws and then cantilever correction can begin (▶ Fig. 14.7). It is important to progressively push the rod down to each vertebra and then secure each rod at each vertebral level using sublaminar wires or screws and not to use the fixation to pull the rod to the spine, which may cause loss of fixation (either wires cutting through the laminae or pedicle screw pullout). This process of securing the rod to the fixation at each level begins at the L5 vertebral level and progresses gradually up to the T2 or T1 vertebral level. The pelvis, which is typically posteriorly tilted, is also corrected during cantilever correction.

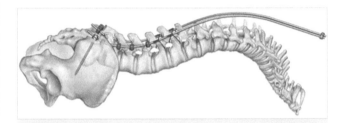

Fig. 14.7 In lumbar and thoracolumbar kyphosis, a distal to proximal cantilever correction is performed, first fixing the rod to distal vertebrae and then pushing down (anterior) on the rod after the rod is anchored to the apical vertebrae. The sagittal placement of the rod should initially parallel the precorrected sagittal alignment of the sacrum, which is tilted posterior along with the pelvis in kyphosis. As the rod is moved to the spine using cantilever correction, the sagittal alignment of the pelvis and spine will correct to the sagittal contour of the rod.

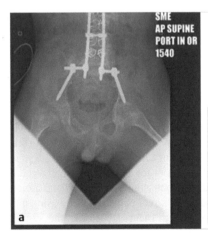
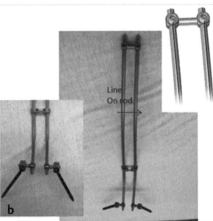

Fig. 14.6 Pelvic fixation is performed first with any distal-to-proximal cantilever correction. (a) The pelvic screws are placed as shown in this anteroposterior radiograph. (b) The construct is then assembled from distal to proximal, securing the rods to the pelvic screws using the rodded connectors shown if using a traditional PSIS entrance into the pelvis. A proximal closed connector and cross-link at the thoracolumbar junction connect the two precontoured rods, which should parallel one another.

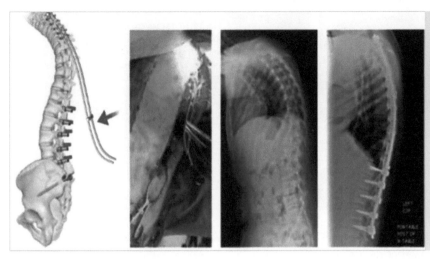

Fig. 14.8 It is difficult to cantilever thoracic kyphosis using the unit rod due to insufficient lever arm. This diagram shows a proximal-to-distal cantilever technique that can be used for thoracic kyphosis. The rod is preassembled and secured proximally and then delivered into lumbar pedicle screws if there is no pelvic sagittal malalignment. Preoperative and postoperative radiographs are shown.

14.8.2 Thoracic Kyphosis

Kyphosis in the thoracic region is more difficult to correct with distal-to-proximal cantilever correction. In such cases, starting distally at the pelvis or in the lumbar spine leaves a short lever arm above the apex at the proximal end of the rod by the time one reaches fixation in the thoracic spine. This makes it very difficult to adequately correct a more proximal kyphosis. Accordingly, this type of curvature is very difficult to correct with the traditional unit rod since the unit rod requires distal fixation into the pelvis first. With this type of curvature, a reverse cantilever (proximal to distal) can be performed using the more modular system (▶ Fig. 14.8). After exposing the spine and pelvis, pelvic screws and sublaminar wires are placed as previously described. The precontoured rods are connected using the proximal closed rod connector at the top and placing a cross-connector in the lumbar region. The rods should be parallel from proximal to distal with respect to their contour. Next, the top of the rod construct is secured using sublaminar wires from T1 down to the apex of the curvature. After the apical vertebrae is secured to the rod, cantilever correction can be performed by gradually pushing the rod down to the next more distal vertebrae, tightening the sublaminar wire or securing to the pedicle screw, performing the same maneuver progressively down the spine until the pelvic screws are reached. The fixed, rodded lateral connectors are then utilized to connect the rod to the pelvic screws in patients who are nonambulators. In some ambulatory patients without pelvic deformity, the instrumentation and fusion can be stopped short of the pelvis and secured to pedicle screws, usually at the L4 or L5 vertebra (▶ Fig. 14.8). Using this "proximal-to-distal" cantilever correction allows for a better lever arm to correct thoracic kyphosis. In thoracic kyphosis, it is critical that fixation be completed up to at least the T1 vertebral level and occasionally the C7 level to prevent "drop-off" at the cervicothoracic junction. Firm fixation at the proximal-most end with two wires, hooks, or screws is recommended.

14.8.3 Hyperlordosis

Neuromuscular lumbar hyperlordosis does occur in isolation but is more frequently seen in combination with scoliosis or

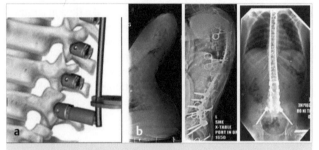

Fig. 14.9 (a) Correction of hyperlordosis can be achieved using pedicle screws with reduction posts in the hyperlordotic region of the deformity after pelvic fixation of the rod is done. **(b)** Preoperative and postoperative photographs are shown.

thoracic kyphosis. Pedicle screws with reduction posts are placed in the region of the hyperlordosis (usually the lumbar spine) (▶ Fig. 14.9a, b).[6] After securing the precontoured rods to the pelvis with pelvic screws as described, the rods are pushed down into the reduction posts and secured with the set screw. Reduction of the hyperlordosis is achieved by gradually screwing down the set screws (▶ Fig. 14.9a, b). Great care is taken to notice any evidence of posterior plowing of the screws. Maximizing the diameter of the screws may help with improved pedicle fixation. In addition, the supplementation of sublaminar wires can be placed at the same level for additional fixation to reduce the risk of screw pullout. Once the hyperlordosis is reduced, the remainder of the spinal instrumentation is completed more proximally.

14.8.4 Rigid Hyperkyphotic and Hyperlordotic Deformity

Rigid thoracic and thoracolumbar kyphosis, like other rigid spinal deformities, are difficult to correct using posterior spinal fusion with instrumentation alone. Multiple level posterior-only (Ponte, vertebral, or Smith-Petersen) osteotomies with posterior instrumentation with or without anterior diskectomies as a first stage in the area of maximum deformity decrease excessive forces to correct the deformity and allow for

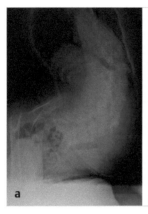
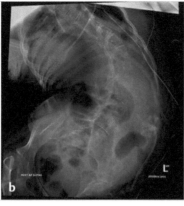
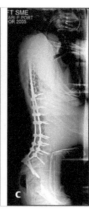

Fig. 14.10 **(a)** Severe lordoscoliosis (with primary lordosis) which underwent **(b)** a staged anterior vertebrectomy, followed by **(c)** posterior completion to a total vertebrectomy with posterior instrumentation and fusion.

shortening of the vertebral column.[7,29,30,31] Halo-femoral traction has also been recommended instead of anterior release in rigid spinal deformities, specifically scoliosis.[32] Little is written about halo-femoral traction and its use in sagittal plane deformity. However, it should be noted that if a flexion contracture of the hip exists, traction on the lower extremities may accentuate the lumbar lordosis. Rigid hyperlordotic deformity may require staged anterior release (multiple anterior diskectomies) around the rigid apex of the deformity followed by posterior spinal fusion with instrumentation.[1,6] In severely rigid hyperlordotic and hyperkyphotic deformity, vertebral column resection can produce excellent curve correction and restoration of sitting balance[33,34] (▶ Fig. 14.10a–c).

14.9 Evidence-Based Outcomes

Lipton et al[1] described 24 patients with cerebral palsy who had isolated sagittal plane spinal deformity (8 with hyperlordotic deformity, 14 with kyphotic deformity, and 2 with both) and underwent posterior spinal fusion and cantilever correction with unit rod instrumentation. Indications for surgery included seating problems despite wheelchair modifications, severe back pain, and superior mesenteric artery syndrome refractory to conservative treatment (in two patients with hyperlordosis). The mean preoperative hyperkyphosis of 93.8 degrees was corrected to a mean postoperative kyphosis of 35.8 degrees in children with kyphosis, while the mean preoperative hyperlordosis of 91.8 degrees was corrected to a mean postoperative lordosis of 43.6 degrees in children with hyperlordosis. Caregivers reported improvements in physical appearance, sitting balance, head control, and pain relief. All seating problems and back pain improved or resolved postoperatively. Both cases of superior mesenteric artery syndrome resolved postoperatively.

Karampalis and Tsirikos[2] described 13 patients with lumbar hyperlordosis and lordoscoliosis who underwent posterior spinal fusion with instrumentation. The mean lumbar lordosis was corrected from 108 to 62 degrees postoperatively. Sacral slope (horizontal sacral inclination) improved from 79 to 50 degrees. Sagittal imbalance was improved from a mean of ▯8 to ▯1.8 cm. Preoperative lumbar lordosis and sacral slope were associated with increased perioperative morbidity. Reduced lumbar lordosis and increased thoracic kyphosis were each associated with improved sagittal balance at follow-up. Postoperative questionnaires at final follow-up indicated improvements in physical appearance, function, and relief of severe preoperative back

pain. There were also improvements in head control, breathing, and hand use.

Sink et al[14] looked at a retrospective case series of 41 patients with spinal deformity, of whom 24 patients had preoperative hyperkyphosis, focusing on who maintained sagittal plane spinal correction. Preoperative thoracic, thoracolumbar, and lumbar hyperkyphosis were risk factors for loss of proximal and distal sagittal correction. As these authors state, increased forces at the proximal- and distal-most ends of the instrumentation during kyphosis correction result in the greatest potential for failure. Reinforcing these ends with stronger fixation is recommended. Distal loss of correction included loss of the pelvic portion of Galveston fixation. We prefer to use the largest diameter pelvic screw fixation, which, in our experience, is less likely to pull out compared to the unit rod or Galveston fixation. Proximal loss of correction occurred in 11 patients who developed a junctional kyphosis. As mentioned earlier, securing fixation proximally with two wires, screws, or hooks may provide more secure proximal fixation.

References

[1] Lipton GE, Letonoff EJ, Dabney KW, Miller F, McCarthy HC. Correction of sagittal plane spinal deformities with unit rod instrumentation in children with cerebral palsy. J Bone Joint Surg Am. 2003; 85-A(12):2349–2357

[2] Karampalis C, Tsirikos AI. The surgical treatment of lordoscoliosis and hyperlordosis in patients with quadriplegic cerebral palsy. Bone Joint J. 2014; 96-B (6):800–806

[3] McCarthy JJ, Betz RR. The relationship between tight hamstrings and lumbar hypolordosis in children with cerebral palsy. Spine. 2000; 25(2):211–213

[4] Shapiro F, Zurakowski D, Bui T, Darras BT. Progression of spinal deformity in wheelchair-dependent patients with Duchenne muscular dystrophy who are not treated with steroids: coronal plane (scoliosis) and sagittal plane (kyphosis, lordosis) deformity. Bone Joint J. 2014; 96-B(1):100–105

[5] Lipton GE, Miller F, Dabney KW, Altiok H, Bachrach SJ. Factors predicting postoperative complications following spinal fusions in children with cerebral palsy. J Spinal Disord. 1999; 12(3):197–205

[6] Dabney KW, Miller F, Lipton GE, Letonoff EJ, McCarthy HC. Correction of sagittal plane spinal deformities with unit rod instrumentation in children with cerebral palsy. J Bone Joint Surg Am. 2004; 86-A(Pt 2) Suppl 1:156–168

[7] Diab MG, Franzone JM, Vitale MG. The role of posterior spinal osteotomies in pediatric spinal deformity surgery: indications and operative technique. J Pediatr Orthop. 2011; 31(1) Suppl:S88–S98

[8] Takeshita K, Lenke LG, Bridwell KH, Kim YJ, Sides B, Hensley M. Analysis of patients with nonambulatory neuromuscular scoliosis surgically treated to the pelvis with intraoperative halo-femoral traction. Spine. 2006; 31 (20):2381–2385

[9] Jain A, Njoku DB, Sponseller PD. Does patient diagnosis predict blood loss during posterior spinal fusion in children? Spine. 2012; 37(19):1683–1687

[10] Sponseller PD, LaPorte DM, Hungerford MW, Eck K, Bridwell KH, Lenke LG. Deep wound infections after neuromuscular scoliosis surgery: a multicenter study of risk factors and treatment outcomes. Spine. 2000; 25(19):2461–2466

[11] Bell DF, Moseley CF, Koreska J. Unit rod segmental spinal instrumentation in the management of patients with progressive neuromuscular spinal deformity. Spine. 1989; 14(12):1301–1307

[12] Dias RC, Miller F, Dabney K, Lipton G, Temple T. Surgical correction of spinal deformity using a unit rod in children with cerebral palsy. J Pediatr Orthop. 1996; 16(6):734–740

[13] Rinsky LA. Surgery of spinal deformity in cerebral palsy. Twelve years in the evolution of scoliosis management. Clin Orthop Relat Res. 1990(253):100–109

[14] Sink EL, Newton PO, Mubarak SJ, Wenger DR. Maintenance of sagittal plane alignment after surgical correction of spinal deformity in patients with cerebral palsy. Spine. 2003; 28(13):1396–1403

[15] Dearolf WW, III, Betz RR, Vogel LC, Levin J, Clancy M, Steel HH. Scoliosis in pediatric spinal cord-injured patients. J Pediatr Orthop. 1990; 10(2):214–218

[16] Samdani AF, Belin EJ, Bennett JT, et al. Major perioperative complications after spine surgery in patients with cerebral palsy: assessment of risk factors. Eur Spine J. 2016; 25(3):795–800

[17] Brenn BR, Theroux MC, Dabney KW, Miller F. Clotting parameters and thromboelastography in children with neuromuscular and idiopathic scoliosis undergoing posterior spinal fusion. Spine. 2004; 29(15):E310–E314

[18] Dhawale AA, Shah SA, Sponseller PD, et al. Are antifibrinolytics helpful in decreasing blood loss and transfusions during spinal fusion surgery in children with cerebral palsy scoliosis? Spine. 2012; 37(9):E549–E555

[19] DiCindio S, Theroux M, Shah S, et al. Multimodality monitoring of transcranial electric motor and somatosensory-evoked potentials during surgical correction of spinal deformity in patients with cerebral palsy and other neuromuscular disorders. Spine. 2003; 28(16):1851–1855

[20] Sees JP, Sitoula P, Dabney K, et al. Pamidronate treatment to prevent reoccurring fractures in children with cerebral palsy. J Pediatr Orthop. 2016; 36 (2):193–197

[21] Mohamed Ali MH, Koutharawu DN, Miller F, et al. Operative and clinical markers of deep wound infection after spine fusion in children with cerebral palsy. J Pediatr Orthop. 2010; 30(8):851–857

[22] Sponseller PD, Shah SA, Abel MF, Newton PO, Letko L, Marks M. Infection rate after spine surgery in cerebral palsy is high and impairs results: multicenter analysis of risk factors and treatment. Clin Orthop Relat Res. 2010; 468 (3):711–716

[23] Sponseller PD, Jain A, Shah SA, et al. Deep wound infections after spinal fusion in children with cerebral palsy: a prospective cohort study. Spine. 2013; 38(23):2023–2027

[24] Borkhuu B, Borowski A, Shah SA, Littleton AG, Dabney KW, Miller F. Antibiotic-loaded allograft decreases the rate of acute deep wound infection after spinal fusion in cerebral palsy. Spine. 2008; 33(21):2300–2304

[25] Vitale MG, Riedel MD, Glotzbecker MP, et al. Building consensus: development of a Best Practice Guideline (BPG) for surgical site infection (SSI) prevention in high-risk pediatric spine surgery. J Pediatr Orthop. 2013; 33 (5):471–478

[26] Miller F, Moseley C, Koreska J. Pelvic anatomy relative to lumbosacral instrumentation. J Spinal Disord. 1990; 3(2):169–173

[27] Chang TL, Sponseller PD, Kebaish KM, Fishman EK. Low profile pelvic fixation: anatomic parameters for sacral alar-iliac fixation versus traditional iliac fixation. Spine. 2009; 34(5):436–440

[28] Sponseller PD, Zimmerman RM, Ko PS, et al. Low profile pelvic fixation with the sacral alar iliac technique in the pediatric population improves results at two-year minimum follow-up. Spine. 2010; 35(20):1887–1892

[29] Dorward IG, Lenke LG. Osteotomies in the posterior-only treatment of complex adult spinal deformity: a comparative review. Neurosurg Focus. 2010; 28(3):E4

[30] Geck MJ, Macagno A, Ponte A, Shufflebarger HL. The Ponte procedure: posterior only treatment of Scheuermann's kyphosis using segmental posterior shortening and pedicle screw instrumentation. J Spinal Disord Tech. 2007; 20 (8):586–593

[31] Modi HN, Suh SW, Hong JY, Yang JH. Posterior multilevel vertebral osteotomy for severe and rigid idiopathic and nonidiopathic kyphoscoliosis: a further experience with minimum two-year follow-up. Spine. 2011; 36(14):1146–1153

[32] Keeler KA, Lenke LG, Good CR, Bridwell KH, Sides B, Luhmann SJ. Spinal fusion for spastic neuromuscular scoliosis: is anterior releasing necessary when intraoperative halo-femoral traction is used? Spine. 2010; 35(10):E427–E433

[33] Helenius I, Serlo J, Pajulo O. The incidence and outcomes of vertebral column resection in paediatric patients: a population-based, multicentre, follow-up study. J Bone Joint Surg Br. 2012; 94(7):950–955

[34] Sponseller PD, Jain A, Lenke LG, et al. Vertebral column resection in children with neuromuscular spine deformity. Spine. 2012; 37(11):E655–E661

15 Spinal Deformity Associated with Neurodegenerative Disease in Adults

Dana L. Cruz, Shaleen Vira, Virginie Lafage, Themistocles Protopsaltis, and Thomas J. Errico

Abstract

Neurodegenerative disease is an important, though often overlooked, etiology of spinal deformity in adults. Due to the complex etiology of their deformity and presence of comorbidities, these patients often have high complication and failure rates when surgical intervention is pursued. This chapter provides an overview of the clinical features and management strategies used to treat spinal deformity in patients with neurodegenerative conditions such as Parkinson's and Alzheimer's diseases.

Keywords: adult spinal deformity, Alzheimer's disease, antecollis, camptocormia, Parkinson's disease, Pisa syndrome

15.1 Introduction

Neurodegenerative diseases represent a small but important portion of patients undergoing spinal deformity surgery. From 2001 to 2010, there were 1,347,359 patients who underwent thoracolumbar spinal fusion surgery (ICD9 8104–8108, 8134–8138) in the U.S. National Inpatient Sample (NIS) database, representing 20% of weighted U.S. hospitalizations. Of these patients, 146,268 (10.9%) were diagnosed with Parkinson's disease, just one of the myriad of neurodegenerative disorders. Degenerative diseases of the central nervous system are characterized by a progressive loss of neurons with associated secondary changes in white matter tracts. The pattern of neuronal loss is selective, and symptoms can arise in patients with no history of neurologic deficits and without any clear inciting event.[1] Neurodegenerative diseases encompass a wide range of pathologies and thus are often grouped by affected anatomic regions of the central nervous system.

Degenerative diseases affecting the cerebral cortex manifest with dementia, a loss of cognitive function independent of the state of attention. These include Alzheimer's disease (the most common neurodegenerative disease in adults), frontotemporal dementias including Pick's disease, progressive supranuclear palsy, corticobasal degeneration, frontotemporal dementias without tau pathology, multi-infarct dementia, Creutzfeldt–Jakob disease, and neurosyphilis. Degenerative diseases of the basal ganglia and brainstem are characterized by pathological movements including rigidity, abnormal posturing, and chorea. These include Parkinson's disease, multiple system atrophy, and Huntington's disease. Spinocerebellar degenerative diseases are characterized by motor and sensory ataxia, spasticity, and sensorimotor peripheral neuropathy. This heterogeneous group of diseases includes spinocerebellar ataxias. Finally, degenerative diseases affecting motor neurons result in muscle denervation from loss of lower motor neuron input, including amyotrophic lateral sclerosis (ALS), bulbospinal atrophy (Kennedy's syndrome), and spinal muscular atrophy.

Management of spinal deformity in patients with neurodegenerative disease, be it medical or operative, differs significantly from that of a patient with chronic degenerative disease. Patients with neurodegenerative disorders such as Parkinson's and Alzheimer's diseases present unique challenges and considerations to all aspects of care, including medical optimization, operative intervention, and rehabilitation. Given the complexity and importance of tailoring treatment to each patient, the goal of this chapter is to highlight the overarching principles and considerations when approaching spinal deformity in patients with neurodegenerative disease.

15.2 Etiology and Pathogenesis

A common deficiency among patients with neurodegenerative disease is a loss of the normal cellular mechanisms of degradation,[1] resulting in the development of cytotoxic protein aggregates characteristically recognized as inclusion bodies. In Huntington's disease, an expanded polyglutamine repeat results in an aberrant form of the huntingtin protein. In Alzheimer's disease, abnormal aggregates of the transmembrane protein Aβ elicit neurotoxic responses from astrocytes and microglia. Parkinson's disease is characterized by an unexplained alteration of a normal cellular protein (α-synuclein) forming the hallmark protein aggregates known as Lewy's bodies. In ALS, dysfunction of copper–zinc superoxide dismutase gene results in periodic acid–Schiff (PAS)-positive cytoplasmic inclusions of autophagic vacuoles. Each of these disease processes ultimately results in the loss of neuronal transmission, causing muscular spasticity or atrophy. The subsequent loss of muscular balance caused by these disorders finally culminates in those axial skeletal changes diagnosed as coronal and sagittal deformity.

15.3 Disease-Specific Deformity Characteristics and Comorbidities

A wide range of spinal deformities are seen in neurodegenerative conditions, including antecollis, lateral axial dystonia (LAD), camptocormia, and scoliosis.

15.3.1 Antecollis

In 1817, James Parkinson first described the disease that bears his name as "a propensity to bend the trunk forward" along with the following physical exam finding: "the chin is now almost immovably bent down upon the sternum."[2,3,4] Later in 1886, Gerlier used the term "vertigeparalysant" to refer to the phenomenon of a dropped head associated with torticollis and pain of the occipital muscles that spread to the shoulders.[5] Meanwhile, in Japan, Miura in 1897 described "kubisagari," or attacks of dropped head with weakness of the upper and lower extremities.[4] These represent the earliest descriptions of antecollis.

Antecollis is defined as significant (minimum of 45 degrees) neck flexion which may be partially overcome by voluntary or passive movement. Severity is variable, with some patients presenting with an inability to fully extend the neck against gravity but able to exert force against the resistance of the examiner's hand.[6,7] Antecollis occurs in Parkinson's disease resulting from dystonia of flexor neck muscles or weakness of extensor neck muscles.[4] Antecollis develops in 5 to 6% of patients with Parkinson's disease,[3,4,8] yet it is also occasionally a component of multiple system atrophy, with shorter intervals between the onset of motor symptoms and antecollis.[7]

15.3.2 Lateral Axial Dystonia

LAD is a general term used to describe the laterally flexed posture caused by extensor truncal dystonia, also known as pleurothotonus and Pisa syndrome.[9,10] First described by Ekbom et al in 1972 as a constellation of physical exam findings associated with neuroleptic therapy,[11] Pisa syndrome, reminiscent of the well-known Italian structure, is defined by significant (minimum of 10 degrees) lateral flexion, often with a component of backward axial rotation, that can be alleviated by passive mobilization or supine positioning.[12] LAD is characterized by continuous electromyography (EMG) activity of ipsilateral paraspinal muscles while standing or seated, though EMG activity is absent while recumbent.[9] Despite the often interchanging use of these terms, there is some controversy among authors regarding the etiology of these conditions (i.e., tardive neuroleptic syndromes vs. idiopathic primary dystonia) and possibility that they represent more than one clinical entity.

Pisa syndrome has been described among patients with Alzheimer's disease,[13,14] multiple system atrophy,[15] Parkinson's disease,[6,16] and ALS,[17] as well as in patients with dementia treated with cholinesterase inhibitors.[9,18] One series of 1,400 patients with Parkinson's disease demonstrated 1.9% with classic features of Pisa syndrome,[9] which may be a precursor to the development of scoliosis in these patients.[6,9] Though there are documented cases of idiopathic Pisa syndrome, most cases are associated with the use of neuroleptic medications and respond well to adjustments or withdrawal of offending agents.[19,20]

15.3.3 Camptocormia

In 1818, Sir Benjamin Collins Brodie described a "functionally bent back," referring to what would later be called bent spine syndrome.[21,22,23] Camptocormia, derived from the Greek words "camptos" (bent) and "kormos" (trunk), is also known as the bent spine syndrome.[21,24,25] Camptocormia is defined as significant (minimum of 45 degrees) thoracolumbar flexion in the sagittal plane, with almost complete resolution in the supine position.[26,27] These patients frequently report a gradual, though occasionally subacute, sensation of being "pulled forward" with worsening of posture and pain after prolonged activity. Originally thought to be a psychogenic disorder, camptocormia is now considered to be of idiopathic origin or secondary to neuromuscular disease, including Parkinson's disease, ALS, polymyositis, inclusion body myositis, muscular dystrophies, myasthenia gravis, and cervical dystonia. An associated condition is proximal myotonic myopathy characterized by progressive painful paraspinal muscle weakness exaggerated by

exercise.[28] Other unusual cases of camptocormia have been reported in the literature and observed by these clinicians as well (► Fig. 15.1a, b). In a 2010 Japanese case report, for example, a patient is illustrated with postherpetic abdominal wall paresis resulting in pseudohernia and 40-degree right convex deformity from T12 to L4.[29]

Camptocormia in Parkinson's disease is caused by myopathy resulting in axial dystonia,[30] resulting in an imbalance of spinal flexion and extension. Camptocormia secondary to neurodegenerative or neuromuscular disorder can be diagnosed by EMG, which reveals weakness of the paravertebral muscles and elevated creatinine kinase levels. Muscle biopsy in patients with Parkinson's disease reveals disorganized myofibrils with intrafascicular fibrosis and fatty degeneration.[31] Magnetic resonance imaging (MRI) findings include early edema and swelling followed by fatty infiltration of paravertebral muscles.[32,33] Camptocormia occurs in 3 to 17.6% of patients with Parkinson's disease.[24,25,34,35]

15.3.4 Scoliosis

The earliest identification of spinal deformities including scoliosis dates back to Hippocrates, who described spinal curves in

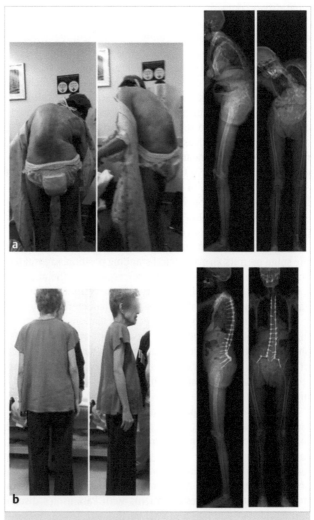

Fig. 15.1 (a) Postherpetic scoliosis (preoperative). (b) Postherpetic scoliosis (postoperative).

his book *On Bones and Joints*.[36,37] Traditional definitions of scoliosis summarize the vastly encompassing term as "lateral flexion not relieved by voluntary or passive movement, and lateral curvature of the spine of at least 10° as measured by the Cobb method with evidence of axial vertebral rotation on radiograph."[38] Scoliosis should be differentiated from the previously described postural deformities including camptocormia, antecollis, and Pisa syndrome as a rigid deformity.

The vertebral column serves to provide support and balance to the human body. Specifically, the spine is the primary means by which the body maintains an upright posture and a horizontal gaze. Dubousset described a theoretical conus within which the whole body maintains an upright posture. His conus ranges from the narrower "cone of economy," representing minimal exertion, to the "cone of maximum work," which is the upper limit of energy expenditure.[39,40] Dubousset visualized a conus of balance for the standing position, in which the feet are located within a zone referred to as the "polygon of sustentation," and the body, under the influence of muscle function and ligamentous support, can move in a conical fashion without moving the feet. The body adapts to changes in balance in order to regulate the center of gravity over the smallest perimeter possible.[41] This fundamental tendency toward equilibrium is what drives compensatory changes in the spine as it attempts to adapt to pathological processes either inherent to the spine or external to the spinal column such as neurodegenerative diseases.

Antecollis, camptocormia, and lateral truncal dystonia are postural deformities that can lead to rigid deformities including scoliosis. Specifically, the use of the term scoliosis pertaining to adult patients with neuromuscular diseases such as Parkinson's disease is restricted to those spinal deformities not related to medical treatment such as L-dopa and not related to any clinical manifestations of the neuromuscular or neurodegenerative disease. Additionally, the direction of the convexity must not be related to the laterality of initial parkinsonian symptoms.[42] Scoliosis is more common in patients with Parkinson's disease (ranging from 43 to 90%[42,43,44]) compared to an age-matched population (ranging from 6 to 30%[45,46]).

While sagittal alignment reflects how the anatomic shape of the spine permits an economical standing position, sagittal balance is a dynamic parameter and corresponds to the ability of the subject to maintain stability of the standing position. Patients with Parkinson's disease have characteristically poor stability, often presenting with greater oscillations in the standing position and a significantly greater risk of fall.[47] In 2005, Sinaki et al demonstrated that patients with hyperkyphosis also present with significant loss of spinal erector muscles (erector spinae) and a compromised gait, leading to trunk shift and a higher risk of falling.[48]

With regard to spinopelvic malalignment, patients with Parkinson's disease present with a pattern of flexion of the spine, hips, and knees. Abnormal neuromuscular activation patterns can result in a greater tendency to forward bend, which can lead to global sagittal malalignment, a powerful driver of pain and disability.[49] Oh et al evaluated the incidence of sagittal malalignment in a series of patients with Parkinson's disease and found that 42% had a sagittal vertical axis (SVA) measurement of greater than 50 mm. Furthermore, 51% of patients had spinopelvic mismatch (pelvic incidence minus lumbar lordosis

[PI-LL]) greater than 10 degrees, suggesting that the severity of the Parkinson symptoms affects the ability to compensate with pelvic retroversion.[50,51] Lastly, it is important to note that some patients with Parkinson's disease may present with de novo or progression of idiopathic scoliosis independent of their neurodegenerative pathology.

An emerging concept with respect to the etiology of spinal pathologies is that there are subclinical changes in the neuromuscular quality of the soft tissues that cause progressive deformity through a mechanism that has not yet been elucidated.

It is not known whether muscle degeneration leads to sagittal imbalance, or whether sagittal malalignment is the premise for muscle degeneration that then drives pain and disability. Further study of the role of "soft tissues" would improve our understanding of compensatory mechanisms (knee flexion, pelvic retroversion, hip hyperextension) that are used to maintain posture in adults with spinal deformity. Future aims to surgically address deformity must take into account this complex pathophysiology in addition to each of these compensatory mechanisms. In summary, understanding the nonbony factors that drive adult neurodegenerative disease will deepen our understanding of adult spinal conditions and optimize treatment strategies.

15.4 Disorder-Specific Techniques

15.4.1 Nonoperative Treatment

An appropriate history, physical exam, and imaging workup must be obtained for any patient with a neurodegenerative disorder prior to treatment of a spinal deformity. Caution must be taken to rule out other disorders, such as inflammatory myopathies, that are capable of resembling neurodegenerative disorders such as Parkinson's disease. Moreover, these conditions can similarly be related to the development of spinal deformity, though their responses to treatment differ enormously. This possibility demands the accurate diagnosis prior to intervention. Accordingly, consultation with a neurologist is reasonable to ensure the diagnosis whenever in question and to optimize medical treatment.

Conservative treatment begins with treatment of the primary neurodegenerative condition. While there are no curative treatments for neurodegenerative diseases, various medications have been developed to temporize symptoms and maximize function in these patients.[1] As consultant physicians, spine specialists must appreciate the risks and benefits of proposed medications with respect to spinal pathologies. For example, L-dopa is effective for the treatment of Parkinson symptoms such as rigidity and akinesia but may exacerbate camptocormia.[25,26] With respect to treating spinal pathology, nonoperative treatments may include bracing, physical therapy, and injections, with possible adjunctive use of more recently developed technologies such as deep brain stimulation (DBS).

15.4.2 Operative Treatment

Traditionally, the goals of surgical correction of scoliosis involve restoration of coronal and sagittal alignment.[52] Specific correction of sagittal malalignment can offer major improvements in quality and functionality in adult spinal deformity patients[53,54,55]; however, there are many considerations when contemplating surgical treatment in these patients. Moreover, the management of deformity in adult patients with neuromuscular diseases such as cerebral palsy remains challenging with little empiric evidence to support guidelines for operative treatment.[56] Despite the absence of studies suggesting optimal spinopelvic parameters in patients with neurodegenerative disease, experience of these clinicians suggests goals similar to those of degenerative scoliosis as follows: pelvic tilt (PT) < 25 deegrees,[57] C7–S1 SVA < 50 mm,[49,58] PI-LL < 10 degrees,[54,57,59] and T1 pelvic angle < 20 degrees.[60]

Technical Considerations

Patients with neurodegenerative disease often have major deformities localized to the thoracolumbar region. These deformities make alignment goals more difficult to define in the setting of limited reserve, combined with both coronal and sagittal malalignment. These patients have a limited ability to compensate through pelvic retroversion or thoracic hypokyphosis,[61] thereby highlighting the importance of obtaining optimal SVA, PT, and PI-LL with correction. On the other hand, long fusions of the spine may create an unfavorable biomechanical state with the introduction of a long lever arm that may compromise the compensatory mechanisms used to recover the center of mass above the feet. This can reduce the width of the cone of stability of these patients and contribute to fall risk. A long fusion in patients with an intrinsic loss of stability, such as in cases of neurodegenerative disease, can result in correct alignment but poor balance and gross instability, ultimately leading to repeated falls. This sacrifice of stability should be taken into account when treating neurodegenerative patients with sagittal malalignment.[51]

Perioperative and Postoperative Considerations

Surgeons must carefully consider the risks involved in pursuing operative intervention in patients with neurodegenerative scoliosis. These medically fragile patients are susceptible to the most common risks of surgery, in addition to higher rates of medical complications such as postoperative delirium, epidural hematomas, pulmonary emboli, cardiac events, and transfusion-related events as well as surgical complications such as instrumentation failure, proximal junction kyphosis (PJK), and adjacent segment disease. Because of the numerous risks and potential complications associated with operative treatment in the setting of neurodegenerative disorder, indications for surgery are generally limited to highly motivated patients who are capable of participating in rehabilitation. In some instances, patients with progressive myelopathy or severe radiculopathy failing nonoperative interventions are indicated for surgery. Nonetheless, the decision to proceed with operative intervention is one that must carefully balance the patient's medical status and response to pharmacologic therapy as well as potential for disease progression. Risk of perioperative and postoperative complications, for example, increases with deformity severity, further complicating the decision making regarding timing of intervention. The surgical indication then often defaults to

progression of curvature and pain, often in tandem. Lastly, the decision to perform short versus long fusions with or without decompression must consider comorbid conditions and other patient factors that will undoubtedly impact efficacy and risk.

Due to inherent fragility of these patients, it is important to define perioperative monitoring guidelines to optimize outcomes. For example, Bourghli et al recommend the use of transcranial motor evoked potentials, somatosensory evoked potentials, free running EMG of the lower extremities, and evoked EMGs with pedicle screw stimulation.[62]

In addition, patients with Parkinson's disease are more susceptible to immobility, postoperative dysphagia, respiratory dysfunction, and urinary retention.[63] These issues lead to higher rates of pneumonia, urinary tract infections, deconditioning, and falls compared to patients without Parkinson's disease, as well as prolonged hospital stays and a greater need for posthospitalization rehabilitation. With these rates in mind, Katus and Shtilbans recommend limiting nil per os (NPO) status duration, alternative routes of drugs administration during NPO, careful avoidance of drug interactions and medications that can worsen Parkinson's disease, assessing swallowing ability frequently, encouraging incentive spirometry, performing frequent bladder scans, avoiding indwelling catheters, and providing aggressive physical therapy.[64] In a similar effort, Bourghli et al recommend close monitoring in the ICU for at least 48 hours to minimize the risk of postoperative pulmonary and cardiac complications.[62]

Furthermore, in light of the increased risk of postoperative complications, patients with Parkinson's disease who undergo spinal fusion surgery require long-term rehabilitation. These patients are well known to have an inherent festinating gait, making postoperative rehabilitation difficult. Patients and physicians report a lack of motivation to ambulate in this population.[62] Nevertheless, aggressive physical therapy and ambulation in the postoperative period is advisable to allow for acclimation to new spinal alignment and to maximize recovery. Exercise has the potential to benefit both motor (gait, balance, strength) and nonmotor (depression, apathy, fatigue, constipation) aspects of Parkinson's disease as well as secondary complications of immobility (cardiovascular, osteoporosis).[64] The increased prevalence of osteoporosis within this patient population,[45] however, must be considered before initiating aggressive rehabilitation. Bourghli et al, for example, recommend bracing with a thoracolumbosacral orthosis for 3 months to avoid screw pullout.[62]

Finally, exacerbation of primary neurodegenerative pathology can occur at any point during the postoperative course. Appropriate consultation with neurology and intensive care services is required not only to optimize these patients preoperatively but also to appropriately manage neurodegenerative exacerbations and comorbidities throughout the postoperative course.

Despite these risks, operative treatment can offer significant functional benefits. Operative treatment is generally divided into long versus short thoracic fusion. Long decompression and fusion may be indicated in patients with camptocormia with myelopathy or radiculopathy without motor fluctuations.[62] Longer constructs may also be necessary in older patients with osteoporosis as mentioned previously. Short decompression and fusion is recommended in select cases. Upadhyaya et al, for example, recommend short fusion for unmotivated patients with camptocormia without motor fluctuations.[65]

15.5 Evidence-Based Outcomes

15.5.1 Nonoperative Treatment

Despite the summaries of evidence-based outcomes that follow, these authors agree on the necessity to preface the findings with a note on their limitations. While most spine clinicians recognize the modest but important proportion of patients affected by neurodegenerative diseases, the diversity of disorders and complexity of their treatment is reflected in the scarcity of literature on the topic. The literature regarding postural deformity in patients with neurodegenerative disease is sparse with very few poorly powered studies, most of which are retrospective utilizing patients with Parkinson's disease. In the future, we hope for an increase in interinstitutional collaboration in order to produce more robust studies including larger sample sizes, more uniform methods of comparison, and patient populations that span the full spectrum of neurodegenerative disease.

Bracing

Bracing for neurodegenerative deformity has been attempted in an effort to emulate the success in idiopathic scoliosis but with moderate efficacy at best. In a recent Korean case report of a patient with camptocormia associated with Parkinson's disease, investigators report resolution of symptoms, improved ambulatory ability, and overall improved patient satisfaction in just 3 months with the use of a cruciform anterior spinal hyperextension (CASH) brace combined with exercise. According to this study, after 5 months of CASH bracing, the patient was able to maintain corrected posture even without the brace.[66] Similarly, in one prospective case series of 15 patients (6 of whom were diagnosed with Parkinson's disease) with camptocormia treated with a thoracopelvic anterior distraction orthosis, patients benefited from a decrease in mean SVA from 18.3 to 7 ($p < 0.01$), a reduced visual analog scale (VAS) of 70% ($p < 0.01$), and an increased VAS scale of 92% ($p < 0.01$) at 90 days.[67] Likewise, a French prospective study of 15 patients with camptocormia treated with orthosis and exercise found an average increase in lumbar lordosis of 10.1 and 12.5 degrees after 30 and 90 days, respectively ($p < 0.05$), a 7-degree increase in thoracic kyphosis after 90 days ($p < 0.05$), and an average of 70% reduction in pain after 90 days.[68] Despite reported benefits of bracing, patients often have difficulty with compliance.

Rehabilitation

Although the role of rehabilitation for the treatment of postural disorders is rarely investigated, a number of therapies such as physiotherapy, hydrotherapy, yoga, Pilates, and intensive exercise have been proposed as potential strategies.[6] In a 2014 study of patients with Parkinson's disease with postural abnormalities, patients were randomized to one of two treatment groups receiving a prescribed postural rehabilitation program with or without kinesio taping and a control group. At the conclusion of the study period, all patients treated with postural rehabilitation showed a significant improvement in global sagittal alignment with respect to baseline. Furthermore, treated patients demonstrated improved gait and balance, as illustrated by enhanced functional measures Timed Up and Go and Berg Balance Scale, supporting the role of the rehabilitation protocol in the treatment of neurodegenerative postural deformities.[69]

Botulin Toxin Injections

Early studies of patients with primary or tardive neuroleptic dystonia treated with botulinum toxin demonstrate substantial improvement in pain and range of motion with minimal adverse risk[70,71]; however, similar trials for camptocormia,[72] LAD,[9] and antecollis[73] show variable results. In a series observing 16 patients with Parkinson's disease and camptocormia, 4 of 9 patients who received botulinum toxin A into the rectus abdominis demonstrated notable improvement in camptocormia; however, a quantitative change in posture is not provided.[74] In a 2007 blinded crossover trial of nine patients with LAD related to Parkinson's disease, six (67%) patients treated with botulinum toxin A demonstrated improvement in function, pain, and grading of LAD, while no adverse outcomes were observed.[9] Finally, in another study evaluating efficacy of botulinum toxin injection for the treatment of antecollis, investigators report a subjective patient response of "excellent" in 13.3% of cases, "good" in 33.3%, "mild" in 26.7%, and no response in 26.7% of cases.[73]

Similar studies have attempted to deliver botulinum toxin more accurately using imaging modalities such as ultrasound and CT guidance. In a 2009 study by Fietzek et al, injection of iliopsoas or rectus abdominis muscles of patients with camptocormia associated with Parkinson's disease failed to reach any patient-identified therapeutic goals despite confirmation of muscular atrophy by ultrasound examination.[75] In a separate study evaluating the efficacy of ultrasound-guided botulinum toxin A injection of the iliopsoas, assessment of all patients failed to show improvement in posture and, in fact, resulted in complaints secondary to hip flexor weakness.[76] Given the conflicting response to treatment and few rigorous studies, the use of botulinum toxin in the management of camptocormia is designated a level "U" recommendation (Level U: inadequate or conflicting data; treatment is unproven).[77]

Lidocaine Injections

Previous attempts to reduce abnormal truncal flexion using lidocaine injection have shown modest success.[78,79] In the premier study of five patients with camptocormia treated with lidocaine injections, Furusawa et al demonstrated improved posture following injection of the external oblique muscles, but improved posture was not observed with injection to the rectus abdominis or internal obliques.[78] In their follow-up study, 12 patients with Parkinson's disease and camptocormia were treated with repeated lidocaine injections into the external oblique, beginning with a single injection, followed by repeated injections (once a day for 4–5 days). Despite subsidence of effect after several days, 8 of 12 patients demonstrated significant improvement (as exhibited by a decrease in mean flexion angle from 62.1 to 54 degrees, $p = 0.018$) in posture after a single injection. Meanwhile, 9 of 12 showed improvement (mean flexion angle decreased with repeated injections from 62.1 to 49 degrees, $p = 0.005$) over a 90-day observation period following repeated injections.[79]

Deep Brain Stimulation

Deep brain stimulation (DBS) is accomplished through the surgical implantation of electrodes that modulate specific targets in the brain for the treatment of various neurologic diseases. Successful use of DBS has been demonstrated for a number of movement disorders, most notably Parkinson's disease and dystonia, resulting in significant improvements in functional status.[80] Targets of DBS electrodes include the thalamus, subthalamic nucleus (STN), and the globus pallidus internus, depending on the disorder of interest.[81]

In one review of 67 patients with Parkinson's disease and camptocormia treated with DBS (from 13 studies), 61% of patients were observed to have an effective outcome.[30] Given the inconsistent results of DBS in this population, study authors Schulz-Schaeffer et al sought to identify prognostic factors for the effect of DBS on camptocormia. Multifactorial analysis of 25 patients who underwent bilateral neurostimulation of the STN revealed the duration of camptocormia prior to neurostimulation to be the relevant factor in predicting outcome. For example, of 13 patients who demonstrated an improvement of at least 50% of bending angle, all were determined to have camptocormia for less than 1.5 years. Concomitantly, patients who demonstrated symptoms between 1.5 and 3 years prior to neurostimulation showed mixed results, while no patients suffering from camptocormia for longer than 40 months showed improvement following DBS.[30] In light of these optimistic results and the comparatively low risks associated with DBS, several authors recommend that all patients meeting criteria for DBS be considered for neurostimulation prior to operative intervention for postural deformity.[65]

15.5.2 Operative Treatment

Mechanical Outcomes

Multiple challenges and outcomes have been addressed in the surgical treatment of patients with neurological disease and scoliosis, though additional technical challenges exist. Bone anchorage is often an issue due to a high rate of osteoporosis; one study found that 34% of patients with Parkinson's disease were osteoporotic.[45] Instrumentation failure may be due to any combination of the iatrogenic effect of the fusion, age-related osteoporosis, and disk degeneration, and/or the neuromuscular disease itself.[62] Studies show that 29 to 33.3%[62,82] of these patients may experience this complication. PJK may be due to any combination of elderly age, osteoporosis, and/or the neuromuscular disease itself. This complication may be experienced by 16.7 to 17.6% of patients with Parkinson's disease.[61,62] To reduce the risk of PJK, authors suggest particular care in preserving the supraspinous and interspinous ligaments between T1 and T2 to avoid destabilization of the cervicothoracic junction following long posterior fusion.[83]

When considering the surgical approach to postural deformity in a patient with neurodegenerative disease, one must consider that these patients can suffer from a range of postural or fixed deformities including scoliosis. Additionally, the estimated etiology of these deformities must be considered. For example, in a patient found to have camptocormia in the presence of truncal dystonia, the muscular pathology is more likely to place additional stress on instrumented levels and adjacent segments compared to a similar patient with extensor muscle weakness. Moreover, when considering alignment objectives as mentioned previously, postural goals may differ significantly between patients with varying degrees of deformity and severity of neurodegenerative disease.

Given these challenges, revisions may be performed for non-fusion, instrumentation failure or pullout, PJK, adjacent level instability, epidural hematomas, and infection. Based on these indications, 50 to 79% of these patients may require reoperations.[61,62,82] These issues are highlighted in a retrospective review by Babat et al of 14 patients with Parkinson's disease who underwent lumbar/lumbosacral (8), thoracolumbar (2), and cervical (4) spinal surgery. The authors reported a very high reoperation rate associated with technical complications. Of the 14 patients, 12 (86%) required additional surgery, either for instability and/or implant failure or pullout.[82] Despite these findings, the development of modern techniques and instruments, combined with added operative experience, is likely to yield more favorable outcomes in future studies.

Medical Outcomes

Patients with neurological disorders are especially susceptible to the already high risks of major spine surgery. Koller et al conducted a retrospective review of 23 patients with Parkinson's disease treated surgically for spinal disorders. Medical complications were seen in 30.4% during the perioperative course and included appendicitis (1), postoperative delirium (3), liver decompensation with temporary hepatic encephalopathy (1), pneumothorax (1), akinetic crisis indicating intensive neurologic care (1), decompensation of insulin-dependent diabetes mellitus (1), and decompensation of kidney insufficiency (1). Postoperative complications included adjacent segment collapse or fractures (17.6%), PJK (17.6%), and reoperation (58.8%).[61]

Neurodegenerative pathology can expectedly complicate the postoperative surgical course. For example, postoperative delirium is a common and potentially serious condition within this patient population. In a study evaluating patients with Parkinson's disease undergoing T2–pelvis posterior fusion, 66.7% developed postoperative delirium[62] compared to an incidence of 8.4 per 1,000 lumbar spine procedures performed in the general population.[84] To illustrate the potential implications of this complication, one study reported that in the general population postoperative delirium increases risk of postoperative complications ($p = 0.01$), resulting in worse postoperative mood and an increased length of stay by about 1.5 days in patients undergoing orthopaedic procedures.[85] Another study found that delirious patients are less likely to improve in function at 6 months when compared with preoperative baseline HAQ ($t = 6.43$, $p < 0.001$).[63]

Operative Benefits

Despite the risk of complications reiterated previously, there are also many benefits derived from operative treatment. In a 2015 review of the literature, Sarkiss et al identified 95 patients with Parkinson's disease who underwent spinal surgery across six studies published between 2000 and 2013. From this subset of patients, 63% were judged to have satisfactory results.[86] In a retrospective review by Bourghli et al, investigators analyzed 12 patients with Parkinson's disease with spinal deformity undergoing long segment posterior spinal fusion (T2–sacrum) with iliac screws and autologous graft (with bone morphogenetic protein if revision surgery).[62] In this analysis, patients demonstrated improved global alignment: SVA decreased from 15.2 to 0.5 cm, C7 PL decreased from 8.9 to 3.2 cm, PI-LL decreased from 34 to ⬚3 degrees, and PT decreased from 31.6 to 19.1 degrees.[64] Additionally, functional results were assessed postoperatively with the SRS-30 demonstrating a mean function score of 24/35, mean pain score of 24/30, mean patient satisfaction score of 12.5/15, and mean total score of 114/150 (76%). Similarly, from the Koller et al review of postoperative outcomes among 23 patients with Parkinson's disease who underwent spinal surgery, 11 patients were satisfied, 6 were very satisfied, 2 were neither satisfied nor dissatisfied, and 2 were not satisfied (in 2 patients clinical outcome data were not available).[61]

15.6 Case Presentation

A 64-year-old woman with Parkinson's disease presents with leg pain (left worse than right) along with back pain for many years. Her pain is worse with standing, better with sitting. To date, the Parkinson's disease has been well managed with medications and DBS. On exam, she had weakness of the left quadriceps and diminished reflexes at the left patella and Achilles. Romberg's test was positive and tandem gait walking was unsteady. She had a left lumbar trunk shift. Full-body X-rays and MRI (▶ Fig. 15.2a, b) revealed lumbar scoliosis with left-sided concavity, anterior sagittal malalignment, and nerve root compression at the left L3 and L4 foramina with lateral listhesis at several levels.

She underwent T10–pelvis posterior spinal fusion with L5–S1 transforaminal lumbar interbody fusion, L3–L4 and L4–L5 hemilaminectomy and foraminotomies for decompression of the L3 and L4 nerve roots, and iliac fixation (▶ Fig. 15.2c, d).

Postoperatively, she developed arrhythmias, which were managed medically, as well as deep vein thromboses and pulmonary emboli, for which she was treated with inferior vena cava filter placement. Her hospital course was also complicated by episodes of confusion and hallucinations that were managed medically. She was discharged on postoperative day 9 to an acute rehab facility.

At 1-month follow-up in the office, the patient reported improvement in back and leg symptoms and was able to walk up to half a mile. At 3- and 6-month follow-up visits, she continued to have nearly complete resolution of pain with some residual numbness around the left knee. At 10-month follow-up, the patient reported recurrence of right leg pain with limitation in walking and balance. X-rays (▶ Fig. 15.2e, f) showed adequate alignment across the fused segments with maintained PI-LL but increased thoracic kyphosis above the fusion, potentially representing PJK. The patient was managed medically with adjustment of pain medications after consultation with her primary neurologist. In summary, this case illustrates that good clinical results can be achieved in patients with Parkinson's disease; however, these patients are prone to the development of perioperative and long-term postoperative complications as well as progression of degenerative spinal pathology.

15.7 Conclusion

The complex pathophysiology of neurodegenerative diseases in adults makes surgical treatment of spinal deformity challenging. An appreciation of the complications in the peri- and postoperative period is required. Based on the nonoperative and operative strategies presented here, intervention by spine surgeons can afford improved functionality and quality of life. To optimize outcomes for these patients, seamless cooperation from the entire health care team including nursing, neurology, anesthesiology, rehabilitation, and internal medicine is of utmost importance. Future work lies in robust prospective studies that can guide the development of treatment guidelines and protocols in these challenging cases.

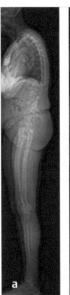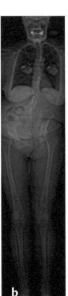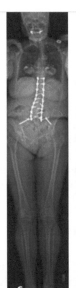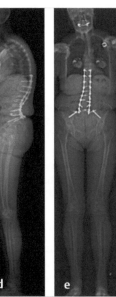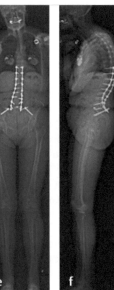

Fig. 15.2 (a, b) (Preoperative lateral and PA) A 64-year-old woman with Parkinson's disease presents with lumbar scoliosis with left-sided concavity, anterior sagittal malalignment, and nerve root compression at the left L3 and L4 foramina with lateral listhesis at several levels. **(c, d)** (Postoperative PA and lateral) T10–pelvis posterior spinal fusion with L5–S1 transforaminal lumbar interbody fusion, L3–L4 and L4–L5 hemilaminectomy and foraminotomies for decompression of the L3 and L4 nerve roots, and iliac fixation. **(e, f)** (PA and lateral at 10 months postoperative) Adequate alignment across the fused segments with maintained PI-LL but increased thoracic kyphosis above the fusion, potentially representing PJK.

References

[1] Frosch MP, Anthony DC, De Girolami U. The central nervous system. In: Kumar V, Abbas AK, Fausto N, eds. Robbins and Cotran Pathologic Basis of Disease. 7th ed. Philadelphia, PA: Elsevier Saunders; 2005:1374–1419

[2] Parkinson J. An essay on the shaking palsy. 1817. J Neuropsychiatry Clin Neurosci. 2002; 14(2):223–236, discussion 222

[3] Kashihara K, Ohno M, Tomita S. Dropped head syndrome in Parkinson's disease. Mov Disord. 2006; 21(8):1213–1216

[4] Fujimoto K. Dropped head in Parkinson's disease. J Neurol. 2006; 253 Suppl 7:VII21–VII26

[5] Gerlier EF. Une epidemie de vertige paralysant. Rev Med Suisse Romande. 1887; 7:5–29

[6] Doherty KM, van de Warrenburg BP, Peralta MC, et al. Postural deformities in Parkinson's disease. Lancet Neurol. 2011; 10(6):538–549

[7] van de Warrenburg BPC, Cordivari C, Ryan AM, et al. The phenomenon of disproportionate antecollis in Parkinson's disease and multiple system atrophy. Mov Disord. 2007; 22(16):2325–2331

[8] Ashour R, Jankovic J. Joint and skeletal deformities in Parkinson's disease, multiple system atrophy, and progressive supranuclear palsy. Mov Disord. 2006; 21(11):1856–1863

[9] Bonanni L, Thomas A, Varanese S, Scorrano V, Onofrj M. Botulinum toxin treatment of lateral axial dystonia in Parkinsonism. Mov Disord. 2007; 22 (14):2097–2103

[10] Fichtner CG. Pleurothotonus and the Pisa syndrome. Biol Psychiatry. 1992; 31 (5):534

[11] Ekbom K, Lindholm H, Ljungberg L. New dystonic syndrome associated with butyrophenone therapy. Z Neurol. 1972; 202(2):94–103

[12] Uemura T, Kasai Y, Araki K, Uchida A. Pisa syndrome. J Spinal Disord Tech. 2008; 21(6):455–457

[13] Patel S, Tariot PN, Hamill RW. Pisa syndrome without neuroleptic exposure in a patient with dementia of the Alzheimer type. J Geriatr Psychiatry Neurol. 1991; 4(1):48–51

[14] Davidson M, Powchik P, Davis KL. Pisa syndrome in Alzheimer's disease. Biol Psychiatry. 1988; 23(2):213

[15] Colosimo C. Pisa syndrome in a patient with multiple system atrophy. Mov Disord. 1998; 13(3):607–609

[16] Di Matteo A, Fasano A, Squintani G, et al. Lateral trunk flexion in Parkinson's disease: EMG features disclose two different underlying pathophysiological mechanisms. J Neurol. 2011; 258(5):740–745

[17] Deriu M, Murgia D, Paribello A, Marcia E, Melis M, Cossu G. Pisa syndrome as presenting symptom of amyotrophic lateral sclerosis. J Neurol. 2011; 258 (11):2087–2089

[18] Cossu G, Melis M, Melis G, et al. Reversible Pisa syndrome (pleurothotonus) due to the cholinesterase inhibitor galantamine: case report. Mov Disord. 2004; 19(10):1243–1244

[19] Villarejo A, Camacho A, García-Ramos R, et al. Cholinergic-dopaminergic imbalance in Pisa syndrome. Clin Neuropharmacol. 2003; 26(3):119–121

[20] Hung T-H, Lee Y, Chang Y-Y, Chong M-Y, Lin P-Y. Reversible Pisa syndrome induced by clozapine: a case report. Clin Neuropharmacol. 2007; 30(6):370–372

[21] Ponfick M, Gdynia H-J, Ludolph AC, Kassubek J. Camptocormia in Parkinson's disease: a review of the literature. Neurodegener Dis. 2011; 8(5):283–288

[22] Cooper A. Sir Benjamin Collins Brodie (1783–1862). JAMA. 1967; 200 (4):331–332

[23] Hawkins C. The Works of Sir Benjamin Collins Brodie. London: Longman, Green, Longman, Roberts, & Green; 1865

[24] Tiple D, Fabbrini G, Colosimo C, et al. Camptocormia in Parkinson disease: an epidemiological and clinical study. J Neurol Neurosurg Psychiatry. 2009; 80 (2):145–148

[25] Abe K, Uchida Y, Notani M. Camptocormia in Parkinson's disease. Parkinsons Dis. 2010

[26] Marinelli P, Colosimo C, Ferrazza AM, et al. Effect of camptocormia on lung volumes in Parkinson's disease. Respir Physiol Neurobiol. 2013; 187(2):164–166

[27] Sato M, Sainoh T, Orita S, et al. Posterior and anterior spinal fusion for the management of deformities in patients with Parkinson's disease. Case Rep Orthop. 2013; 2013:140916

[28] Serratrice G. Axial myopathies: an elderly disorder. Acta Myol. 2007; 26 (1):11–13

[29] Tashiro S, Akaboshi K, Kobayashi Y, Mori T, Nagata M, Liu M. Herpes zoster-induced trunk muscle paresis presenting with abdominal wall pseudohernia, scoliosis, and gait disturbance and its rehabilitation: a case report. Arch Phys Med Rehabil. 2010; 91(2):321–325

[30] Schulz-Schaeffer WJ, Margraf NG, Munser S, et al. Effect of neurostimulation on camptocormia in Parkinson's disease depends on symptom duration. Mov Disord. 2015; 30(3):368–372

[31] Wrede A, Margraf NG, Goebel HH, Deuschl G, Schulz-Schaeffer WJ. Myofibrillar disorganization characterizes myopathy of camptocormia in Parkinson's disease. Acta Neuropathol. 2012; 123(3):419–432

[32] Lenoir T, Guedj N, Boulu P, Guigui P, Benoist M. Camptocormia: the bent spine syndrome, an update. Eur Spine J. 2010; 19(8):1229–1237

[33] Margraf NG, Rohr A, Granert O, Hampel J, Drews A, Deuschl G. MRI of lumbar trunk muscles in patients with Parkinson's disease and camptocormia. J Neurol. 2015; 262(7):1655–1664

[34] Seki M, Takahashi K, Koto A, et al. Keio Parkinson's Disease Database. Camptocormia in Japanese patients with Parkinson's disease: a multicenter study. Mov Disord. 2011; 26(14):2567–2571

[35] Lepoutre AC, Devos D, Blanchard-Dauphin A, et al. A specific clinical pattern of camptocormia in Parkinson's disease. J Neurol Neurosurg Psychiatry. 2006; 77(11):1229–1234

[36] Marketos SG, Skiadas P. Hippocrates. The father of spine surgery. Spine. 1999; 24(13):1381–1387

[37] The Genuine Works of Hippocrates. Hippocrates. Charles Darwin Adams. New York. Dover. 1868.

[38] Schwab FJ, Smith VA, Biserni M, Gamez L, Farcy J-PC, Pagala M. Adult scoliosis: a quantitative radiographic and clinical analysis. Spine. 2002; 27(4):387–392

[39] Dubousset J. Three-dimensional analysis of the scoliotic deformity. In: Weinstein SL, ed. The Pediatric Spine: Principles and Practices. New York, NY: Raven Press; 1994:479–496

[40] Dubousset J, Challier V, Farcy J-P, Schwab FJ, Lafage V. Spinal alignment versus spinal balance. In: Haid RW, Shaffrey CI, Schwab FJ, Youssef JA, eds. Global Spinal Alignment: Principles, Pathologies, and Procedures. St. Louis, MO: Quality Medical Publishing; 2015

[41] Tang JA, Scheer JK, Smith JS, et al. ISSG. The impact of standing regional cervical sagittal alignment on outcomes in posterior cervical fusion surgery. Neurosurgery. 2012; 71(3):662–669

[42] Baik JS, Kim JY, Park JH, Han SW, Park JH, Lee MS. Scoliosis in patients with Parkinson's disease. J Clin Neurol. 2009; 5(2):91–94

[43] Duvoisin RC, Marsden CD. Note on the scoliosis of Parkinsonism. J Neurol Neurosurg Psychiatry. 1975; 38(8):787–793

[44] Grimes JD, Hassan MN, Trent G, Halle D, Armstrong GW. Clinical and radiographic features of scoliosis in Parkinson's disease. Adv Neurol. 1987; 45:353–355

[45] Robin GC, Span Y, Steinberg R, Makin M, Menczel J. Scoliosis in the elderly: a follow-up study. Spine. 1982; 7(4):355–359

[46] Vanderpool DW, James JI, Wynne-Davies R. Scoliosis in the elderly. J Bone Joint Surg Am. 1969; 51(3):446–455

[47] Maetzler W, Mancini M, Liepelt-Scarfone I, et al. Impaired trunk stability in individuals at high risk for Parkinson's disease. PLoS One. 2012; 7(3):e32240

[48] Sinaki M, Brey RH, Hughes CA, Larson DR, Kaufman KR. Balance disorder and increased risk of falls in osteoporosis and kyphosis: significance of kyphotic posture and muscle strength. Osteoporos Int. 2005; 16(8):1004–1010

[49] Glassman SD, Bridwell K, Dimar JR, Horton W, Berven S, Schwab F. The impact of positive sagittal balance in adult spinal deformity. Spine. 2005; 30 (18):2024–2029

[50] Oh JK, Smith JS, Shaffrey CI, et al. Sagittal spinopelvic malalignment in Parkinson disease: prevalence and associations with disease severity. Spine. 2014; 39(14):E833–E841

[51] Diebo BG, Henry J, Lafage V, Berjano P. Sagittal deformities of the spine: factors influencing the outcomes and complications. Eur Spine J. 2015; 24 Suppl 1:S3–S15

[52] Fu K-MG, Bess S, Shaffrey CI, et al. International Spine Study Group. Patients with adult spinal deformity treated operatively report greater baseline pain and disability than patients treated nonoperatively; however, deformities differ between age groups. Spine. 2014; 39(17):1401–1407

[53] Djurasovic M, Glassman SD. Correlation of radiographic and clinical findings in spinal deformities. Neurosurg Clin N Am. 2007; 18(2):223–227

[54] Bess S, Schwab F, Lafage V, Shaffrey CI, Ames CP. Classifications for adult spinal deformity and use of the Scoliosis Research Society-Schwab Adult Spinal Deformity Classification. Neurosurg Clin N Am. 2013; 24(2):185–193

[55] Terran J, Schwab F, Shaffrey CI, et al. International Spine Study Group. The SRS-Schwab adult spinal deformity classification: assessment and clinical correlations based on a prospective operative and nonoperative cohort. Neurosurgery. 2013; 73(4):559–568

[56] Kalen V, Conklin MM, Sherman FC. Untreated scoliosis in severe cerebral palsy. J Pediatr Orthop. 1992; 12(3):337–340

[57] Schwab F, Ungar B, Blondel B, et al. Scoliosis Research Society-Schwab adult spinal deformity classification: a validation study. Spine. 2012; 37(12):1077–1082

[58] Lafage V, Schwab F, Patel A, Hawkinson N, Farcy J-P. Pelvic tilt and truncal inclination: two key radiographic parameters in the setting of adults with spinal deformity. Spine. 2009; 34(17):E599–E606

[59] Smith JS, Klineberg E, Schwab F, et al. International Spine Study Group. Change in classification grade by the SRS-Schwab Adult Spinal Deformity Classification predicts impact on health-related quality of life measures: prospective analysis of operative and nonoperative treatment. Spine. 2013; 38 (19):1663–1671

[60] Protopsaltis T, Schwab F, Smith JS, et al. The T1 pelvic angle (TPA), a novel radiographic measure of sagittal deformity, accounts for both pelvic retroversion and truncal inclination and correlates strongly with HRQOL. In: Scoliosis Research Society (SRS); September 18–21, 2013; Lyon, France

[61] Koller H, Acosta F, Zenner J, et al. Spinal surgery in patients with Parkinson's disease: experiences with the challenges posed by sagittal imbalance and the Parkinson's spine. Eur Spine J. 2010; 19(10):1785–1794

[62] Bourghli A, Guérin P, Vital JM, et al. Posterior spinal fusion from T2 to the sacrum for the management of major deformities in patients with Parkinson disease: a retrospective review with analysis of complications. J Spinal Disord Tech. 2012; 25(3):E53–E60

[63] Katus L, Shtilbans A. Peri-operative management of patients with Parkinson's disease. Am J Med. 2014; 127(4):275–280

[64] van der Kolk NM, King LA. Effects of exercise on mobility in people with Parkinson's disease. Mov Disord. 2013; 28(11):1587–1596

[65] Upadhyaya CD, Starr PA, Mummaneni PV. Spinal deformity and Parkinson disease: a treatment algorithm. Neurosurg Focus. 2010; 28(3):E5

[66] Ye BK, Kim H, Kim YW. Correction of camptocormia using a cruciform anterior spinal hyperextension brace and back extensor strengthening exercise in a patient with Parkinson disease. Ann Rehabil Med. 2015; 39(1):128–132

[67] de Sèze M-P, Creuzé A, de Sèze M, Mazaux J-M. An orthosis and physiotherapy programme for camptocormia: a prospective case study. J Rehabil Med. 2008; 40(9):761–765

[68] De Sèze M, Creuzé A. Background summary: a new brace for the treatment of camptocormia. Scoliosis. 2009; 4 Suppl 1:O70

[69] Capecci M, Serpicelli C, Fiorentini L, et al. Postural rehabilitation and Kinesio taping for axial postural disorders in Parkinson's disease. Arch Phys Med Rehabil. 2014; 95(6):1067–1075

[70] Comella CL, Shannon KM, Jaglin J. Extensor truncal dystonia: successful treatment with botulinum toxin injections. Mov Disord. 1998; 13(3):552–555

[71] Nuzzo RM, Walsh S, Boucherit T, Massood S. Counterparalysis for treatment of paralytic scoliosis with botulinum toxin type A. Am J Orthop. 1997; 26 (3):201–207

[72] Bertram KL, Stirpe P, Colosimo C. Treatment of camptocormia with botulinum toxin. Toxicon. 2015; 107 Pt A:148–153

[73] Papapetropoulos S, Tuchman A, Sengun C, Russell A, Mitsi G, Singer C. Anterocollis: clinical features and treatment options. Med Sci Monit. 2008; 14(9): CR427–CR430

[74] Azher SN, Jankovic J. Camptocormia: pathogenesis, classification, and response to therapy. Neurology. 2005; 65(3):355–359

[75] Fietzek UM, Schroeteler FE, Ceballos-Baumann AO. Goal attainment after treatment of parkinsonian camptocormia with botulinum toxin. Mov Disord. 2009; 24(13):2027–2028

[76] von Coelln R, Raible A, Gasser T, Asmus F. Ultrasound-guided injection of the iliopsoas muscle with botulinum toxin in camptocormia. Mov Disord. 2008; 23(6):889–892

[77] Mills R, Bahroo L, Pagan F. An update on the use of botulinum toxin therapy in Parkinson's disease. Curr Neurol Neurosci Rep. 2015; 15(1):511

[78] Furusawa Y, Mukai Y, Kobayashi Y, Sakamoto T, Murata M. Role of the external oblique muscle in upper camptocormia for patients with Parkinson's disease. Mov Disord. 2012; 27(6):802–803

[79] Furusawa Y, Mukai Y, Kawazoe T, et al. Long-term effect of repeated lidocaine injections into the external oblique for upper camptocormia in Parkinson's disease. Parkinsonism Relat Disord. 2013; 19(3):350–354

[80] Nandi D, Parkin S, Scott R, et al. Camptocormia treated with bilateral pallidal stimulation: case report. Neurosurg Focus. 2002; 12(2):ECP2

[81] Lang AE. Deep brain stimulation for dystonia. Mov Disord. 2011; 26 Suppl 1: S3–S4

[82] Babat LB, McLain RF, Bingaman W, Kalfas I, Young P, Rufo-Smith C. Spinal surgery in patients with Parkinson's disease: construct failure and progressive deformity. Spine. 2004; 29(18):2006–2012

[83] Kretzer RM, Hu N, Umekoji H, et al. The effect of spinal instrumentation on kinematics at the cervicothoracic junction: emphasis on soft-tissue response in an in vitro human cadaveric model. J Neurosurg Spine. 2010; 13(4):435–442

[84] Fineberg SJ, Nandyala SV, Marquez-Lara A, Oglesby M, Patel AA, Singh K. Incidence and risk factors for postoperative delirium after lumbar spine surgery. Spine. 2013; 38(20):1790–1796

[85] Rogers MP, Liang MH, Daltroy LH, et al. Delirium after elective orthopedic surgery: risk factors and natural history. Int J Psychiatry Med. 1989; 19(2):109–121

[86] Sarkiss CA, Fogg GA, Skovrlj B, Cho SK, Caridi JM. To operate or not?: A literature review of surgical outcomes in 95 patients with Parkinson's disease undergoing spine surgery. Clin Neurol Neurosurg. 2015; 134:122–125

Part III

Surgical Techniques

16 Sacropelvic Fixation Techniques   114

17 Comparison of Unit Rods with Modular
    Constructs in Cerebral Palsy   122

18 Halo-Gravity Traction: An Adjunctive
    Treatment for Severe Spinal Deformity   126

19 Osteotomies: Ponte and Vertebral
    Column Resection   132

20 Growing Spine Options for
    Neuromuscular Scoliosis   136

21 Anterior Approaches to the Spine for
    Neuromuscular Spinal Deformity   143

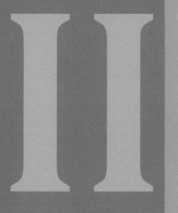

16 Sacropelvic Fixation Techniques

Suken A. Shah

Abstract

Considerable flexion moments and cantilever forces at the transitional area of the lumbosacral junction necessitate strong distal fixation to allow control and correction of deformity and avoid pseudarthrosis and implant failure. This chapter will discuss the biomechanics and various techniques of sacral and pelvic screw fixation with an emphasis on contemporary techniques to achieve better fusion rates, improve fixation, neutralize forces, and avoid failure and other complications.

Keywords: iliac screws, sacropelvic fixation, S2 alar iliac screw fixation

16.1 Introduction

Indications for sacropelvic fixation include long spinal fusions for scoliosis, high-grade spondylolisthesis, pelvic obliquity correction, sagittal plane deformity correction, sacral fractures, and lumbosacral fusions in patients with poor bone quality and osteoporosis. Each of these indications requires strong distal fixation to resist significant flexion moments and cantilever forces in this transitional area. Despite many advances and developments in spinal instrumentation techniques, fixation failure at the lumbosacral junction continues to be a challenge.

Due to the significant biomechanical forces across this junction and relatively poor sacral cancellous bone quality, fusion at the lumbosacral junction has been associated with rates of pseudarthrosis as high as 33 to 39%,[1,2] loss of lordosis,[1,2] and instrumentation failure, especially with historical methods such as body casting and Harrington and Luque instrumentation. Cotrel–Dubousset (CD) instrumentation and the Galveston technique were introduced in the 1980s, and although pseudarthrosis rates were lower, there were instrumentation-related complications with the CD system[3] and technical difficulties with rod contouring, insertion in the ilium, and rod loosening with the Galveston technique.

16.2 Biomechanics

McCord et al pointed out the importance of the lumbosacral pivot point, which was defined as the point at the middle osteoligamentous column between the last lumbar vertebra and the sacrum. The farther the implants extend anterior to this point, the greater the stiffness of the construct. Various instrumentation models (iliac fixation, S1 fixation, and S2 fixation) were tested. The two constructs that withstood the greatest load before failure had caudad iliac (rod or screw) fixation, and they concluded that crossing the sacroiliac (SI) joint is warranted if instrumentation extends anterior to the pivot point.[4]

O'Brien identified three distinct zones of the sacropelvic region: zone 1 consists of the S1 vertebral body and the cephalad margins of the sacral alae; zone 2 consists of the inferior margins of the sacral alae, S2, and the area extending to the tip of the coccyx; and zone 3 consists of both ilia. Fixation strength improves progressively from zone 1 to zone 3. Zone 3 offers the greatest biomechanical fixation strength to counter the pullout forces and bending moments at the lumbosacral junction. Also, in agreement with McCord, iliac fixation with pelvic screws or iliac rods allows placement of implants more anteriorly beyond the lumbosacral pivot point than any other implant type.[5]

Lebwohl and colleagues performed a biomechanical comparison of lumbosacral fixation in a calf spine model and noted that supplementary fixation distal to S1 pedicle screws provides a benefit over S1 fixation alone, and iliac fixation was superior to a second point of fixation in the sacrum.[6]

Cunningham et al studied ex vivo porcine spines biomechanically to ascertain the value of anterior column support compared with that of iliac fixation in lumbosacral fusions. When tested to failure, the authors found that iliac screws significantly reduced lumbosacral motion, particularly with axial rotation, flexion–extension, and lateral bending. Iliac fixation was found to be more protective of S1 screws and more resistive of motion than anterior interbody cages.[7]

However, other investigators have argued in favor of anterior column support, particularly at L4–L5 and L5–S1, in long fusions to the sacrum.[8,9] Anterior lumbar interbody fusions place the bone graft ventral to the instrumentation and the lumbosacral pivot point, and the graft is placed in compression to optimize fusion and stability.[9] This procedure improves the overall chance of fusion, decreases the strain on caudad pedicle screws, and has a definite role in long fusions to the sacrum, especially in adults and other patients at risk for pseudarthrosis.

Various contemporary techniques of sacropelvic fixation have been described to achieve better fusion rates, improve bone purchase, neutralize forces, avoid pullout, ease difficulty, and reduce complications. In this chapter, we will cover the key components of surgical techniques for the majority of iliac fixation options. This will include the following: (1) Galveston and unit rod technique; (2) iliac bolts/screws with and without offset connections to the longitudinal rods; (3) double iliac bolts; (4) iliac screws in an alternative, anatomic pathway; and (5) S2 alar iliac (S2AI) screw fixation

16.2.1 Galveston and Unit Rod Technique

The Galveston technique allows for the incorporation of the ilium into the foundation of the construct *via* the insertion of rods between the inner and outer tables of the ilium, which provides a broader base and a more biomechanically advantageous position.[1,4] The transverse portions of the rods are inserted under a large muscle flap and enter the ilium at the posterosuperior iliac crest. The orientation is approximately 30 to 35 degrees caudally and 20 to 25 degrees laterally. The rods may cross the SI joint, and contouring can be difficult.[10] The technique lowers the pseudarthrosis rate of long fusions to the sacrum,[11,12] but it is also associated with a moderate incidence of loosening secondary to micromotion at the rod tips within the ilium, despite lumbosacral fusion.[13] Radiographically, this is described as a windshield-wiper effect and may be associated with pain and the need for implant removal,[13,14] but in our long-term experience of unit rod fixation in patients with cerebral palsy, this has not been a common symptomatic issue requiring reoperation.[15] Lonstein and his colleagues published their results and complications of 93 patients with cerebral palsy and scoliosis who underwent posterior-only spinal fusion with Luque–Galveston instrumentation with an average follow-up of 3.8 years.[14] Coronal curve correction was 50% and pelvic obliquity correction was 40% at latest follow-up. The late complication rate was 47% and included the windshield-wiper sign, junctional kyphosis, pseudarthrosis (7.5%), and implant problems including breakage, dislodgement, and prominence. Seven patients required reoperation, most commonly for pseudarthrosis and/or failed implants.

The unit rod, by virtue of its precontoured unibody construction, provides rigid control of spinal deformities involving pelvic obliquity and allows for a cantilever mechanism to correct the pelvic obliquity and the scoliosis simultaneously.[16] See ▶ Fig. 16.1 for an example of a patient with severe thoracolumbar scoliosis and pelvic obliquity treated with a unit rod. The rods are available in various lengths with corresponding thoracic, lumbar, and pelvic contours. The specific technique of unit rod insertion follows.[17]

At the inferior margin of the incision, the outer wing of the ilium is subperiosteally exposed down to the sciatic notch and sponges packed out over the pelvis to maintain hemostasis. The right and left drill guides for the unit rod are placed in the respective sciatic notch; care should be taken to ensure that the drill guide is as inferior as possible along the posterosuperior iliac spine (PSIS). The handles of the drill guide are the reference points for alignment: the lateral handle should be parallel with the pelvis and the axial handle parallel with the sacrum. The drill hole is next made utilizing the guide using a 3/8-inch drill to the predetermined depth directed toward the anteroinferior iliac spine (AIIS); the hole is then palpated with a ball-tipped feeler to confirm that there has been no breach of the cortical bone of the inner or outer pelvic table. Alternatively, after establishing the landmarks, the pedicle gearshift can be used to cannulate the cancellous bone of the iliac pathway, either freehand or with fluoroscopic guidance. Gelfoam should be inserted into the drill holes to control cancellous bone bleeding. After the proper length unit rod is selected, the pelvic limbs of the rod are crossed and inserted into their respective drill holes. Each limb should be advanced alternatively in 1-cm increments with an impactor. Care must be taken to maintain control of the rod and insure that it does not penetrate either table of the pelvis. In the setting of hyperlordosis, the marked anterior inclination of the pelvis increases the risk of the pelvic limb perforating the inner cortex during insertion. The pelvic ends of the rod need to be directed in a more posterior direction to accommodate this angulation; rod placement is facilitated by manual correction of the lordosis prior to rod insertion. In instances of marked lordosis, the pelvic limbs of the rod may be cut and inserted separately and then attached to the rod with rod-to-rod connectors.

In our series of surgical correction of scoliosis in pediatric patients with cerebral palsy using unit rod instrumentation,[15]

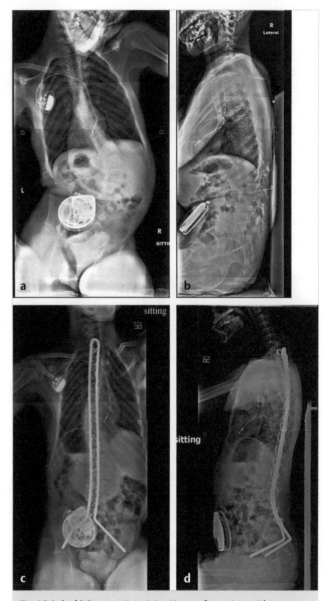

Fig. 16.1 (a, b) Preoperative sitting X-rays of a patient with severe thoracolumbar scoliosis and pelvic obliquity. **(c, d)** Postoperative sitting X-rays of the patient after posterior spinal fusion with the unit rod.

241 patients were observed for more than 2 years and had an average coronal curve correction of 68% and pelvic obliquity correction of 71% with a very cost-effective implant system. Intraoperative complications with pelvic fixation occurred in 17 patients; sagittal plane deformities, especially lumbar hyperlordosis, were a risk factor. Late postoperative complications occurred in 12 patients: 3 pseudarthroses, 3 deep infections, and 6 prominent proximal implant issues.

Although the unit rod provides excellent correction of pelvic obliquity and resistance to flexion moments, there is little resistance to axial pullout and torsion by virtue of the rods being smooth and immediate micromotion of the iliac construct after insertion. These concerns can be mitigated by adding a transverse connector distally to improve torsional rigidity and adding lumbar pedicle screws distally at L5 to significantly improve axial pullout, strength, and stiffness.[18]

16.2.2 Iliac Screws—Standard Technique

The difficult learning curve associated with rod contouring and insertion into the ilium using the Galveston technique has been resolved with the use of iliac screws, which permits screws of variable length and diameter to be inserted into each ilium separately. Simpler fixation to the pelvis with screws may also mitigate the potential complications of the Galveston technique, which was up to 62% in Gau et al's series[11] and 47% in Lonstein et al's series.[14] The screws can then be connected to the main construct by various connectors. This technique has simplified the process of obtaining iliac fixation, especially in patients with significant pelvic asymmetry or hyperlordotic lumbar deformities while improving pullout strength through better interdigitation of the threaded implant within the iliac cortical and cancellous bone.[19,20] See ▸ Fig. 16.2 for an example of a patient

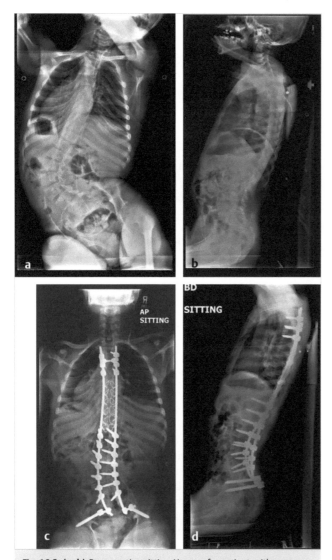

Fig. 16.2 (a, b) Preoperative sitting X-rays of a patient with severe thoracolumbar scoliosis and pelvic obliquity. **(c, d)** Postoperative sitting X-rays of the patient 3 years after posterior spinal fusion with precontoured rods and a proximal transverse connector from the Expedium Neuromuscular Set and iliac screws with offset connectors from the Sacropelvic Collection (DePuy Synthes Spine, Raynham, MA).

with severe thoracolumbar scoliosis and pelvic obliquity treated with segmental instrumentation and iliac screws.

When placing iliac screws in lieu of smooth Galveston pelvic fixation, the starting point is similar—1 to 2 cm inferior to PSIS. To decrease implant prominence, a notch in the ilium can be used to bury the head of the screw below the contour of the cortical bone. A pedicle gearshift or drill is used to cannulate the cancellous bone between the inner and outer tables of the ilium, directed toward the AIIS, 1 cm above the sciatic notch. The pathway is then palpated with a ball-tipped probe and tapped to increase purchase and size the diameter and length of the screw. The exposure of the PSIS can be made through the same incision, elevating the paraspinal lumbosacral musculature and soft tissues, with a subperiosteal dissection of the PSIS and a portion of the outer table or through a separate, small oblique fascial incision by retracting the skin over the iliac crest. Alternatively, using a technique described by Wang and colleagues[21] with the Viper Screw System (DePuy Synthes Spine, Raynham, MA), iliac screws can be inserted with a fluoroscopically guided percutaneous technique to avoid the morbidity and complications associated with such a large muscle dissection and soft-tissue devitalization.

Every effort should be made to insert the largest diameter, longest screws that can be safely accommodated to achieve favorable biomechanics. Screws should extend past McCord's sacropelvic pivot point at the anterior edge of the L5/S1 disk at a minimum.[4] The farther anteriorly and laterally the screws extend, the better control of pelvic flexion, extension, obliquity, and rotation. Even in smaller patients, we have been successful in implanting screws of 7.5 to 8 mm in diameter and 65 to 80 mm in length. Larger patients can accommodate screws of up to 10 mm × 100 mm. Large taps are available to enlarge the entry site and size the screws by using insertional torque. These various options are all available in the Expedium Neuromuscular and Pelvic Fixation Set (DePuy Synthes Spine, Raynham, MA) in closed and open screw head options along with offset connections that will allow modular, rigid connections to the longitudinal rods up to the spinal implants. Since the typical iliac pathway starting at the PSIS is 1 to 2 cm lateral to the pedicular line, offset connectors are frequently needed and options in the set are fixed or variable axis, open or closed connectors that can be customized for length, or short-throw rod contour and attached to the rod with slip strengths equal to Expedium pedicle screw connections. Alternatively, the longitudinal rods can be contoured laterally in the coronal plane distal to the L5 or S1 screws to connect directly to the iliac screws either prior to rod insertion or with in situ benders.

A retrospective, single-center cohort study comparing two groups of 20 patients (flaccid and spastic paralytic scoliosis) each with Luque–Galveston constructs and iliac screws showed similar maintenance of pelvic obliquity and scoliosis correction, but the iliac screw techniques avoids the complex lumbosacral three-dimensional rod bends and had less haloing around the pelvic implants with minimal implant complications. The Galveston group had four broken rods and two reoperations and the iliac screw group had one broken screw and no reoperations.[22]

A larger multicenter retrospective study of 157 patients with virtually equal distribution compared the unit rod to "custom-bent" rods with iliac screw fixation and found that although the unit rod had better pelvic obliquity correction, mean surgical time, blood loss, hospital stay, infection rate, and proximal fixation problems were significantly higher in the patients with unit rods.[23]

16.2.3 Double Iliac Screws

Occasionally, double iliac screw fixation is needed to overcome challenges of osteoporosis, fractures involving the sacropelvis, or tumor resections/reconstructions to impart better biomechanical stability. Phillips et al provide an overview of their technique and experience in 50 patients with neuromuscular scoliosis who were treated with Luque instrumentation techniques modified with the addition of iliac screw anchorage, 20 of whom had 2 iliac screws in each pelvic wing (4 in total). The patients with two screws in each ilium had a lower complication rate; conversely, patients with single iliac screws had a 2.5 times greater incidence of rod disengagement and sevenfold greater prevalence of implant failure cephalad to the pelvis.[24]

Their technique involves a muscle-splitting approach to the standard PSIS starting point, exposure of the outer table of the pelvis to the sciatic notch to identify the trajectory, and cannulation of the cancellous bone between the inner and outer tables, aiming for the AIIS. The first screw is placed approximately 2 cm superior to the PSIS, with a second screw placed 2 cm further superiorly. Average curve correction was 48% and average pelvic tilt correction was 59%.[24]

16.2.4 Iliac Screws—Anatomic Technique

Placement of iliac screws using the traditional standard technique described earlier requires the use of offset connectors and may devascularize and denervate the iliac muscles. An alternative technique described by Harrop et al provides for the screw heads to be inserted in a more anatomic position aligning with the rods without the detachment of the erector spinae muscles.[25] The erector spinae muscles are carefully dissected medial to lateral, but are not detached distally to maintain muscle viability. The authors point out that disconnection of

the midline muscles on exposure with the ensuing dissection of the medial iliac crest causes the muscles to contract, leaving a void; consequently, this can result in a hematoma, possible infection, and morbidity. A second fascial incision is made over the soft tissues that attach to the lateral iliac crest wall; gluteal muscle is subperiosteally dissected off the lateral ilium to allow finger palpation of the sciatic notch. The starting point for this screw is located along the medial border of the PSIS at its junction with the sacrum. A pedicle probe is used to develop the screw path 20 degrees lateral to the midsagittal plane and 30 to 35 degrees caudal to the transverse plane toward the anterior superior iliac spine, 1.5 to 2 cm above the sciatic notch. This places the iliac screw tulip head in line with the longitudinal rods without the need for an offset connector, does not require bone resection, and is less prominent than a screw starting at the PSIS.

16.2.5 S2 Alar Iliac Screws for Pelvic Fixation

The S2AI technique, described by Chang et al,[26] Kebaish,[27] and Sponseller et al[28] has become my preferred technique for various reasons. Since the starting point is 1.5 cm deeper than the traditional iliac entry from the PSIS, decreased implant prominence is the main advantage. The starting point and, consequently, the screw head are in line with L5 and S1 pedicle screws, thus avoiding an offset connection from the longitudinal rod (see ▶ Fig. 16.3). This point is easily found, requires little muscle dissection, and can even be performed in a minimally invasive fashion.[29] The starting point for the screw is 2 to 4 mm lateral and 4 to 8 mm inferior to the S1 foramen; minimal muscle stripping and dissection are needed (see ▶ Fig. 16.4). A sharp awl or burr is used to mark the starting point and penetrate the cortical bone. Then, a drill or pedicle gearshift is used to enter the cancellous bone of the sacrum directed toward the dorsal aspect of the SI joint, into the ilium. Even in osteopenic bone, the screw can obtain decent fixation, since multiple cortical layers are penetrated. I find palpation of the ipsilateral greater trochanter of the proximal femur as a valuable virtual target (see ▶ Fig. 16.5). The trajectory is lateral (approximately

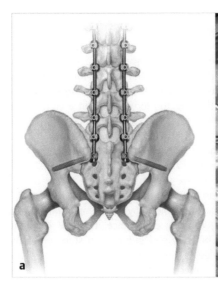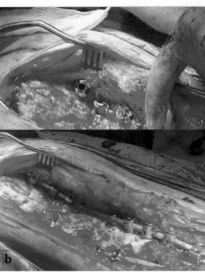

Fig. 16.3 (a) The S2AI pathway allows the iliac screw to line up with the lumbar and sacral pedicle screws so no offset connection is needed when securing the longitudinal rods. **(b)** Intraoperative photos of the screw arrangement and alignment.

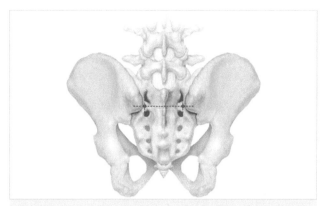

Fig. 16.4 The starting point of the SAI screw is a point between the S1 and S2 foramen, along the lateral border, in line with an S1 pedicle screw.

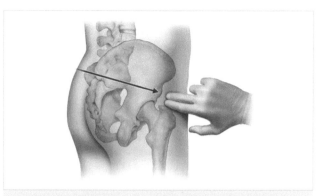

Fig. 16.5 From the starting point, one should aim for the AIIS, palpating the tip of the ipsilateral greater trochanter.

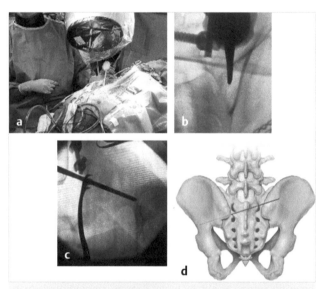

Fig. 16.6 (a–c) Intraoperative photos illustrating use of a cannulated gearshift from the VIPER SAI Screw Set (DePuy Synthes Spine, Raynham, MA) used to cannulate the S2AI pathway under fluoroscopy and then use of a guidewire to tap and implant the SAI screw. Minimal muscle dissection is required and the technique is very efficient. **(d)** Illustration of guidewire placement in the S2AI pathway.

40 degrees to the horizontal plane) and 20 to 30 degrees caudal (this depends on pelvic tilt), and fluoroscopy is helpful to guide this trajectory. The anteroposterior projection shows the pelvis and sciatic notch. The teardrop view helps ensure that the pathway is in the thickest part of the ilium without a cortical breach (see ▶ Fig. 16.6). Once in the ilium, the pathway is 1 to 2 cm above the sciatic notch directed toward the AIIS. A polyaxial screw, typically 80 to 90 mm long, is used and adults can accommodate diameters of 8 to 10 mm; screw diameters of 7 to 8 mm can be used in smaller patients.

The Expedium SAI screw (DePuy Synthes Spine, Raynham, MA) has novel features that are desirable for use in this capacity: a favored angled polyaxial head for added tilt and ease of rod attachment, a smooth shank for enhanced outer diameter and strength at the proximal part of the screw, large thread form for cancellous bone purchase, and a diverse variety of sizes

for all types of patients. Kebaish and colleagues reported on a group of 52 patients (adult and pediatric) followed over 2 years using this technique and reported lower complication rates than other techniques with no adverse effect on the SI joint and only one patient that required implant removal.[30] Sponseller et al described excellent results in a cohort study of pediatric patients (predominantly with scoliosis secondary to cerebral palsy) with the S2AI technique compared to screws inserted into the ilium from the traditional starting point of the PSIS. Patients with S2AI screws had better restoration of pelvic obliquity and fewer complications: no deep infections, prominent implants, or anchor migration compared to three patients with infections and three instances of implant prominence, skin breakdown, or anchor migration in the PSIS group.[28]

The S2AI screw technique can also be performed minimally invasively using existing Expedium instruments and its cannulated components (see ▶ Fig. 16.7 and ▶ Fig. 16.8). This technique saves operative and fluoroscopy time after placement of the guidewire down the pathway with either a drill or cannulated gearshift.

16.3 Complications and Avoidance

Complications associated with sacropelvic fixation include injuries to the adjacent structures (bladder, colon, iliac or gluteal vessels) due to misplacement, cortical bone breach, implant prominence and loosening, wound problems, infections, and implant failure and nonunion.

S1 pedicle screws placed in a convergent manner may injure the middle sacral artery or veins. Diverging S1 screws or alar screws that are placed bicortically and are too long may cause injury to the common or internal iliac artery/vein or lumbosacral trunk. S2 screws that are too long placed in a convergent trajectory may injure the inferior hypogastric plexus or colon. Iliac screws violating the sciatic notch may injure the superior gluteal artery and those that violate the medial ilium may injure the internal iliac artery/vein or lumbar plexus, causing an iliacus hematoma, or violate the hollow viscera of the pelvis. Iliac screws that are too long anteriorly may violate the acetabulum. Misplacement can be avoided by becoming familiar with the anatomy at risk, cadaver experience, the use of blunt probes, confirmation of bony end point at all steps of screw placement, and knowledge about the fluoroscopic X-ray views to confirm proper screw placement.

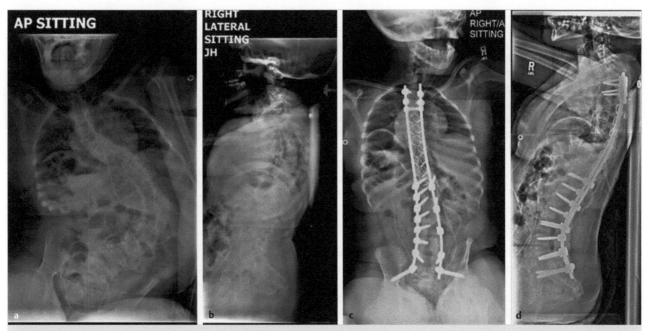

Fig. 16.7 (a,d) Pre- and postoperative sitting X-rays of a patient with neuromuscular scoliosis after posterior fusion and instrumentation with precontoured rods and a proximal transverse connector from the Expedium Neuromuscular Set and pelvic fixation using the VIPER SAI screw via the S2AI pathway.

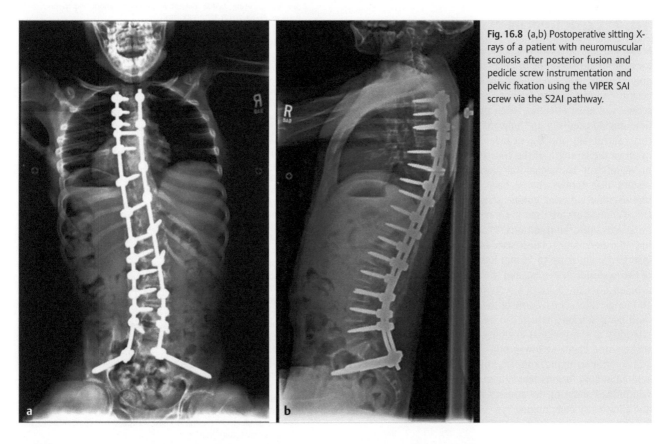

Fig. 16.8 (a,b) Postoperative sitting X-rays of a patient with neuromuscular scoliosis after posterior fusion and pedicle screw instrumentation and pelvic fixation using the VIPER SAI screw via the S2AI pathway.

Implant prominence is cited as a frequent cause of removal; for example, in one series of 36 patients with iliac screw fixation, 8 required subsequent removal,[31] but this can be mitigated by resecting the top of the iliac crest, forming a notch for the screw head to lie deeper within the ilium, or using the S2AI technique, which allows the screw head to be almost 15 mm deeper than traditional iliac screws.[26] Kebaish et al's series of 52 adult patients with S2AI fixation listed only 1 patient that needed subsequent removal.[30]

The infection rate seems lower with this technique as well, perhaps since less dissection is needed for this technique, and combined with soft-tissue preservation and lower profile, this technique seems ideally suited even for our malnourished neuromuscular patients. In Sponseller et al's report of 32 patients with cerebral palsy and scoliosis and 2-year follow-up from surgery, there were no infections, prominent implants, or failures of the S2AI screws.[28] The infection rate associated with iliac fixation alone is difficult to compare from the literature because iliac fixation is performed in conjunction with other procedures. However, in a thorough 2-year follow-up study of patients treated with iliac fixation, Kuklo et al[19] reported an infection rate of 4% (3 of 81 patients). Those authors also noted iliac screw back-out in three patients, all of whom had spondylolisthesis; however, no pseudarthrosis occurred in these patients.

Nonunion and implant failure typically occur together and host biology as well as strength of fixation may play a role. Proper workup to rule out a pseudarthrosis must be undertaken prior to implant removal to allow for proper preparation in the operating room. Again, consideration of anterior interbody support is important, especially in the face of pseudarthrosis. At L5/S1, an anterior structural graft is biomechanically favorable since it is loaded in compression and anterior to the pivot point; this can optimize fusion and stability.[9]

16.4 Conclusion

Many sacropelvic fixation techniques have been described historically to aid surgeons in long constructs to the sacrum, but only a few are still widely used, including sacral screws, the Galveston technique, iliac screws, and S2AI screws. S1 pedicle screws are most effective when placed with "tricortical" fixation, angled medially and upward toward the sacral promontory. Sacral ala and S2 pedicle screws have been used to improve the strength of the construct, but studies have shown no significant biomechanical alteration or improved clinical results. Iliac screws (bolts) have been shown to protect S1 screws, have superior pullout strength, and high fusion rates. Offset connectors are used to connect the screws to the longitudinal rods with the traditional PSIS starting point. S2AI screws have the advantages of decreased implant prominence since the insertion point is up to 15 mm lower than the prominent part of the posterior iliac crest, and the use of an offset connector is avoided since the point of insertion is in line with the S1 screw and longitudinal rods. Some of these techniques are associated with complications, which can be minimized by paying close attention to the regional anatomy, minimizing soft-tissue dissection, and choosing low-profile implants and techniques. To add anterior structural support, anterior fusions should be considered in long fusions that extend to the thoracic spine, which will offload some of the stresses from the posterior implants and allow early bony union.

References

[1] Devlin VJ, Boachie-Adjei O, Bradford DS, Ogilvie JW, Transfeldt EE. Treatment of adult spinal deformity with fusion to the sacrum using CD instrumentation. J Spinal Disord. 1991; 4(1):1–14

[2] Balderston RA, Winter RB, Moe JH, Bradford DS, Lonstein JE. Fusion to the sacrum for nonparalytic scoliosis in the adult. Spine. 1986; 11(8):824–829

[3] Camp JF, Caudle R, Ashmun RD, Roach J. Immediate complications of Cotrel-Dubousset instrumentation to the sacro-pelvis. A clinical and biomechanical study. Spine. 1990; 15(9):932–941

[4] McCord DH, Cunningham BW, Shono Y, Myers JJ, McAfee PC. Biomechanical analysis of lumbosacral fixation. Spine. 1992; 17(8) Suppl:S235–S243

[5] O'Brien MF. Sacropelvic fixation in spinal deformity. In: DeWald RL, ed. Spinal Deformities: The Comprehensive Text. New York, NY: Thieme; 2003:601–614

[6] Lebwohl NH, Cunningham BW, Dmitriev A, et al. Biomechanical comparison of lumbosacral fixation techniques in a calf spine model. Spine. 2002; 27 (21):2312–2320

[7] Cunningham BW, Lewis SJ, Long J, Dmitriev AE, Linville DA, Bridwell KH. Biomechanical evaluation of lumbosacral reconstruction techniques for spondylolisthesis: an in vitro porcine model. Spine. 2002; 27(21):2321–2327

[8] Ogilvie JW, Schendel M. Comparison of lumbosacral fixation devices. Clin Orthop Relat Res. 1986(203):120–125

[9] Crock HV. Anterior lumbar interbody fusion: indications for its use and notes on surgical technique. Clin Orthop Relat Res. 1982(165):157–163

[10] Allen BL, Jr, Ferguson RL. The Galveston technique of pelvic fixation with L-rod instrumentation of the spine. Spine. 1984; 9(4):388–394

[11] Gau YL, Lonstein JE, Winter RB, Koop S, Denis F. Luque-Galveston procedure for correction and stabilization of neuromuscular scoliosis and pelvic obliquity: a review of 68 patients. J Spinal Disord. 1991; 4(4):399–410

[12] Allen BL, Jr, Ferguson RL. L-rod instrumentation for scoliosis in cerebral palsy. J Pediatr Orthop. 1982; 2(1):87–96

[13] Broom MJ, Banta JV, Renshaw TS. Spinal fusion augmented by Luque-rod segmental instrumentation for neuromuscular scoliosis. J Bone Joint Surg Am. 1989; 71(1):32–44

[14] Lonstein JE, Koop SE, Novachek TF, Perra JH. Results and complications after spinal fusion for neuromuscular scoliosis in cerebral palsy and static encephalopathy using Luque Galveston instrumentation: experience in 93 patients. Spine. 2012; 37(7):583–591

[15] Tsirikos AI, Lipton G, Chang WN, Dabney KW, Miller F. Surgical correction of scoliosis in pediatric patients with cerebral palsy using the unit rod instrumentation. Spine. 2008; 33(10):1133–1140

[16] Bell DF, Moseley CF, Koreska J. Unit rod segmental spinal instrumentation in the management of patients with progressive neuromuscular spinal deformity. Spine. 1989; 14(12):1301–1307

[17] Dabney KW, Miller F, Lipton GE, Letonoff EJ, McCarthy HC. Correction of sagittal plane spinal deformities with unit rod instrumentation in children with cerebral palsy. J Bone Joint Surg Am. 2004; 86-A(Pt 2) Suppl 1:156–168

[18] Erickson MA, Oliver T, Baldini T, Bach J. Biomechanical assessment of conventional unit rod fixation versus a unit rod pedicle screw construct: a human cadaver study. Spine. 2004; 29(12):1314–1319

[19] Kuklo TR, Bridwell KH, Lewis SJ, et al. Minimum 2-year analysis of sacropelvic fixation and L5-S1 fusion using S1 and iliac screws. Spine. 2001; 26 (18):1976–1983

[20] Schwend RM, Sluyters R, Najdzionek J. The pylon concept of pelvic anchorage for spinal instrumentation in the human cadaver. Spine. 2003; 28(6):542–547

[21] Wang MY, Ludwig SC, Anderson DG, Mummaneni PV. Percutaneous iliac screw placement: description of a new minimally invasive technique. Neurosurg Focus. 2008; 25(2):E17

[22] Peelle MW, Lenke LG, Bridwell KH, Sides B. Comparison of pelvic fixation techniques in neuromuscular spinal deformity correction: Galveston rod versus iliac and lumbosacral screws. Spine. 2006; 31(20):2392–2398

[23] Sponseller PD, Shah SA, Abel MF, et al. Harms Study Group. Scoliosis surgery in cerebral palsy: differences between unit rod and custom rods. Spine. 2009; 34(8):840–844

[24] Phillips JH, Gutheil JP, Knapp DR, Jr. Iliac screw fixation in neuromuscular scoliosis. Spine. 2007; 32(14):1566–1570

[25] Harrop JS, Jeyamohan SB, Sharan A, Ratliff J, Vaccaro AR. Iliac bolt fixation: an anatomic approach. J Spinal Disord Tech. 2009; 22(8):541–544

[26] Chang TL, Sponseller PD, Kebaish KM, Fishman EK. Low profile pelvic fixation: anatomic parameters for sacral alar-iliac fixation versus traditional iliac fixation. Spine. 2009; 34(5):436–440

[27] Kebaish KM. Sacropelvic fixation: techniques and complications. Spine. 2010; 35(25):2245–2251

[28] Sponseller PD, Zimmerman RM, Ko PS, et al. Low profile pelvic fixation with the sacral alar iliac technique in the pediatric population improves results at two-year minimum follow-up. Spine. 2010; 35(20):1887–1892

[29] O'Brien JR, Matteini L, Yu WD, Kebaish KM. Feasibility of minimally invasive sacropelvic fixation: percutaneous S2 alar iliac fixation. Spine. 2010; 35 (4):460–464

[30] Kebaish KM, Pull ter Gunne AF, Mohamed AS, et al. A new low profile sacropelvic fixation using S2 alar iliac (S2AI) screws in adult deformity fusion to the sacrum: a prospective study with minimum 2-year follow-up. Presented at: the North American Spine Society Annual Meeting; November 10–14, 2009; San Francisco, CA

[31] Emami A, Deviren V, Berven S, Smith JA, Hu SS, Bradford DS. Outcome and complications of long fusions to the sacrum in adult spine deformity: Luque-Galveston, combined iliac and sacral screws, and sacral fixation. Spine. 2002; 27(7):776–786

17 Comparison of Unit Rods with Modular Constructs in Cerebral Palsy

Mark Shasti and Paul D. Sponseller

Abstract

This chapter compares unit rods with modular instrumentation constructs for neuromuscular scoliosis surgery. Unit rods and modular or "custom-contoured" systems are both frequently used for surgery, but each method has its own risks and benefits. Unit rods cost less than precontoured products and yield nearly "automatic" correction of pelvic obliquity, but can be quite difficult to tailor for use in patients with lumbar hyperlordosis and intrapelvic rotation. They work by cantilever moment arm correction and transverse approximation. Modular systems allow incorporation of additional correction mechanics, including compression, distraction, derotation, and separate pelvic obliquity correction. The corrective maneuvers can be adjusted as needed, and asymmetry of the pelvis can be accommodated. This greater versatility has resulted in increased use of modular systems and a relative decline in the use of unit rods. Nevertheless, the standards for complete pelvic obliquity correction, as well as the power of the cantilever maneuver, are permanent lessons taught by the unit rod. Both historical data and contemporary results are presented in this chapter to provide the reader with an in-depth understanding of both techniques.

Keywords: modular construct, pedicle screw, pelvic obliquity, posterior spinal fusion, scoliosis, sublaminar wires, unit rod

17.1 Introduction and Background

The unique nature of scoliosis in children with cerebral palsy (CP) presents many challenges for treatment. Instrumented spinal arthrodesis effectively corrects spinal deformity and spinopelvic obliquity in these patients.[1,2] The decision to pursue surgical correction in children with CP can be difficult. The indications for surgical correction are: (1) scoliosis that exceeds 50 degrees; (2) major impairment (current or predicted) of the patient's ability to function; or (3) presence of substantial pain.[3] The goal of operative management should be to achieve the greatest improvement of scoliotic deformity and pelvic obliquity possible without compromising safety. Sitting posture can be improved dramatically with simultaneous correction of pelvic obliquity by including the pelvis in the fusion.[4] Techniques for posterior spinal fusion have evolved over the past 30 years: early Harrington instrumentation and the later development of Luque rods, modified for the Galveston technique, have been major achievements in the operative treatment of neuromuscular scoliosis. However, the problems associated with each of these techniques led to development of the unit rod and modular constructs.

17.2 Unit Rod Construct

Galveston rod fixation consisted of paired Luque rods bent so they could be anchored in the ilium.[5] Differential migration of the two rods was partially solved by adding cross-links and, later, by joining the two rods together at the top as one unit in an inverted "U." This innovation by Moseley, in 1989, resulted in a one-piece, precontoured system of instrumentation that, when combined with sublaminar wires, followed the principles of the Luque–Galveston technique.[6] It allowed for stable, segmental fixation of the spine and pelvis. This produced better correction of spinal and pelvic deformity, as well as restoration of coronal and sagittal trunk balance.[6] Once the distal ends had been inserted and seated into the iliac wings, the proximal end of the rod could be cantilevered toward the midline, forcing the pelvis into a horizontal position. The curve of the spine could then be further corrected by transverse approximation of the apex of the curve to the rod with tightening of the sublaminar wires into the fixed vertical plane of the rod (▶ Fig. 17.1).[7]

In their review of the literature on degree of correction obtained using the unit rod, Tsirikos et al[2] analyzed a series of 287 children and adolescents with severe CP treated with the unit rod technique. They reported an excellent major curve correction of 68% and pelvic obliquity correction of 71%, with good lateral balance of the spine and a low rate of complications. The authors stated that the unit rod was the preferred system for the treatment of patients with CP for several reasons: its relative ease of use, lower cost compared with all–pedicle screw instrumentation, comparable deformity correction, low rate of loss of correction, and low rates of reoperation and complications. An earlier study by Bulman et al[7] found similar results, validating the use of the unit rod.

The unit rod produces near-automatic correction of pelvic obliquity. However, several drawbacks are notable. First, it is not optimal for correction of proximal thoracic curves because insertion must start from the pelvis and the cantilever mode of correction becomes less efficient the more proximal the deformity. Second, it is unable to compress the posterior column and correct major thoracic kyphosis for the same reasons. Third, developmental asymmetry of the pelvis in patients with CP may not match the typical pelvic anatomy on which the unit rod relies. Fourth, the many required laminotomies and passage of sublaminar wires contribute to increased bleeding. Fifth, lumbar hyperlordosis virtually necessitates that the unit rod be cut, recontoured, and reconnected with multiple connectors at the thoracolumbar junction. Because of these limitations, other modular systems developed to treat neuromuscular scoliosis have gained popularity.

17.3 Modular Constructs

All–pedicle -screw constructs have been used extensively in patients with adolescent idiopathic scoliosis. The convex rod can be placed first, and alignment is achieved through a cantilever maneuver combined with vertebral compression, translation, and derotation using the screws and the rods. The concave rod is placed second to augment the construct. Or, alternatively,

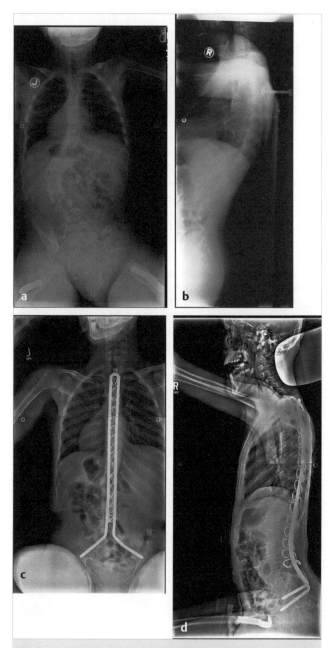

Fig. 17.1 A 13-year-old boy with cerebral palsy and scoliosis treated with unit rod. Radiographs showing (a) preoperative anteroposterior view; (b) preoperative lateral view; (c) postoperative anteroposterior view; and (d) postoperative lateral view. (These images are provided courtesy of the Harms Study Group database.)

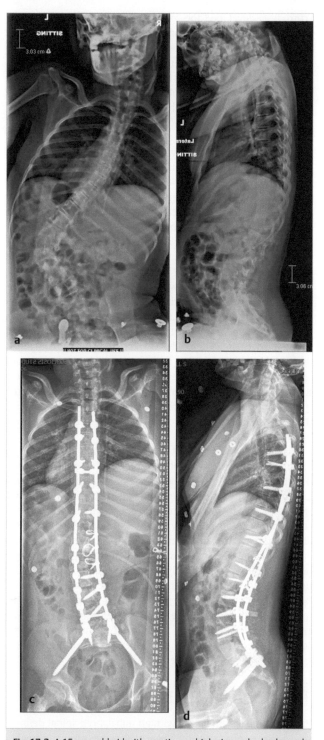

Fig. 17.2 A 15-year-old girl with spastic quadriplegic cerebral palsy and scoliosis treated with modular construct. Radiographs showing (a) preoperative anteroposterior view; (b) preoperative lateral view; (c) postoperative anteroposterior view; and (d) postoperative lateral view. (These images are provided courtesy of the Harms Study Group database.)

the concave rod can be placed first, the apex translated medially and dorsally, distracted to obtain kyphosis in the thoracic spine, and the convex rod placed to cantilever the apex to the midline and correct the rib prominence. The correction can be individually tailored to the patient. The development of modular constructs using screws, wires, and hooks has been advantageous in treating patients with neuromuscular scoliosis (▶ Fig. 17.2).

Tsirikos and Mains[8] reviewed 45 consecutive patients with severe CP (Gross Motor Function Classification System [GMFCS] level 5) who underwent spinal arthrodesis using pedicle screw/

rod instrumentation. They reported mean correction of 74% for scoliosis and 83% for pelvic obliquity, with loss of only 2.5 degrees of correction at a mean 3.5-year follow-up. None of their patients treated by posterior or anteroposterior spinal arthrodesis developed the "crankshaft" phenomenon, possibly because of the three-column fixation provided by segmental pedicle screws. (The crankshaft phenomenon, described by Dubousset et al,[9] occurs when posterior spinal fusion stops longitudinal growth in the posterior elements but the vertebral bodies continue to grow anteriorly and result in progressive angulation and rotation of the spine.) They reported no problems related to positioning of the iliac bolts or pelvic fixation of the construct, in contrast to the unit rod technique. Placement of the iliac screws was always performed after exposure of the pelvis and under direct visualization. They reported that, in patients with lumbar hyperlordosis and marked anterolateral pelvic tilt, it is easier and safer to place iliac screws than the pelvic legs of the unit rod, which can cut out from the osteopenic iliac bed. In their study, complications included one deep and five superficial wound infections treated with surgical debridement and antibiotics. There were no detected pseudarthroses and only one reoperation for prominent instrumentation. Their results compared favorably with their previous unit rod study,[2] in which 3 nonunions requiring revision surgery and 12 reoperations for prominent implants occurred more than 3 years after combined anteroposterior spine arthrodesis in 45 patients. In their 2012 study, Tsirikos and Mains[8] concluded that spinal correction using segmental pedicle screw/rod constructs can be performed safely and with fewer major complications and a lower reoperation rate compared with the traditional unit rod. After 3.5 years of postoperative follow-up, they reported that correction of spinopelvic imbalance was maintained.

In a similar study, Modi et al[10] reported on 52 patients with CP and various degrees of neurological involvement who underwent scoliosis correction through posterior-only spinal arthrodesis with pedicle screw instrumentation and mean follow-up of 3 years. Mean scoliosis correction was 63%. Overall correction of pelvic obliquity was 56% postoperatively and 43% at 3 years of follow-up. Compared with the study by Tsirikos and Mains,[8] in which all patients had quadriplegia with major pelvic obliquity, in the study by Modi et al, 20 patients had diplegia or hemiplegia, which explains the smaller degree of pelvic deformity.[10] They reported a 33% complication rate, including two perioperative deaths, one neurological deficit caused by screw penetration in the canal, one prominent pelvic screw that required removal, and several respiratory complications but no deep wound infections.

17.4 Pelvic Fixation

Progressive pelvic obliquity with an unbalanced spinal deformity adversely affects sitting balance, skin pressure, and quality of life.[11,12,13,14,15] Pelvic fixation is used in spinal deformity surgery for three purposes: (1) to improve correction of deformity, especially if the apex is in the lumbar spine; (2) to stabilize the lumbosacral junction to facilitate arthrodesis; and (3) to prevent add-on of the deformity in the lumbosacral area and improve sitting posture in a neurologically compromised patient with poor truncal control. Screws in the sacral vertebrae can provide fixation but these anchors cannot always withstand the loads applied, since the sacrum is largely cancellous bone. The use of long anchors projecting into the ilium past the "pivot point" has been shown by McCord et al[16] to provide the most

mechanically effective form of pelvic fixation because the moment of the anchors extends far anterior and lateral to the spine. Galveston and unit rods, as described earlier, were early applications of this. Recently, "modular" assemblies have become more popular, with screws individually placed into the ilia and joined to long rods, sometimes with connectors. This technique requires subfascial dissection to the posterior superior iliac spine, which may compromise the muscle flap. In addition, the anchors inserted through the posterior superior iliac spine are more prominent than those in the remainder of the implant and can loosen. For this reason, Chang et al[17] developed a trajectory to insert iliac screws through a sacral starting point using the widest screw possible (▶ Fig. 17.3). This starting point is immediately caudal to the starting point of S1 screws, at the top of the S2 ala, extending into the thickest portion of the ilium just above the sciatic notch. It traverses the fibrous or the articular portion of the sacroiliac joint (▶ Fig. 17.4). The trajectory allows a length nearly equal to that of traditional iliac screws, and the more oblique angle prevents them from backing out. The implant is in line with all of the other spinal anchors so that no connector is needed. The length and width of the implant allow pelvic obliquity to be corrected even in the presence of osteopenic bone. In a study with minimum 2-year follow-up, Sponseller et al[18] reviewed 32 consecutive pediatric patients who underwent sacral–alar–iliac (SAI) screw fixation compared with 27 patients with traditional pelvic fixation using sacral or iliac screws. In the SAI group, pelvic obliquity was corrected to less than 10 degrees in most cases. There were no cases of vascular or neurologic complications, deep infections, implant prominence, late skin breakdown, or anchor migration with SAI screw insertion. With the use of SAI or buried iliac screws, technical complications of pelvic fixation have become less common.

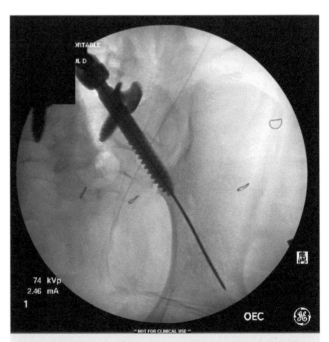

Fig. 17.3 Intraoperative fluoroscopic image of the starting point of sacral–alar–iliac screw insertion, which is immediately caudal to the starting point of S1 screws, at the top of the S2 ala.

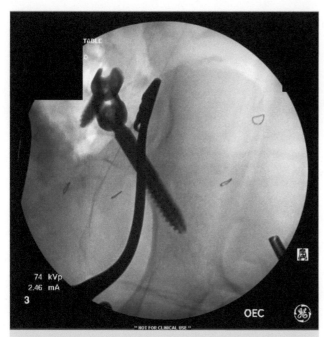

Fig. 17.4 Intraoperative fluoroscopic image of sacral–alar–iliac screw extending into the thickest portion of the ilium, just above the sciatic notch. It traverses the fibrous or the articular portion of the sacroiliac joint.

17.5 Blood Loss

Blood loss is a major risk in scoliosis surgery for patients with CP. This risk is especially high in patients in a hypocoagulable state caused by comorbidities or medication. Thomson and Banta[19] reported that patients taking antiseizure medications have greater blood loss perioperatively when undergoing scoliosis corrective surgery compared with patients not taking antiseizure medications. When comparing unit rod with modular construct fixation, Sponseller et al[20] reported that patients undergoing unit rod surgery did not have significantly more blood loss (2,124 vs. 1,885 mL, $p = 0.3$). Tsirikos and Mains,[8] in their prospective series of patients with CP treated with pedicle screw/rod instrumentation, compared surgical outcomes against a historical series of patients treated with unit rods or third-generation instrumentation and found that greater preoperative curve magnitudes correlated with greater intraoperative blood loss ($r = 0.56$). Furthermore, greater intraoperative blood loss was correlated with longer stays in the hospital ($r = 0.44$) or intensive care unit ($r = 0.53$). They also reported that greater preoperative pelvic obliquity was correlated with longer surgical time ($r = 0.58$), greater intraoperative blood loss ($r = 0.34$), and longer stays in the hospital ($r = 0.22$) or intensive care unit ($r = 0.44$). Teli et al[21] reported that blood loss was correlated with the degree of pelvic obliquity ($r = 0.29$) and number of operated levels. Various strategies employed by surgeons to reduce intraoperative bleeding are the following: reduced mean arterial pressure during the exposure only, antifibrinolytic use, and decreased operative time with two surgeons.

References

[1] Tsirikos AI. Development and treatment of spinal deformity in patients with cerebral palsy. Indian J Orthop. 2010; 44(2):148–158

[2] Tsirikos AI, Lipton G, Chang WN, Dabney KW, Miller F. Surgical correction of scoliosis in pediatric patients with cerebral palsy using the unit rod instrumentation. Spine. 2008; 33(10):1133–1140

[3] Lonstein JE, Akbarnia A. Operative treatment of spinal deformities in patients with cerebral palsy or mental retardation. An analysis of one hundred and seven cases. J Bone Joint Surg Am. 1983; 65(1):43–55

[4] Allen BL, Jr, Ferguson RL. The Galveston technique for L rod instrumentation of the scoliotic spine. Spine. 1982; 7(3):276–284

[5] Allen BL, Jr, Ferguson RL. The Galveston technique of pelvic fixation with L-rod instrumentation of the spine. Spine. 1984; 9(4):388–394

[6] Bell DF, Moseley CF, Koreska J. Unit rod segmental spinal instrumentation in the management of patients with progressive neuromuscular spinal deformity. Spine. 1989; 14(12):1301–1307

[7] Bulman WA, Dormans JP, Ecker ML, Drummond DS. Posterior spinal fusion for scoliosis in patients with cerebral palsy: a comparison of Luque rod and unit rod instrumentation. J Pediatr Orthop. 1996; 16(3):314–323

[8] Tsirikos AI, Mains E. Surgical correction of spinal deformity in patients with cerebral palsy using pedicle screw instrumentation. J Spinal Disord Tech. 2012; 25(7):401–408

[9] Dubousset J, Herring JA, Shufflebarger H. The crankshaft phenomenon. J Pediatr Orthop. 1989; 9(5):541–550

[10] Modi HN, Hong JY, Mehta SS, et al. Surgical correction and fusion using posterior-only pedicle screw construct for neuropathic scoliosis in patients with cerebral palsy: a three-year follow-up study. Spine. 2009; 34(11):1167–1175

[11] Dubousset J. Pelvic obliquity: a review. Orthopedics. 1991; 14(4):479–481

[12] Larsson EL, Aaro S, Normelli H, Oberg B. Weight distribution in the sitting position in patients with paralytic scoliosis: pre- and postoperative evaluation. Eur Spine J. 2002; 11(2):94–99

[13] Murans G, Gutierrez-Farewik EM, Saraste H. Kinematic and kinetic analysis of static sitting of patients with neuropathic spine deformity. Gait Posture. 2011; 34(4):533–538

[14] Patel J, Walker JL, Talwalkar VR, Iwinski HJ, Milbrandt TA. Correlation of spine deformity, lung function, and seat pressure in spina bifida. Clin Orthop Relat Res. 2011; 469(5):1302–1307

[15] Smith RM, Emans JB. Sitting balance in spinal deformity. Spine. 1992; 17(9):1103–1109

[16] McCord DH, Cunningham BW, Shono Y, Myers JJ, McAfee PC. Biomechanical analysis of lumbosacral fixation. Spine. 1992; 17(8) Suppl:S235–S243

[17] Chang TL, Sponseller PD, Kebaish KM, Fishman EK. Low profile pelvic fixation: anatomic parameters for sacral alar-iliac fixation versus traditional iliac fixation. Spine. 2009; 34(5):436–440

[18] Sponseller PD, Zimmerman RM, Ko PS, et al. Low profile pelvic fixation with the sacral alar iliac technique in the pediatric population improves results at two-year minimum follow-up. Spine. 2010; 35(20):1887–1892

[19] Thomson JD, Banta JV. Scoliosis in cerebral palsy: an overview and recent results. J Pediatr Orthop B. 2001; 10(1):6–9

[20] Sponseller PD, Shah SA, Abel MF, et al. Harms Study Group. Scoliosis surgery in cerebral palsy: differences between unit rod and custom rods. Spine. 2009; 34(8):840–844

[21] Teli M, Elsebaie H, Biant L, Noordeen H. Neuromuscular scoliosis treated by segmental third-generation instrumented spinal fusion. J Spinal Disord Tech. 2005; 18(5):430–438

18 Halo-Gravity Traction: An Adjunctive Treatment for Severe Spinal Deformity

Joshua M. Pahys and Amer F. Samdani

Abstract

Halo-gravity traction (HGT) has evolved from halo-femoral and halo-pelvic traction to become a safe and effective adjunctive tool in the treatment of severe spinal deformity in ambulatory and nonambulatory patients. HGT has been shown to potentially reduce the need for vertebral column resections as well as provide a means of optimizing a patient from a medical and nutritional standpoint prior to spinal surgery. HGT can be applied either before spinal surgery or between stages of a multistage procedure, with traction weight calculated based on a patient's total body weight. The timing and duration of HGT is surgeon-specific and is typically based on curve severity and rigidity, as well as the health of the patient. The indications for pre- and/or perioperative HGT include severe scoliosis or kyphosis > 100 degrees with limited flexibility (< 20%). Relative contraindications are cervical kyphosis and/or stenosis, ligamentous laxity, and open fontanelles. Complications during HGT are typically minor and include pin site irritation or infection, which can be treated with pin care, antibiotics, or pin removal. Neurologic injury, although extremely rare with HGT, has been reported. Studies on patients with HGT commonly involve a heterogeneous patient population; thus, it is challenging to reach a definitive consensus on indications and treatment protocols. However, a growing number of reports are substantiating the potential benefits of HGT for severe spinal deformity.

Keywords: halo-gravity traction, kyphosis, scoliosis, severe spinal deformity, vertebral column resection

18.1 Overview

Since the late 1950s, various forms of halo traction have been utilized as an adjunctive form of treatment in spinal deformity. Perry and Nickel[1] revised Bloom's fascial traction device to an aluminum tiara fixed to the skull with threaded pins. This was initially indicated for cervical paralysis related to poliomyelitis, but was later expanded to include severe scoliosis.[2] Several forms of halo traction have been described to date including halo femoral,[3,4] halo tibial,[5] halo pelvic,[6] and, more recently, halo gravity.[7,8,9]

Halo-femoral traction was utilized by Kane and colleagues[3] in 30 patients with scoliosis in whom the average curve was reduced from 112 to 58 degrees after final correction. Bonnett and colleagues[4] later reported a 53% correction with halo-femoral traction for patients with paralytic scoliosis. However, 28 of 37 patients sustained fractures after treatment was completed, 17 of which involved the femurs during simple range-of-motion exercises posttreatment. This study highlighted the potential significant complications associated with halo-femoral traction and bed rest as it relates to the loss of bone mineral density.

Halo-gravity traction (HGT) was then introduced building on work by Klaus Zielke and Pierre Stagnara.[7] HGT offers a distinct advantage over the previous treatments in that it affords significantly more versatility. HGT may be applied in a bed, a wheelchair, and/or a walking frame, allowing the patient to be upright and out of bed during treatment[8] (▶ Fig. 18.1).

There are several published series on HGT for severe spinal deformity.[7,8,9,10,11,12] The study by Sponseller and colleagues[9] is the lone level III study of the existing literature on HGT in which a retrospective, multicenter, nonrandomized comparison study of pediatric patients with severe scoliosis was performed. In this study, patients were treated with or without HGT based on surgeon preference. The study found no statistically significant difference between the HGT and the non-HGT groups with

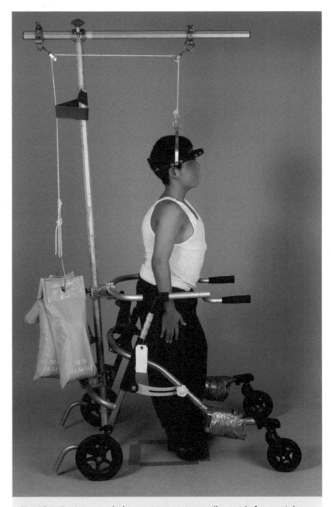

Fig. 18.1 Patient in a halo-gravity traction walker with free weights applied through a pulley system. A fold-down seat allows the patient to be seated while remaining in upright traction for rest and during mealtimes. A similar setup is utilized in wheelchair for nonambulatory patients.

regard to final curve correction, spinal length gain, blood loss, operating time, or complications. However, in this study, patients who underwent HGT required significantly fewer vertebral column resection procedures compared to patients who did not undergo HGT (3 vs. 30%, respectively; $p = 0.015$).

Rinella and colleagues[8] retrospectively reviewed 33 patients with severe scoliosis at a single center and demonstrated a 46% curve correction after HGT and spinal fusion with no neurologic deficits. No mention was made of curve correction while the patients were in HGT. Sink and colleagues[7] retrospectively reviewed 19 pediatric patients with severe scoliosis treated with HGT for 6 to 21 weeks and reported an average Cobb's correction of 35%. Watanabe and colleagues[10] reported a single-center retrospective review of 21 consecutive pediatric patients with scoliosis > 100 degrees. The study reported the greatest improvement in Cobb angle correction after 1 week of HGT (17.5%) and plateaued at 23.3% correction after 3 weeks of HGT. The reported final curve correction after fusion and HGT was 51.3%. No significant improvements in correction of the Cobb angle were noted with > 3 weeks of HGT.

Koller and colleagues[13] retrospectively reviewed 45 adult and pediatric patients with severe scoliosis and/or kyphosis treated with HGT. An improvement of only 8 and 7 degrees, respectively, was achieved in the coronal and sagittal planes with preoperative HGT, while a 9% improvement in forced vital capacity (FVC) was noted during preoperative HGT. Bogunovic and colleagues[11] reported an average deformity correction of 35%, with the majority of the correction occurring in the first 3 to 4 weeks of HGT (average HGT weight: 35.4% of total body weight [TBW]). Pulmonary function (FVC and forced expiratory volume 1 [FEV1]) similarly improved an average of 9% during HGT in this study.

Nemani et al[12] reported on 29 patients with an average coronal curve of 131 degrees who underwent HGT for an average of 107 days prior to definitive posterior spinal fusion or placement of growing rods. They reported an average major curve correction of 31% after HGT and a final correction of 56% postoperatively, with deformity correction plateauing at 63 days.

18.2 Preprocedure Planning

18.2.1 Indications and Contraindications for HGT

Radiographic indications for consideration of HGT vary considerably among studies and institutions; however, a coronal and/or sagittal Cobb angle of ≥ 90 to 110 degrees is typical. Curve flexibility has also been shown to play a role in consideration of HGT. Sponseller et al[9] utilized HGT for curves > 90 degrees with < 25% flexibility, while Watanabe et al[10] used the criteria of a Cobb angle > 100 degrees and < 20% curve flexibility as an indication for HGT. True contraindications have also not been fully agreed upon, but generally cervical kyphosis, cervical stenosis, ligamentous laxity, and/or open fontanelles are considered relative contraindications to HGT.

A head computed tomography (CT) or skull radiograph can be performed prior to halo placement, although this is not the standard practice at the authors' institution unless there are

specific concerns. Approximately 50% of respondents in a survey of spinal deformity surgeons obtain pre–halo placement imaging of the skull.[14] One must be acutely aware of prior surgery, especially the placement of ventriculoperitoneal (VP) shunts, as fracturing of these devices has been reported in HGT.[15]

18.2.2 Equipment

Halo Application

At our institution, we do not typically obtain studies prior to halo placement for evaluation of the skull. However, if the patient has undergone any cranial surgery (VP shunt), has poor bone density (osteogenesis imperfecta), or is very young (potentially open fontanelles), a head CT scan or skull radiographs should be obtained prior to halo placement.[16]

The most common determining factor for the number of pins used in HGT is the patient's age, followed by underlying diagnosis. Typically, in children younger than 8 years, four anterior pins are used, and for children 8 years and older, two anterior pins are used. Similarly, six posterior pins are utilized for children younger than 5 years, four to six pins for children 6 to 8 years of age, and four pins for children older than 8 years. In patients who have reached skeletal maturity, a total of four pins (two anterior and two posterior) may be sufficient.

The halo is applied under conscious sedation with local anesthesia in the operating room or procedure room. The halo is placed slightly below the equator of the skull, but above the orbits and superior aspect of the pinnae.[12] The ideal pin torque is also based on patient age and underlying diagnosis. We recommend the use of an adjustable torque wrench during halo placement starting at 2 inch-pounds (in-lb) and progressing in 1 to 2 in-lb increments. A goal of at least 4 in-lb is ideal. The greater the skull density, the more torque may be applied, to a maximum of 8 in-lb. If only a lower amount of torque is tolerated, the surgeon must then place additional pins to distribute the forces. The surgeon must be aware of avoiding the medial half of the orbits anteriorly so as not to injure the supraorbital nerve. Furthermore, avoiding pin placement in the temporal fossa is critical as this can injure the temporalis muscle, and the bone of this portion of the skull is relatively thin[16,17,18] (▶ Fig. 18.2).

Halo-Gravity Traction Apparatus

A modified walker for ambulatory patients or wheelchair for nonambulatory patients is utilized when the patient is out of bed. The walker device ideally has a fold-down seat so that the patient may remain in the traction walker for the entire day including meals and limit the number of necessary traction devices. The authors utilize free weights with a pulley system (▶ Fig. 18.1). Other institutions have reported the use of a calibrated spring/tension device (e.g., fish scale). A similar traction setup is used when the patient is in bed. The head of the bed should be elevated and/or the patient will need to be placed in reverse Trendelenburg to minimize cephalad migration overnight. The authors do not typically reduce the traction weight during sleeping hours,[12] but reducing the nighttime HGT weight by up to 50% has been reported.[11,19]

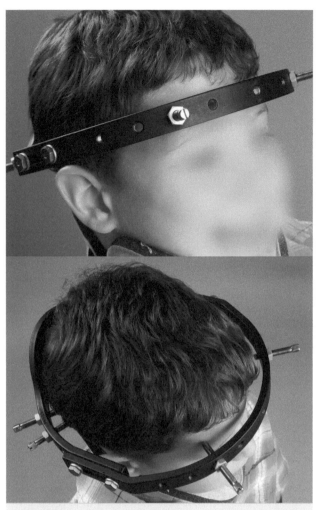

Fig. 18.2 The proper placement of halo pins is in the lateral one-third of the orbit anteriorly and above the pinnae posteriorly. The halo ring sits just below the equator of the skull.

18.2.3 Setup

Halo Weight Application and Management

The typical starting weight for HGT is 5 to 10 pounds based on the patient's age and weight. The goal HGT weight ranges from 33 to 50% of the patient's TBW.[9,11,12] Some studies have reported increasing the HGT weight until the patient is "barely touching" or "slightly off" the chair of their traction walker/wheelchair.[8]

The HGT weight can be increased once or twice a day. An increase of 2 to 5 pounds per day is typically reasonably well tolerated by patients. The authors have found that adding a smaller amount of weight, but doing so twice per day (e.g., 1–3 pounds added morning and afternoon) has improved patient comfort and decreased the timing to achieve the goal traction weight. Increases in HGT weight is dependent on patient comfort and continued thorough neurologic examinations. Goal traction weight can typically be achieved in 1 to 2 weeks, but may take as long as 4 weeks for larger patients.[12,14]

Duration of HGT

There are no clear guidelines or agreement regarding the optimum length of HGT. The decision is multifactorial and based on patient diagnosis and curve size/rigidity as well as pulmonary and nutritional status. The duration of HGT has been reported to be between 2 and 28 weeks.[7,9,11,12,19] Several studies have also reported on the efficacy of an additional 2 to 8 weeks of perioperative HGT if a staged release (anterior or posterior) procedure is performed.[8,10,19] Watanabe et al[10] reported a plateau in curve correction with HGT after 3 weeks. Park et al[20] found that 66% of the maximal coronal correction was achieved by 2 weeks of HGT, 88% by 3 weeks, and 96% by 4 weeks. Bogunovic et al[11] demonstrated maximal curve correction after an average of 42.6 days of HGT. Finally, Nemani et al[12] did not see a plateau in correction until 2 months of HGT. These differences are all likely due to the significant heterogeneity of the patients that are included in these studies as well as variations in technique and traction weight. The authors typically utilize HGT for 3 to 6 weeks prior to surgical intervention. If a staged procedure with anterior or posterior releases is planned, we typically do not utilize perioperative HGT for longer than 3 weeks between stages (▶ Fig. 18.3a–g).

Several studies[7,10,11] state that the duration of HGT was also dependent on the maximization of the patient's pulmonary and nutritional status. Bogunovic et al[11] reported an improvement in pulmonary function in 19 of 22 patients during HGT prior to surgical correction. Koller et al[13] demonstrated a 9% improvement in FVC% with HGT and recommended definitive surgical intervention after FVC% has improved or plateaued, typically around 2 weeks of HGT. Rizzi et al[21] noted a strong positive correlation between degree of curve correction and improvement in pulmonary function, while Zhang et al[22] demonstrated a trend toward increased postoperative complications in patients with poorer preoperative pulmonary function.

Imaging During HGT

The authors obtain weekly full-length biplanar radiographs from skull to pelvis during periods of HGT. This allows for assessment of the sagittal and coronal deformity as well as evaluation of the cervical spine. Dedicated cervical spine radiographs can be performed if there are any changes in the neurologic examination or if the patient's cognition limits his or her ability to undergo a complete neurologic examination.

18.2.4 Challenges and Complications

Patient Discomfort and Achieving Goal Traction Weight

Increasing HGT weight can be challenging for pediatric patients and families who are understandably going through physical and emotional discomfort as they acclimate to the treatment. As stated earlier, the authors prefer to spread out traction weight increases to twice a day to allow for less weight added at one time, reducing the potential that the patient will be cognizant of any changes. Patients typically complain of neck

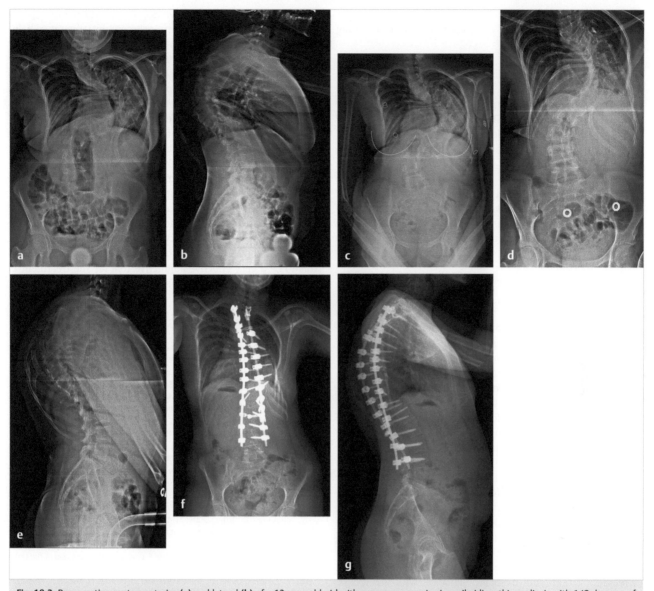

Fig. 18.3 Preoperative posteroanterior **(a)** and lateral **(b)** of a 13-year-old girl with severe progressive juvenile idiopathic scoliosis with 142 degrees of scoliosis and 102 degrees of kyphosis. The patient underwent 4 weeks of HGT and the coronal curve improved to 115 degrees **(c)**. This was followed by anterior diskectomies from T5–T11 and an additional 2 weeks of HGT with a subsequent coronal curve reduction to 100 degrees **(d)** and modest improvement in kyphosis **(e)** prior to the final surgery. Final postoperative posteroanterior **(f)** and lateral **(g)** radiographs after T2–L4 instrumented posterior spinal fusion with a main coronal Cobb of approximately 67 degrees and thoracic sagittal Cobb of 63 degrees.

discomfort initially with HGT. This has been well managed at our institution with small doses of benzodiazepines and/or low-dose narcotics. The authors have found that limited medications, if any, are required for discomfort after 1 to 2 weeks of HGT. The authors also stress the importance of involving additional hospital resources such child life services to assist the patient and family during the often-lengthy treatment time.

Neurologic Examinations

Scheduled formal neurologic examinations including cranial nerves as well as extremity motor and sensation are paramount during HGT. The frequency of exams in the literature ranges from every 4 to 24 hours during periods of HGT weight increase. After goal HGT weight is achieved, most studies agree

that neurologic examinations can be performed on a daily basis. The authors perform neurologic checks every 8 hours during periods of HGT weight increase. Only after the patient is comfortable at their goal HGT weight and demonstrates a stable neurologic examination do we reduce the frequency of neurologic checks to once daily.[11,12] The authors also regularly measure the distance from the pinnae and the tip of the nose to the halo ring to assess for migration of the device.

Pin Care

Pin care is performed at our institution once per day with soap and water. In a survey of surgeons who use HGT, pin care was performed by 83% of respondents, and five different solutions were used.[14] Diluted hydrogen peroxide has also been described as a common pin care solution.[7,19] Several studies have also reported that they do not use any pin care during HGT.[8,10,11]

Pin Site Infection

Pin site infection and/or loosening is the most frequently reported complication for HGT, ranging from 19 to 38%.[11,12,19] This is typically treated with local wound care with or without the addition of oral antibiotics. For pin tract infections that continue despite conservative measures, the pin should be removed and relocated if an additional safe insertion site is available. The pin sites should also be assessed to determine if any loosening has occurred, as the pins may need to be retightened. Some studies retorque the pins on a weekly basis during HGT,[12] while others retorque the pins only if there is evidence of loosening.[11]

Neurologic Injury

As stated earlier, it is critical to perform regular cranial nerve and motor/sensory examinations during HGT. Neurologic changes including transient nystagmus, oral numbness, cranial nerve palsies (notably cranial nerves VI and XII), brachial plexus palsy, and paralysis have been reported with HGT.[7,8,23,24,25] It has been felt that the most common problem leading to neurologic injury was excessive traction applied too rapidly. The benefit of HGT is that it allows for the gradual correction of the spinal deformity and stretching of the spinal cord in an awake patient who can provide continuous feedback.[12]

If any neurologic deficits arise, the first step is to reduce the traction weight immediately to the previous weight that was well tolerated by the patient. If there is no immediate improvement in the neurologic deficit, the weight is reduced by 50%, and then to zero if the deficit persists. Imaging of the spine with magnetic resonance imaging (MRI) and/or CT of skull is then necessary. While catastrophic complications such as paralysis have been reported, they are rare. Surgeons should exercise increased caution and maintain vigilance with neurologic exams in patients whose cognition limits their ability to communicate.

Craniocervical Complications

Fracture of a VP shunt has been reported with placement of HGT.[15] Therefore, preoperative imaging and discussion with the neurosurgeon is paramount prior to placing a halo ring for these patients. Although rare, there have also been reports of more severe complications related to halo placement such as osteomyelitis of the skull and extradural abscess as a result of pin tract infection.[26,27] Increased cervical degenerative changes postoperatively secondary to the potential loss of cervical lordosis during HGT have also been postulated.[28]

Additional Techniques Specific to Neuromuscular Scoliosis

Increased curve rigidity and severe pelvic obliquity are encountered in patients with neuromuscular scoliosis, specifically those with spastic quadriplegic cerebral palsy (CP). As with any severe deformity, perioperative HGT can be utilized to improve curve magnitude before or during surgery. Intraoperative halo-femoral traction has been reported to provide improved curve correction and significant reduction in pelvic obliquity for non-ambulatory CP patients. Takeshita et al[29] reported significantly improved main curve and pelvic obliquity correction with patients who had intraoperative halo-femoral traction compared to those who did not. Keeler et al[30] demonstrated similar curve correction when halo-femoral traction was used for a posterior spinal fusion versus anteroposterior spinal fusion.

Building on this principle, Buchowski et al[31,32] described the use of temporary internal distraction as an aid to correct severe scoliosis and/or pelvic obliquity. In the setting of severe pelvic obliquity, the surgeon can place a temporary rod on the concave pelvis and ipsilateral spine and/or ribs to gradually correct the deformity and pelvic obliquity by periodically distracting the temporary rod during the procedure. The authors have found this to be a very effective adjunctive tool for the treatment of severe neuromuscular scoliosis.

References

[1] Perry J, Nickel VL. Total cervical spine fusion for neck paralysis. J Bone Joint Surg Am. 1959; 41-A(1):37–60

[2] Nickel VL, Perry J, Garrett A, Heppenstall M. The halo. A spinal skeletal traction fixation device. J Bone Joint Surg Am. 1968; 50(7):1400–1409

[3] Kane WJ, Moe JH, Lai CC. Halo-femoral pin distraction in the treatment of scoliosis. J Bone Joint Surg Am. 1967; 49:1018–1019

[4] Bonnett C, Brown JC, Perry J, et al. Evolution of treatment of paralytic scoliosis at Rancho Los Amigos Hospital. J Bone Joint Surg Am. 1975; 57(2):206–215

[5] Schmidt AC. Halo-tibial traction combined with the Milwaukee Brace. Clin Orthop Relat Res. 1971; 77(77):73–83

[6] Edgar MA, Chapman RH, Glasgow MM. Pre-operative correction in adolescent idiopathic scoliosis. J Bone Joint Surg Br. 1982; 64(5):530–535

[7] Sink EL, Karol LA, Sanders J, Birch JG, Johnston CE, Herring JA. Efficacy of perioperative halo-gravity traction in the treatment of severe scoliosis in children. J Pediatr Orthop. 2001; 21(4):519–524

[8] Rinella A, Lenke L, Whitaker C, et al. Perioperative halo-gravity traction in the treatment of severe scoliosis and kyphosis. Spine. 2005; 30(4):475–482

[9] Sponseller PD, Takenaga RK, Newton P, et al. The use of traction in the treatment of severe spinal deformity. Spine. 2008; 33(21):2305–2309

[10] Watanabe K, Lenke LG, Bridwell KH, Kim YJ, Hensley M, Koester L. Efficacy of perioperative halo-gravity traction for treatment of severe scoliosis (≥ 100°). J Orthop Sci. 2010; 15(6):720–730

[11] Bogunovic L, Lenke LG, Bridwell KH, Luhmann SJ. Preoperative halo-gravity traction for severe pediatric spinal deformity. Complications, radiographic correction and changes in pulmonary function. Spine Deform. 2013; 1(1):33–39

[12] Nemani VM, Kim HJ, Bjerke-Kroll BT, et al. FOCOS Spine Study Group. Preoperative halo-gravity traction for severe spinal deformities at an SRS-GOP site in West Africa: protocols, complications, and results. Spine. 2015; 40 (3):153–161

[13] Koller H, Zenner J, Gajic V, Meier O, Ferraris L, Hitzl W. The impact of halo-gravity traction on curve rigidity and pulmonary function in the treatment of severe and rigid scoliosis and kyphoscoliosis: a clinical study and narrative review of the literature. Eur Spine J. 2012; 21(3):514–529

[14] Pahys JM, Cahill PJ, D'Amato C, Asghar J, Betz RR. Chest Wall & Spine Deformity Study Group. Indications and treatment protocols for halo gravity traction in severe pediatric scoliosis: a survey of the experts. 47th Scoliosis Research Society Annual Meeting; September 5–8, 2012; Chicago, IL

[15] Blakeney WG, D'Amato C. Ventriculoperitoneal shunt fracture following application of halo-gravity traction: a case report. J Pediatr Orthop. 2015; 35 (6):e52–e54

[16] Wong WB, Haynes RJ. Osteology of the pediatric skull. Considerations of halo pin placement. Spine. 1994; 19(13):1451–1454

[17] Garfin SR, Roux R, Botte MJ, Centeno R, Woo SL. Skull osteology as it affects halo pin placement in children. J Pediatr Orthop. 1986; 6(4):434–436

[18] Chavasiri C, Chavasiri S. The thickness of skull at the halo pin insertion site. Spine. 2011; 36(22):1819–1823

[19] Garabekyan T, Hosseinzadeh P, Iwinski HJ, et al. The results of preoperative halo-gravity traction in children with severe spinal deformity. J Pediatr Orthop B. 2014; 23(1):1–5

[20] Park DK, Braaksma B, Hammerberg KW, Sturm P. The efficacy of preoperative halo-gravity traction in pediatric spinal deformity: the effect of traction duration. J Spinal Disord Tech. 2013; 26(3):146–154

[21] Rizzi PE, Winter RB, Lonstein JE, Denis F, Perra JH. Adult spinal deformity and respiratory failure. Surgical results in 35 patients. Spine. 1997; 22(21):2517–2530, discussion 2531

[22] Zhang JG, Wang W, Qiu GX, Wang YP, Weng XS, Xu HG. The role of preoperative pulmonary function tests in the surgical treatment of scoliosis. Spine. 2005; 30(2):218–221

[23] MacEwen GD, Bunnell WP, Sriram K. Acute neurological complications in the treatment of scoliosis. A report of the Scoliosis Research Society. J Bone Joint Surg Am. 1975; 57(3):404–408

[24] Ginsburg GM, Bassett GS. Hypoglossal nerve injury caused by halo-suspension traction. A case report. Spine. 1998; 23(13):1490–1493

[25] Qian BP, Qiu Y, Wang B. Brachial plexus palsy associated with halo traction before posterior correction in severe scoliosis. Stud Health Technol Inform. 2006; 123:538–542

[26] Humbyrd DE, Latimer FR, Lonstein JE, Samberg LC. Brain abscess as a complication of halo traction. Spine. 1981; 6(4):365–368

[27] Tindall GT, Flanagan JF, Nashold BS, Jr. Brain abscess and osteomyelitis following skull traction. A report of three cases. Arch Surg. 1959; 79:638–641

[28] O'Brien JP, Yau AC, Hodgson AR. Halo pelvic traction: a technic for severe spinal deformities. Clin Orthop Relat Res. 1973(93):179–190

[29] Takeshita K, Lenke LG, Bridwell KH, Kim YJ, Sides B, Hensley M. Analysis of patients with nonambulatory neuromuscular scoliosis surgically treated to the pelvis with intraoperative halo-femoral traction. Spine. 2006; 31(20):2381–2385

[30] Keeler KA, Lenke LG, Good CR, Bridwell KH, Sides B, Luhmann SJ. Spinal fusion for spastic neuromuscular scoliosis: is anterior releasing necessary when intraoperative halo-femoral traction is used? Spine. 2010; 35(10):E427–E433

[31] Buchowski JM, Bhatnagar R, Skaggs DL, Sponseller PD. Temporary internal distraction as an aid to correction of severe scoliosis. J Bone Joint Surg Am. 2006; 88(9):2035–2041

[32] Buchowski JM, Skaggs DL, Sponseller PD. Temporary internal distraction as an aid to correction of severe scoliosis. Surgical technique. J Bone Joint Surg Am. 2007; 89 Suppl 2 Pt.2:297–309

19 Osteotomies: Ponte and Vertebral Column Resection

Scott C. Wagner, Ronald A. Lehman Jr., and Lawrence G. Lenke

Abstract

Performing osteotomies of the spine for the purposes of complex deformity correction is technically demanding and requires advanced surgical knowledge of spinal anatomy and biomechanics. Posterior osteotomies range in complexity from Ponte osteotomies, or segmental removal of the posterior elements, to complete resection of the vertebral column. The extent of the resection for a successful Ponte osteotomy includes resection of the inferior portion of the spinous process, bilateral facet joints, inferior lamina, interspinous ligaments, and ligamentum flavum at each level. A vertebral column resection is complete, 360-degree removal of the spinal column at the intended level. Each osteotomy offers powerful deformity correction capabilities to varying degrees, and careful preoperative planning is essential to decrease the potential for catastrophic complications. Halo traction prior to the procedure can aid in straightening the deformity and allow for gradual stretching of the neural elements, and intraoperative neuromonitoring is mandatory during the surgery. Deformity correction utilizing these techniques has been shown to provide patients with pain relief and improve functional outcomes. While the surgical technique is challenging and associated with significant operative time and blood loss—and revision surgery is likely—patients undergoing this procedure may still expect improved function and satisfaction postoperatively. This chapter will focus on the patient selection process, preparation, and set-up, as well as the techniques to successfully perform these intricate techniques. With careful and diligent methods in all aspects of surgical treatment, successful deformity correction and excellent patient outcomes can be achieved.

Keywords: Ponte osteotomy, posterior osteotomy, scoliosis, spinal deformity, vertebral column resection

19.1 Preprocedure Planning

Posterior osteotomies of the spine and vertebral column resection (VCR) are technically demanding surgical procedures that allow for significant correction of spinal deformity. Vertebrectomy as a surgical technique for scoliosis was originally described in the early twentieth century,[1] though more recent techniques began to appear in the literature in the 1970s and 1980s.[2,3,4] The benefit of these techniques is that a circumferential approach to complex three-dimension deformities allows for better control and improved correction. Pedicle screw and rod constructs have provided for increased stability and the ability to manipulate these deformities, and throughout the 1990s these osteotomy techniques became more widespread in pediatric and adult patients.[5,6] The Ponte-type procedure consists of posterior column disruption via segmental osteotomies, while VCR involves complete resection of the anterior vertebral body, both of which are accomplished via a posterior-only approach.[7,8,9,10,11] In fact, we typically perform all VCR procedures with Ponte osteotomies (POs) as the initial phase of the surgery, which has obviated the requirement for traditional anterior and posterior approaches and provides complete access to the spinal column and spinal cord during the disarticulation process of deformity correction.[12] Most important to note, however, is that these types of severe deformity-correction procedures are technically demanding and are typically performed only by experienced surgical teams.[7,13] The risk of neurologic compromise and injury is very high, related to both the types of spinal deformities undergoing correction and the complete instability of the spinal column inherent with posterior-column osteotomies and VCR.[3,9] Appropriate patient selection, thorough preoperative planning, and comprehensive postoperative management protocols are of utmost importance for successful utilization of POs and VCR procedures. Every patient being considered for surgical management of severe spinal deformity must be counseled for the risk of catastrophic complications, and the operating surgeon must be vigilant in preparation for the procedure.

Unique considerations for preoperative planning in patients with neuromuscular scoliosis must also be included in the preprocedural period.[9,14,15] Proximal muscle weakness and spasticity often lead to development of progressive, severe scoliotic deformities that limit function and lead to sitting discomfort.[14] The goal of surgical intervention in this population therefore has less to do with correction of limited coronal or sagittal deformities, but rather to restore the sitting balance of the patient and minimize the risk of development of pressure sores, or for relief of positional difficulties. For particularly severe deformities in neuromuscular patients requiring restoration of sitting balance, VCR allows for the most significant correction.[14] However, it cannot be overstated that the rate of complications in these patients is also higher than other patient populations, typically due to the high rate of associated comorbidities in patients with neuromuscular scoliosis.[9,14,15] The potential for significant intraoperative blood loss is high with the highest mean percent blood loss typically occurring in patients with higher magnitude coronal and sagittal corrections required.[14] Strategies to minimize surgical time and blood loss are highly important, and it is recommended that various antifibrinolytics be utilized to aid in decreasing overall operative loss. We currently recommend tranexamic acid (TXA) as our intraoperative antifibrinolytic. We administer TXA at a 100 mg/kg loading dose, with a 10 mg/kg maintenance dose throughout the case. Anecdotally, we believe that doing so decreases blood loss 25 to 50% intraoperatively.[16]

19.2 Setup

With the advent of posterior-only techniques like the PO and VCR, intraoperative repositioning is no longer required. Therefore, initial prone positioning on a standard radiolucent orthopaedic table is sufficient for the case. Fluoroscopy is utilized throughout the case. Generally, cranial tongs are placed in the operating room to provide traction if the type and nature of the deformity necessitate doing so; keeping the face and eyes free but the base of the skull anchored in place allows for control of the proximal deformity during correction and protects the face from significant pressure in the prone position. The abdomen hangs free and the arms remain abducted and externally rotated unless contractures do not permit doing so. It is not uncommon for the positioning of the patient to be time-consuming, given the severity of these spinal deformities, but proper positioning can minimize the occurrence of skin injuries or brachial plexopathies and is important for patient safety. When performing complex deformity reduction such as VCR, we employ POs at the periapical region to improve flexibility and exposure of the resection level; thus, any discussion of VCR mandates discussion of the PO technique.

19.2.1 Spinal Cord Monitoring

We recommend complete spinal cord monitoring during all deformity cases requiring PO and/or VCR. Intraoperatively, we employ somatosensory evoked potentials (SSEPs) and transcranial motor evoked potentials (TcMEPs) or neurogenic mixed evoked potentials (NMEPs). Spinal motor conduction can be evaluated by TcMEPs.[17] Upper extremity SSEPs can be used to monitor for any developing brachial plexopathy, while electromyography (EMG) can be used to monitor the activity of lumbar nerve roots in a spontaneous elicited fashion. To evaluate for any violation of the pedicle wall into the canal during placement of pedicle screws, we also use stimulus triggered EMGs of the screws from T6–T12, as well as in the entire lumbar spine to S1. Neuromonitoring changes that necessitate surgical readjustment occur in approximately 10 to 15% of cases with significant deformity.[9,18] If neuromonitoring is not practical or obtainable, such as is the case in patients with previously treated intraspinal anomalies or neurologic conditions like Charcot–Marie–Tooth disease, frequent wake-up tests will be mandatory to corroborate neural integrity. These patients have a recognized higher risk of neurologic deficit postoperatively and should be counseled for such prior to the initiation of any surgical treatment.[13]

19.3 Surgical Technique and Challenges

Complete subperiosteal dissection to the lateral extent of the transverse processes is performed, including all levels that will be included in the posterior instrumentation construct. Depending on the type of the deformity, often exposure of the convex transverse processes of the apical thoracic vertebrae may require medial rib thoracoplasties. We recommend intraoperative fluoroscopic imaging to properly identify the exposed vertebral levels.

19.4 Ponte Osteotomy

The Ponte osteotomy (PO) is a posterior-only procedure, first described by Alberto Ponte in the 1980s, for the treatment of idiopathic kyphosis in skeletally mature patients. The procedure consists of posterior column shortening via segmental resection of posterior elements including the ligamentum flavum and bilateral facet joints.[19,20] Technically, since these procedures may be utilized in unfused segments, an actual surgical osteotomy is not obligatory. However, in patients with complex spinal deformity, autofusion has typically occurred to varying degrees, and because significant osseous removal is required regardless of the site involved, the technicality of the name is generally considered irrelevant. The extent of the resection for a successful PO includes resection of the inferior portion of the spinous process, bilateral facet joints, inferior lamina, interspinous ligaments, and ligamentum flavum at each level.[21] By spreading the resection over many levels, the overall correction achievable is greatly increased. Otherwise, only a few degrees of correction can be achieved with an isolated PO. In addition, because the resection is limited to posterior elements, if there is significant fusion in the middle or anterior columns, any substantial correction would be difficult without a concomitant anterior or circumferential procedure, such as complete VCR. In our experience, performing multilevel POs at the apex of the deformity prior to VCR allows for improved mobility and better correction after completion of the VCR.

Once exposure is complete and the periapical region is appropriately identified, we perform individual notching and excision of approximately 4 mm of the inferior facet at each level. The ligamentum flavum is now exposed and is removed; thus, the superior articulating facets can be removed above the pedicles at the levels involved in the osteotomy. Not only do these multilevel POs increase the flexibility of the periapical region, but they also improve visualization of the pedicles by exposing the medial border of the pedicle walls and protecting the spinal canal. The deformity can be so severe that doing so is the only feasible mechanism by which to safely place pedicle screws in the apical vertebrae; direct palpation of the medial wall allows for placement of the screws under visualization and can prevent intracanal breach of the screw tips. Of note, in patients with very severe angular kyphosis at the apex of the deformity, there exists significant risk for sagging of the spinal column and ventral collapse and crush injury to the spinal cord; in these cases, we place temporary stabilizing rods with pedicle screw fixation prior to resection of the posterior column.

We proceed with placement of pedicle screws after performing POs for all cases in which a VCR is being planned. Segmental fixation, proceeding from distal to proximal, allows for construct stability at the site of the resection. The freehand technique of Kim et al[22] is utilized, which prioritizes anatomical landmarks and employs a blunt gearshift to safely identify the screw tract. As noted previously, placement of an apical concave screw is not attempted unless visualization of the spinal canal and medial pedicle border has been achieved through POs or adjacent laminectomies. However, convex thoracic periapical screws may be placed safely without direct exposure of the medial wall, as the spinal cord typically falls to the contralateral side of the canal. Fluoroscopic guidance is useful at this time to confirm appropriate placement of pedicle screws. Multiaxial reduction screws are placed at the immediately adjacent levels of the resection site and are used for temporary rod placement around the apex and the ends of kyphotic deformities. EMG is performed for all screws placed from T6 caudal to S1 to assess for wall violations.

19.5 Vertebral Column Resection

Complete, subperiosteal exposure of the medial 5 cm of the ribs adjacent to the resection level is required and allows bilateral costotransversectomies to be performed without canal intrusion. Resected ribs may be utilized to fill the laminectomy defects at the end of the procedure and are useful as structural bone graft. Laminectomy then proceeds in the standard fashion, extending from the inferior aspect of the superior pedicles to the superior aspect of the inferior pedicles below the VCR. This maneuver exposes the entire dural sac and all adhesions or intracanal fibrous tissue can be excised. Generally, for a single-level VCR, there will now be a 5-cm laminectomy defect, and the convex thoracic nerve roots are ligated. Temporary clamping of the involved convex roots with continuous spinal cord monitoring prevents inadvertent ligation of spinal cord vasculature, and if there is no change in the monitoring profile the nerve root can be successfully transected as close to the dural sac as possible. Anecdotally, we have found that ligation of multiple thoracic roots unilaterally has not caused any neurologic compromise, nor have we seen any sensory deficit to the chest wall, provided that fewer than three or four roots are ligated. Concave roots are maintained whenever possible, and the lumbar nerve roots are obviously not ligated.

A temporary stabilizing rod is attached to at least two or three pedicle screws both above and below the resection area. Classically, a unilateral rod is used; however, in severe angular kyphotic or kyphoscoliotic deformities, bilateral rods are recommended to prevent subluxation of the spinal column. The pedicles to be resected are encircled, and the vertebral body resection begins by gaining access to its cancellous bone through a lateral pedicle-body entrance. The cancellous bone of the vertebral body is curetted, and all removed bone is saved for graft. For a patient with pure scoliosis or kyphoscoliosis, the majority of the vertebral body will be removed from the convexity of the deformity. Indeed, resecting the apical concave pedicle can be quite challenging. The pedicle encountered during this step tends to be extremely sclerotic, with no cancellous channel, and often the entire dural sac rests on the medial concave pedicle. However, the pedicle on the concavity may not even have an associated ventral vertebral body, as it is often rotated laterally and dorsally on the convexity of the deformity. It is our preference to utilize a small, high-speed burr to carefully remove the cortical bone along the concavity of the deformity while carefully protecting the adjacent dural sac/spinal cord. By performing the concave resection of the pedicle prior to the convexity, bleeding into the dependent concave region is minimized. Doing so also allows the concave dural sac to drift medially, thereby reducing tension on the cord prior to completion of the corpectomy. Following subperiosteal exposure of the lateral portion of the vertebral body and placement of a malleable or "spoon" retractor to protect the adjacent vascular structures and viscera, the entire body is thus removed except for the anterior shell. Maintaining a thin rim of bone on the anterior longitudinal ligament, in theory, improves fusion. However, if the anterior bone is very dense, it must be thinned to allow easy closure of the resection area.

Diskectomies above and below the corpectomy site are now performed. It is important that the endplates of the superior and inferior adjacent vertebral bodies are not violated, as placement of a structural intracorporeal cage may be required. Epidural bleeding must be controlled, and hemostasis can be achieved through the judicious use of bipolar cauterization, topical hemostatic agents and cottonoids. The dural sac must be circumferentially exposed and separated from the epidural venous complex, as well as from the posterior longitudinal ligament. The posterior vertebral wall may then be removed in its entirety with reverse-angled curettes, Kerrison rongeurs, Woodson elevators, or specialized posterior wall impactors. It is imperative that the ventral spinal cord is completely free of any bony prominences to avoid impingement during closure of the osteotomy. Osteophytosis of the adjacent disk levels may cause ventral compression, and careful resection of any bony prominences at these levels must be performed.

The vertebral body resection is now complete. Closure of the resected area always begins with compression forces applied on the convexity, with initial shortening of the spinal column and convex compression as the main correcting vector. In primary cases with good bone stock, this technique is performed with individual pedicle screws. Alternatively, a construct-to-construct closure mechanism utilizing domino connectors at the apex of the resected area may be performed. This method distributes the forces of correction over several vertebral levels and functions in a stepwise fashion by closing the osteotomy from a construct rod above to a construct rod below. It is imperative to compress deliberately and to monitor the dural sac as vertebral subluxation or dural impingement can occur during this step of the operation. If the patient's deformity has any degree of kyphosis, we often place an anterior structural cage to prevent overshortening of the deformity. The cage also acts as a hinge to provide further kyphosis correction. We also prefer to place an intervertebral cage on all posterior VCR procedures to provide shear force stabilization by the interdigitation of the tines of the cage into the endplates above and below and also to procure an anterior fusion. Once the closure has been completed and appropriate correction maneuvers performed, a permanent contralateral rod is placed. The temporary closing rod is removed and a permanent, final rod is placed on the ipsilateral side. Appropriate compression and distraction forces, in situ contouring, and other correction techniques may be performed. Careful and repetitive palpation of the dural sac circumferentially is performed at every iterative step of the correction to confirm that it is free and not under undue tension, impingement, or buckling.

Adequate alignment is confirmed by intraoperative radiographs. Decortication and bone grafting follow, with copious amounts of local graft obtained from the resection procedure. The laminectomy defect is covered with the previously harvested ribs from the costotransversectomy approach. Preferentially, the ribs are cut longitudinally, and the cancellous surface is placed along the entire laminectomy defect. This structural grafting of the laminectomy protects the dura and provides a posterior onlay fusion. The rib is held in place with sutures or a crosslink. Lastly, we always confirm the absence of any dural impingement, final implant security is documented, and intact spinal cord monitoring data are recorded. Per protocol, the wound is closed over suction drains. Final radiographs and an intraoperative wake-up test are performed before exiting the operating room to verify radiographic deformity correction and maintenance of neurologic status prior to extubation, respectively.

19.6 Complications

The overall complication rate of posterior-only VCR has been reported up to 59%,[7,9,14,18,23] related to age older than 60 years, medical comorbidities, and patient body mass index.[24] Despite the relatively high risk of complications postoperatively, overall patient outcomes may improve in the long term.[18]

19.6.1 Neurologic Complications

The spine is rendered highly unstable during these osteotomy procedures, and changes in neuromonitoring are common after the deformity has been corrected.[13,25] Preoperative neurologic deficit is a significant risk factor for neurologic sequelae in the postoperative period and must be carefully considered and discussed with each individual patient.[23] Spinal cord monitoring is mandatory throughout these types of cases, and any changes can be addressed via improvement in the mean arterial pressure, thorough ventral decompression and/or restoration of anterior height. Most neurologic complications are relatively minor and involve transient motor or sensory deficits. Changes in neuromonitoring, as well as neurologic dysfunction documented by intraoperative wake-up test, are commonly encountered.[9] Our institutional experience has suggested that patients with severe kyphoscoliosis are at higher risk for major neurologic compromise postoperatively.[18] Kim et al[23] found a 3.3% rate of permanent neurologic deficit, while a separate series found gait deterioration in 2 of 11 patients postoperatively.[12] Though the risk of major neurologic injury is relatively high, it is plausible that attentive neuromonitoring has allowed for timely intervention during the procedure, and has reduced the incidence of such complications.[9,15]

19.6.2 Non-Neurologic Complications

In addition to the risk of neurologic injury, postoperative pulmonary complications are common and are likely related to the thoracic insufficiency and anatomic deformities present in these patients.[9] Chest tubes may be placed in a prophylactic manner if the risk of pneumothorax is high.[12] In one small series ($N=28$) of patients with thoracic or thoracolumbar deformities greater than 100 degrees, eight patients required chest tube placement, three patients sustained acute pulmonary edema during surgery, and three other patients developed postoperative pneumonia.[26] Posterior wound infection rates have been reported at 4%,[9] though wound infections deep to the fascia are uncommon.[27,28,29] However, a study reported by Papadopoulos et al[12] reported a surgical debridement rate of 8.9% after major posterior spinal deformity surgery. Lastly, the overall revision rate after VCR is as high as 22.2%.[12] Patients must be counseled preoperatively that these risks are significant, and the benefits of surgery must be carefully weighed.

References

[1] MacLennan A. Scoliosis. BMJ. 1922; 2:864–866
[2] Leatherman KD. The management of rigid spinal curves. Clin Orthop Relat Res. 1973(93):215–224
[3] Leatherman KD, Dickson RA. Two-stage corrective surgery for congenital deformities of the spine. J Bone Joint Surg Br. 1979; 61-B(3):324–328
[4] Bradford D, ed. Vertebral column resection. Association of Bone and Joint Surgeons Annual Meeting, Kiawah Island, SC; 1987: Orthop Trans
[5] Boachie-Adjei O, Bradford DS. Vertebral column resection and arthrodesis for complex spinal deformities. J Spinal Disord. 1991; 4(2):193–202
[6] Bradford DS, Tribus CB. Vertebral column resection for the treatment of rigid coronal decompensation. Spine. 1997; 22(14):1590–1599
[7] Suk SI, Chung ER, Kim JH, Kim SS, Lee JS, Choi WK. Posterior vertebral column resection for severe rigid scoliosis. Spine. 2005; 30(14):1682–1687
[8] Suk SI, Chung ER, Lee SM, Lee JH, Kim SS, Kim JH. Posterior vertebral column resection in fixed lumbosacral deformity. Spine. 2005; 30(23):E703–E710
[9] Lenke LG, Newton PO, Sucato DJ, et al. Complications after 147 consecutive vertebral column resections for severe pediatric spinal deformity: a multicenter analysis. Spine. 2013; 38(2):119–132
[10] Dorward IG, Lenke LG. Osteotomies in the posterior-only treatment of complex adult spinal deformity: a comparative review. Neurosurg Focus. 2010; 28(3):E4
[11] Jeszenszky D, Haschtmann D, Kleinstück FS, et al. Posterior vertebral column resection in early onset spinal deformities. Eur Spine J. 2014; 23(1):198–208
[12] Papadopoulos EC, Boachie-Adjei O, Hess WF, et al. Early outcomes and complications of posterior vertebral column resection. Spine J. 2015; 15(5):983–991
[13] Lenke LG, Sides BA, Koester LA, Hensley M, Blanke KM. Vertebral column resection for the treatment of severe spinal deformity. Clin Orthop Relat Res. 2010; 468(3):687–699
[14] Sponseller PD, Jain A, Lenke LG, et al. Vertebral column resection in children with neuromuscular spine deformity. Spine. 2012; 37(11):E655–E661
[15] Lenke LG, O'Leary PT, Bridwell KH, Sides BA, Koester LA, Blanke KM. Posterior vertebral column resection for severe pediatric deformity: minimum two-year follow-up of thirty-five consecutive patients. Spine. 2009; 34(20):2213–2221
[16] Newton PO, Bastrom TP, Emans JB, et al. Antifibrinolytic agents reduce blood loss during pediatric vertebral column resection procedures. Spine. 2012; 37(23):E1459–E1463
[17] Calancie B, Harris W, Broton JG, Alexeeva N, Green BA. "Threshold-level" multipulse transcranial electrical stimulation of motor cortex for intraoperative monitoring of spinal motor tracts: description of method and comparison to somatosensory evoked potential monitoring. J Neurosurg. 1998; 88(3):457–470
[18] Auerbach JD, Lenke LG, Bridwell KH, et al. Major complications and comparison between 3-column osteotomy techniques in 105 consecutive spinal deformity procedures. Spine. 2012; 37(14):1198–1210
[19] Geck MJ, Macagno A, Ponte A, Shufflebarger HL. The Ponte procedure: posterior only treatment of Scheuermann's kyphosis using segmental posterior shortening and pedicle screw instrumentation. J Spinal Disord Tech. 2007; 20(8):586–593
[20] Bergin PF, O'Brien JR, Matteini LE, Yu WD, Kebaish KM. The use of spinal osteotomy in the treatment of spinal deformity. Orthopedics. 2010; 33(8):586–594
[21] Chang KW. Smith-Peterson Osteotomy and Ponte Osteotomy. In: Wang Y, Boachie-Adjei O, Lenke L, ed. Spinal Osteotomy. New York, NY: Springer; 2015:75–109
[22] Kim YJ, Lenke LG, Bridwell KH, Cho YS, Riew KD. Free hand pedicle screw placement in the thoracic spine: is it safe? Spine. 2004; 29(3):333–342
[23] Kim SS, Cho BC, Kim JH, et al. Complications of posterior vertebral resection for spinal deformity. Asian Spine J. 2012; 6(4):257–265
[24] Cho SK, Bridwell KH, Lenke LG, et al. Major complications in revision adult deformity surgery: risk factors and clinical outcomes with 2- to 7-year follow-up. Spine. 2012; 37(6):489–500
[25] Enercan M, Ozturk C, Kahraman S, Sarıer M, Hamzaoglu A, Alanay A. Osteotomies/spinal column resections in adult deformity. Eur Spine J. 2013; 22 Suppl 2:S254–S264
[26] Xie J, Wang Y, Zhao Z, et al. Posterior vertebral column resection for correction of rigid spinal deformity curves greater than 100°. J Neurosurg Spine. 2012; 17(6):540–551
[27] Wang Y, Zhang Y, Zhang X, et al. A single posterior approach for multilevel modified vertebral column resection in adults with severe rigid congenital kyphoscoliosis: a retrospective study of 13 cases. Eur Spine J. 2008; 17(3):361–372
[28] Suk SIKJ, Kim JH, Kim WJ, Lee SM, Chung ER, Nah KH. Posterior vertebral column resection for severe spinal deformities. Spine. 2002; 27(21):2374–2382
[29] Shimode M, Kojima T, Sowa K. Spinal wedge osteotomy by a single posterior approach for correction of severe and rigid kyphosis or kyphoscoliosis. Spine. 2002; 27(20):2260–2267

20 Growing Spine Options for Neuromuscular Scoliosis

Joshua S. Murphy and Burt Yaszay

Abstract

Scoliosis is a common deformity in the neuromuscular population that can interfere with sitting balance as well as pulmonary and gastrointestinal function. Nonoperative treatment has largely been ineffective in controlling neuromuscular spinal deformities. Therefore, they are geared largely toward sitting balance and posture control. Once nonoperative management is no longer effective, a number of surgical techniques have been developed to treat progressive scoliosis in a growing neuromuscular patient including growth-friendly surgery and spinal fusions. Growth-friendly surgeries include traditional growing rods, magnetically controlled growing rods, Shilla procedure, and Vertical Expandable Prosthetic Titanium Rib (VEPTR). Additional modalities include a limited anterior spinal fusion and delayed posterior spinal fusion or an early posterior spinal fusion in appropriate patients. Regardless of technique, there are many variables to consider when treating this patient population including maximizing their preoperative nutritional status and consideration of pulmonary complications and timing of surgery. Furthermore, a high complication rate is associated with growth-friendly surgeries and posterior spinal fusions in the neuromuscular population when compared to patients with idiopathic scoliosis. The surgeon has a multitude of options for treating early-onset scoliosis in the neuromuscular population. It is important to choose the appropriate procedure for each patient as these patients have not only a spinal deformity at a young age, but also other medical comorbidities that put them at risk of complications.

Keywords: early-onset scoliosis, fusion, growing rods, magnetically controlled growing rods, Shilla, vertical expandable prosthetic titanium rib, VEPTER

20.1 Introduction

Neuromuscular scoliosis is defined as an abnormal spinal curvature caused by abnormalities of the brain, spinal cord, and muscular systems. The nervous and musculoskeletal systems are unable to obtain and maintain appropriate balance of the spine and trunk. Based on the Hueter–Volkmann principle, this associated imbalance causes abnormal biomechanical load on the spine, and progressive deformity is thought to be the result of both progressive muscle imbalance and anatomic deformity.

Early-onset scoliosis (EOS) is defined as a spine deformity that is present in a child younger than 10 years of age. It is further broken down into subtypes based on the underlying cause of the deformity. Specifically, neuromuscular EOS is a scoliosis that develops in children with neuromuscular disorders including spinal muscular atrophy (SMA), cerebral palsy, spina bifida, and brain or spinal cord injury.[1] The purpose of this chapter is to highlight the different treatment options in patients with neuromuscular early-onset scoliosis.

20.2 Nonoperative Care

Few nonoperative modalities have been effective in treating neuromuscular scoliosis. Historically, nonoperative treatment has been directed at postural control and maximizing sitting ability. Initially, observation is acceptable treatment of curves that measure 20 degrees or less. If a curve continues to progress, bracing may be an option. Olafsson et al[2] published the results of 90 consecutive patients treated with a prefabricated Boston-type brace for neuromuscular spine deformity. The breakdown of patients consisted of 38 patients with spastic tetraplegia, 24 with syndrome related hypotonia, and 21 with myelomeningocele. The average success rate was 28% with 23 successful cases. They found success related to ambulation and short thoracolumbar or lumbar curves. However, nine patients ultimately underwent operation secondary to curve size, although the curve was unchanged during bracing. In conclusion, bracing was thought to be successful in only a small group of patients including those who are ambulatory, with a thoracolumbar or lumbar curve, and short curve length of approximately 5.7 vertebrae. Long hypotonic curves were found to be difficult to control with an orthosis.[2]

Miller et al reviewed the results of thoracolumbosacral orthosis (TLSO) management in patients with scoliosis and a diagnosis of spastic quadriplegic cerebral palsy. They found no impact on curve or rate of progression when patients were braced 23 hours per day over a mean period of 67 months, compared to a similar cohort that was not braced and followed to spinal fusion.[3] To date, it is generally accepted that bracing in patients with CP will not alter the progression of the curve. However, it is reasonable to utilize a brace to improve muscle balance and sitting. An additional option is the use of chest supports and modular seating systems that utilize 3-point control of the coronal deformity to prop the child up and address sitting balance.[4]

20.3 Operative Care

The decision to proceed with operative care is complex, and there are multiple factors to be considered. In general, operative treatment is considered for curve magnitudes greater than 50 degrees and significant deterioration in function.[5,6,7] The primary goal of surgery is to prevent progression of the spinal curve and in some cases progression of pelvic obliquity. In cases of spinal fusion, additional goals include reestablishing coronal and sagittal alignment of the spine.

20.3.1 Growing Rods

There is a growing interest in the use of growth-friendly techniques in the management of neuromuscular EOS. Historically, many authors recommended against the use of growth-friendly techniques in the neuromuscular scoliosis population secondary to the high risk of complications. However, it is well known that growing rod surgery is a safe and effective treatment for EOS as popularized by Akbarnia et al[8] (▶ Fig. 20.1). Growth assessment in these children can be challenging, as many patients with cerebral palsy and upper motor neuron disease have delayed onset of puberty and delayed bone age. In addition to serial height and weight measurements, evaluation of the triradiate cartilage status and skeletal bone age have been helpful in assessing remaining growth in patients with neuromuscular scoliosis.

Chandran et al investigated a dual growing rod system with pelvic fixation in 11 patients with SMA type 1 or 2. They found a significant improvement of postoperative Cobb angles with 50% correction and no surgical complications or reoperations. However, two patients did have postoperative medical complications including pneumonia and anemia.[9]

In another study, McElroy et al evaluated the use of growing rods in the treatment of SMA and found there was nearly 50%

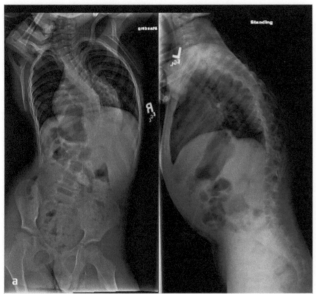
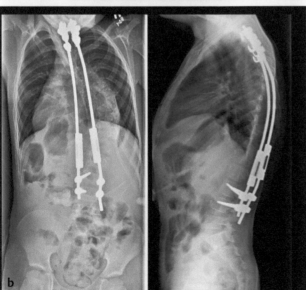

Fig. 20.1 **(a)** Six-year-old male patient with progressive scoliosis. **(b)** Patient underwent placement of traditional growing rods.

correction of the major curve, improved trunk height, and improved space available for the lung ratio at final follow-up. However, they did not find any change in the rib collapse commonly seen in SMA. Additionally, they noted that patients with SMA had longer hospital stays than did patients with idiopathic EOS undergoing the same procedure.[10]

McElroy et al evaluated the use of growing rods in 27 patients with CP with and without pelvic fixation. They found that growing rod constructs with pelvic fixation produced better pelvic obliquity correction ($p < 0.001$). However, the majority of the patients studied had at least one complication, and the cohort had a 30% deep wound infection rate. They recommended sparing use of growing rod constructs in patients with CP.[11]

Currently, we use dual growing rods as described by Akbarnia et al[8] to treat progressive EOS in our patients with neuromuscular deformity, specifically those with CP and SMA. We advise caution in regard to patient selection as these patients must be viewed as a whole in regard to size, magnitude, and location of the curve, medical comorbidities, and, in some cases, soft-tissue coverage. As previously mentioned, these patients are at an increased risk of deep wound infection, and great care must be taken in selecting the appropriate surgery for the patient. The etiology of the deformity has some impact on the rate of complications; those patients with significant spasticity, pelvic obliquity, and kyphosis are at risk of major complications.

20.3.2 Magnetic Growing Rods

In 2014, magnetically controlled growing rods (MCGR) received Food and Drug Administration (FDA) approval for use in the United States after several years of clinical application in Europe and Asia (▶ Fig. 20.2). Yoon et al investigated the effects on pulmonary function in children with EOS using MCGR. With a mean follow-up of 2.5 years, they evaluated six cases and found the average correction to be 34 and 36 degrees for coronal and sagittal deformities, respectively. In addition, mean improvement in postoperative forced vital capacity (FVC) and forced expiratory volume 1 (FEV1) was 14.1 and 17.2%, respectively. Importantly, there were two complications that required reoperation including a prominent rod and one rod breakage. They concluded that early intervention using MCGR was associated with significant improvement in postoperative pulmonary function testing and significant improvement in deformity correction with the added benefits of reducing repeat anesthesia and reducing surgical and psychological distress. The cost–benefit has yet to be determined. However, we believe MCGR to be a viable option in treating the growing spine as it decreases the amount of anesthesia inductions and may decrease the complication rate.[12]

La Rosa et al published their results of 10 patients with EOS and the use of MCGR. They had an improvement in the coronal deformity from 65 to 29 degrees when comparing the preoperative and postoperative radiographs. In this series, they had two complications: one rod breakage and one pullout of the apical hooks. They concluded that MCGR can be effectively used in EOS and may overcome many of the common complications associated with traditional growing rods including fewer anesthesia inductions, fewer surgical scars and surgical site infections, and decreased psychological distress associated with multiple surgeries.[13]

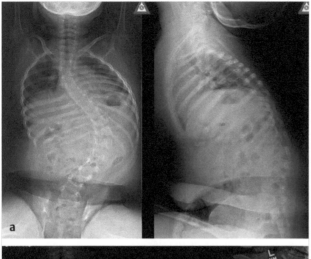

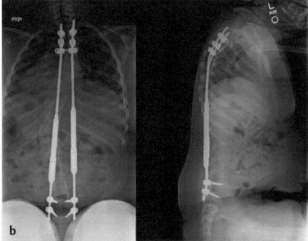

Fig. 20.2 (a) Five-year-old male patient with progressive neuromuscular scoliosis. (b) Patient underwent placement of magnetically controlled growing rods.

However, there is a paucity of literature to date investigating the effectiveness and complication rates associated with MCGRs in the neuromuscular population. The authors believe that MCGR can affect the lives of these patients for the above-mentioned reasons including outpatient lengthening that does not require anesthesia, which may decrease the complication rate and psychological stress for the patient and family. It has yet to be determined if this intervention will be safe and cost-effective for early-onset neuromuscular scoliosis.

20.3.3 Shilla Procedure

The Shilla method is a modern pedicle screw construct described by McCarthy and based on the original Luque trolley system[14,15,16,17,18] (▶ Fig. 20.3). Shilla utilizes an apical fusion with nonlocking polyaxial screws proximally and distally to guide a rod that is purposefully left long to minimize the need for multiple surgical lengthenings. As the spine grows, the rod slides through the nonlocking screws allowing spinal growth of the nonfused segments.

The authors have found the Shilla procedure to be a viable option in treating early-onset neuromuscular scoliosis. This

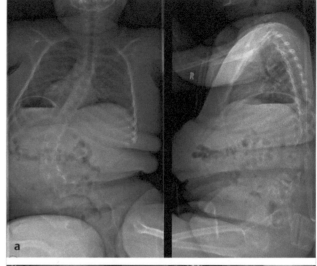

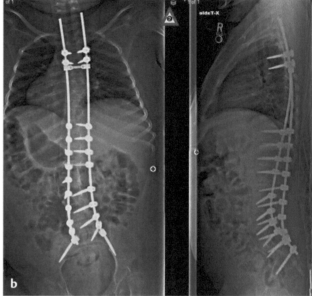

Fig. 20.3 (a) A 6-year-old female patient with spinal muscle atrophy type 2. (b) Patient underwent fusion from T10 to pelvis with placement of Shilla-type instrumentation at T2–T3.

procedure allows one to obtain correction at the apex of the curve with a limited fusion and then allows for continued spinal growth at the remaining unfused segments. This is also a construct that allows continued spinal growth without having to return to the operating room for multiple lengthenings.

20.3.4 Vertical Expandable Prosthetic Titanium Rib (VEPTR)

The pulmonary implications of thoracic insufficiency syndrome (TIS) have been well documented over the past 10 years since it was first characterized.[19] Expansion thoracoplasty was initially described by Campbell in 2003 for the treatment of TIS in skeletally immature patients[20]. However, the indications have continued to evolve to include patients with absent ribs, thoracic constriction related to rib fusion, thoracic hypoplasia, and progressive scoliosis.[21] The VEPTR device has U.S. FDA/

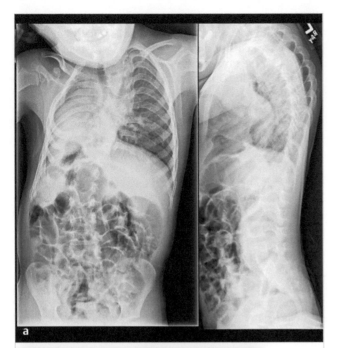

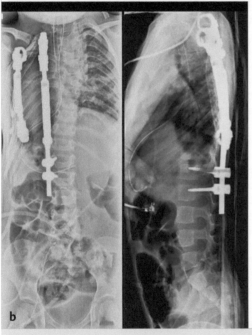

Fig. 20.4 **(a)** A 5-year-old male patient with congenital scoliosis secondary to VATER syndrome. **(b)** Patient underwent a dual VEPTR with rib-to-rib and spine-to-rib implants.

Humanitarian Use Device (HUD) approval for the management of TIS plus the anatomic presence of flail chest, constrictive chest syndrome (includes fused ribs and scoliosis), hypoplastic thorax, neuromuscular scoliosis, and congenital scoliosis without chest wall abnormality. The system utilizes proximal rib-to-distal rib, spine, or pelvis constructs[22] (▶ Fig. 20.4).

White et al studied 14 patients with mean follow-up of 35 months who had VEPTR spine-to-spine dual-rod constructs placed to stabilize spinal deformities for children with TIS and either neuromuscular scoliosis or congenital scoliosis who did not have chest wall deformity. All patients had at least three expansions with an average of five expansions per child. Complications occurred in 6 of 14 patients: 3 rod fractures, 1 superficial infection treated with antibiotics, 1 superficial infection treated with local debridement, and 1 deep infection requiring a local advancement flap after multiple recurrences and rod removal. They found that early preservation of spinal growth and control of spinal deformity using a VEPTR system in combination with conventional spine implants as a spine-to-spine growing construct yield similar results as previously reported in traditional growing rods. However, they do warn that regardless of the system used, a high complication rate persists with multiple procedures in a growing child.[23]

The use of VEPTR has also been supported in the treatment of myelomeningocele, including control of the distal kyphosis (gibbus) deformity. Flynn et al reported on 16 patients with myelomeningocele as part of a multicenter investigational device exemption study. The average age of the patient at time of surgery was 48.6 months with an average of 59-month follow-up. In this study, five patients developed a superficial soft-tissue wound infection treated with local debridement and antibiotics and two patients developed deep wound infections that required removal of implants. They cited that by avoiding midline incisions there were no cases of incisional necrosis. They concluded that within the inherent limitations of the study, VEPTR implantation in patients with spina bifida allows continued thoracic spine growth while controlling the progressive spine deformity. In addition, based on the patients' assisted ventilation rating scores, these data suggested that VEPTR surgery maintained or improved ventilatory status in this patient population. Therefore, it can be used to manage both spinal deformity and respiratory function while maintaining spinal growth in the immature nonambulatory child with myelodysplasia.[24]

Current trends utilize expansion thoracoplasty in the young patient (< 5 years old) so as to minimize autofusion of the spine at a young age and allow for prolonged spinal growth. Careful technique is required in this patient population secondary to the increased risk of infection. In addition, one must be careful to avoid periosteal stripping of the ribs not involved in the proximal rib fixation to minimize rib autofusion. VEPTR implantation may be performed in either the lateral position, when thoracoplasty is planned, or in the prone position when used for rib-to-spine or rib-to-pelvis fixation in the setting of neuromuscular scoliosis with or without pelvic obliquity.[22,25]

20.3.5 Fusion

Varying techniques and instrumentation have been utilized to perform spine surgery in patients with neuromuscular scoliosis. Options include combined anterior and posterior fusion, limited anterior fusion with delayed posterior fusion, and early posterior spinal fusion (PSF). When fusing a skeletally immature patient with neuromuscular scoliosis, there are many factors to consider including pulmonary function, remaining spinal growth, crankshaft phenomenon, and nutritional status. In addition, there are multiple technical options including the use of the Galveston technique with a unit rod and Luque wires, hybrid constructs, and all pedicle screw constructs.

One of the primary goals of scoliosis correction in the early onset population is to maintain and potentially prevent worsening pulmonary function. Karol et al pointed out the importance of spinal growth and its relationship to pulmonary function. They reviewed 28 patients who underwent PSF prior to 9 years of age, with minimum of 5 years of follow-up. Twenty patients had congenital scoliosis, 3 had idiopathic scoliosis, 3 had neurofibromatosis, and 1 had syndromic scoliosis. All patients returned and voluntarily underwent pulmonary function testing. In this non-neuromuscular population, 12 of 28 patients were found to have severe restrictive pulmonary disease. In addition, they measured T1–T12 vertical height and found that the average FVC was 48.2% for patients with less than 18 cm vertical thoracic height. For those patients between 18 and 22 cm, the average FVC was 63% with two patients having an FVC less than 50%. Finally, the average FVC was 85.2% for patients measuring 22 to 28 cm at final follow-up with no patients having an FVC less than 50%. They concluded that patients with a proximal thoracic deformity requiring fusion of greater than four levels, especially with rib anomalies, are at the highest risk of restrictive pulmonary disease. Although this cohort is representative of a non-neuromuscular population, it is reasonable to extrapolate these data to the neuromuscular population, as they are frequently unable to perform pulmonary function tests and routinely have worse pulmonary function than patients with non-neuromuscular deformity.[26]

20.3.6 Limited Anterior with Delayed Posterior Spinal Fusion

As previously mentioned, it is important to allow continued spinal growth, as we know there is a correlation between spinal growth and pulmonary development. In certain instances, large curves develop causing significant pelvic obliquity early in a child's life. When a thoracolumbar curve is greater than 80 degrees and the child is skeletally immature, one technique we utilize is to perform a limited anterior instrumented fusion at the apex of the curve to improve sitting balance and allow for continued pulmonary development and spinal growth. As this is a temporary correction, once the child reaches skeletal maturity we return to the operating room for definitive PSF. The advantage of this approach is it allows continued spinal growth proximal and distal to the apical fusion without having to undergo multiple procedures under anesthesia. However, it is not without complications including progressive deformity cephalad and caudal to the fusion and the complications associated with an anterior fusion.

Tokala et al published their results on a cohort of nine patients with neuromuscular scoliosis that underwent selective anterior single-rod instrumentation for correction of thoracolumbar and lumbar scoliosis. The mean age at surgery was 14 years with a mean follow-up of 2 years. Their group included one patient each with myotonic dystrophy, arthrogryposis, prune belly syndrome, and muscle eye brain syndrome. All patients were ambulatory, and strut grafts were utilized in six patients. Two patients required supplementary PSF. They concluded that there is a role for anterior instrumentation in carefully selected, ambulatory patients with an idiopathic-like neuromuscular scoliosis.[27]

Similarly, Basobas et al published a retrospective review of 21 patients with neuromuscular scoliosis who underwent a selective anterior spinal fusion with anterior instrumentation. The mean age at the time of surgery was 10.5 years with mean follow-up of 5 years. Diagnoses included myelomeningocele, spinal cord injury, cerebral palsy, and other myopathies. At the time of surgery, 15/21 (71.4%) of patients were at least a household ambulator. Three patients went on to require a PSF, with one being anticipated as the anterior procedure was a temporizing measure. From this study, they concluded that anterior instrumentation and fusion is a viable option in the management of neuromuscular scoliosis in select patients.[28]

The authors of this chapter will utilize a staged procedure with an anterior spinal fusion as a temporizing measure to allow for curve correction and improvement of pelvic obliquity, along with continued spinal growth followed by a PSF at a later date for definitive treatment. In large curves in young patients, this is an option that has the benefit of improving their sitting balance and curve progression while allowing the patient's spine to continue to grow and pulmonary function to mature without requiring multiple surgeries as seen with growing rod lengthenings.

20.3.7 Combined Anterior and Posterior Spinal Fusion

For stiff curves or those greater than 90 degrees, anterior release of the apical levels of the curve is indicated to improve the flexibility of the spine to obtain correction. Anterior fusion for the "crankshaft phenomenon" is not necessary, even in young patients, when rigid, segmental instrumentation to the pelvis is utilized such as a unit rod.[29,30,31] However, anterior surgery is known to increase the complication rate and morbidity of spinal surgery, and it is unclear whether to stage the anterior and posterior procedures or to do both procedures on the same day. Evidence exists to support both strategies. It is our practice to perform both procedures on the same day in relatively healthy patients, provided the time under anesthesia and blood loss are not too substantial after anterior release. However, it is not uncommon for the anterior release to be performed on one day and then return to the operating room one week later for PSF and instrumentation.

20.3.8 Early Posterior Spinal Fusion

It is well known that patients with SMA develop large curves well before peak height growth. Zebala et al evaluated the development of major curve progression 5 years after surgery with Luque–Galveston instrumentation from T4 or higher to the sacrum and pelvis in 22 patients with SMA with average of 8.2 years of follow-up. In this study, eight patients showed evidence of major curve progression as defined by progression of the curve of 10 degrees or more. They found that 36% of patients under 8 years of age and those fused short of the pelvis were more likely to progress. Important factors to consider for surgical decision-making in patients with SMA include age, skeletal maturity, curve size and rigidity, ambulatory status, and pelvic obliquity. They concluded that skeletal maturity and length of posterior instrumentation may influence major curve progression in SMA and should be considered during preoperative planning.[32]

Karol et al shed light onto the importance of continued spinal growth and pulmonary development.[26] However, in their study the average age at time of fusion was 3.3 years of age. We do agree that a definitive spinal fusion at this age is too early. However, not every patient must wait until the age of 11 years to undergo this procedure. Yaszay et al reviewed 15 children from a prospective, multicenter registry who underwent a PSF between 8.2 and 10.7 years of age with juvenile cerebral palsy scoliosis and minimum of 2-year follow-up. The mean preoperative curve magnitude and pelvic obliquity was 87 and 28 degrees, respectively. All patients were skeletally immature with open triradiate cartilage. Fourteen patients underwent posterior-only surgery and 1 a combined anterior/posterior fusion. At the most recent follow-up, the curves averaged 29 degrees with a 68% correction rate and pelvic obliquity of 8 degrees with a 71% correction rate. No child required revision surgery for progression and at most recent follow-up the Caregiver Priorities and Child Health Index of Life with Disabilities (CPCHILD) health outcome scores improved from 45 to 58. There were 2 complications reported including 1 deep infection and 1 broken rod that did not require any further intervention. From these findings, the authors concluded that when treating progressive juvenile-onset CP scoliosis, the surgeon must balance the needs for further growth with the risks of progression or repeated surgical procedures. In addition, a definitive fusion in a skeletally immature patient with curves measuring 90 degrees results in significant radiographic and quality-of-life improvement.[33]

Mattila et al compared 70 patients who underwent PSF with either an all pedicle screw construct or a hybrid construct. They found the magnitude of curve correction was significantly greater in the pedicle screw group than in the hybrid cohort ($p = 0.0016$). They also found the mean operative time and estimated blood loss to be significantly lower in the pedicle screw cohort ($p < 0.05$).[34]

20.4 Postoperative Care

Postoperatively, the patient should remain intubated (if necessary) and cared for in an intensive care setting to closely monitor pulmonary function, volume status, and urine output. These patients are frequently coagulopathic; therefore, the hemoglobin should be maintained over 9 g/dL to ensure adequate perfusion and coagulation parameters, and platelet count should be corrected as needed. In patients with poor nutritional status, hyperalimentation should be started intravenously or J-tube feedings can be started if electrolytes are well tolerated.

Due to the increased infection risk in patients with neuromuscular scoliosis, negative pressure therapy has been applied to this population to attempt to reduce infection. This dressing is then removed and replaced by a dressing of gauze and Ioban. It can be removed at 2 weeks postoperatively and then local wound care maintained. In addition, immobilization is not required postoperatively. However, frequently a TLSO is prescribed for patients requiring a Hoyer lift for transfers. Otherwise, these patients are encouraged to be out of bed and into their wheelchair as soon as is medically safe.

Lastly, wheelchairs may require readjustment to accommodate the children's new trunk proportions and pelvic alignment. They may return to school in 3 to 4 weeks when their pain is controlled, sitting tolerance is attained, incisional wounds have healed, and no postoperative restrictions are required. The TLSO may be discontinued for transfers between 4 and 6 weeks postoperatively.

20.5 Complications

Postoperative complications are prevalent in the neuromuscular scoliosis population and should be anticipated after surgery. The incidence of postoperative complications has been documented to range from 18 to 68%.[5,35,36] Infection rates have been reported to be as high as 2 to 15%.[29,35,37] Most early postoperative deep infections respond well to irrigation and debridement with delayed wound closure or negative pressure therapy with intravenous antibiotic therapy and retention of instrumentation. Respiratory complications are frequent, ranging from atelectasis to more severe problems that require prolonged intubation and ventilator support. Postoperative ileus, pancreatitis, superior mesenteric artery syndrome, and cholelithiasis can occur, and the physician and multidisciplinary team must be vigilant in evaluating any clinical abnormalities.[38,39,40]

20.6 Conclusion

Scoliosis is common in children with neuromuscular disorders. The majority of children have progressive spinal deformities that interfere with sitting and other functions, including pulmonary capacity, that will require surgical stabilization to address these problems and facilitate care. The surgeon has a multitude of options for treating early-onset scoliosis in the neuromuscular population. It is important to choose the appropriate procedure for each patient as these patients have not only a spinal deformity at a young age, but also other medical comorbidities that put them at risk of complications.

References

[1] Skaggs DL, Guillaume T, El-Hawary R, et al. Early onset scoliosis consensus statement, SRS Growing Spine Committee, 2015. Spine Deform. 2015; 3 (2):107

[2] Olafsson Y, Saraste H, Al-Dabbagh Z. Brace treatment in neuromuscular spine deformity. J Pediatr Orthop. 1999; 19(3):376–379

[3] Miller A, Temple T, Miller F. Impact of orthoses on the rate of scoliosis progression in children with cerebral palsy. J Pediatr Orthop. 1996; 16(3):332–335

[4] Shah S. Treatment of Spinal Deformity in Cerebral Palsy. In: Akbarnia BA, Yazici M, Thompson GH. The Growing Spine. Berlin: Springer; 2011:229–239

[5] Comstock CP, Leach J, Wenger DR. Scoliosis in total-body-involvement cerebral palsy. Analysis of surgical treatment and patient and caregiver satisfaction. Spine. 1998; 23(12):1412–1424, discussion 1424–1425

[6] Lonstein JE. Spine deformities due to cerebral palsy. In: Weinstein SL, ed. The Pediatric Spine: Principles and Practice. Philadelphia, PA: Lippincott & Wilkins; 2001:797–807

[7] Renshaw T. Cerebral Palsy. In: Morrissy R, ed. Lovell and Winter's Pediatric Orthopaedics. Philadelphia, PA: Lippincott Williams & Wilkins; 2001:563–599

[8] Akbarnia BA, Marks DS, Boachie-Adjei O, Thompson AG, Asher MA. Dual growing rod technique for the treatment of progressive early-onset scoliosis: a multicenter study. Spine. 2005; 30(17) Suppl:S46–S57

[9] Chandran S, McCarthy J, Noonan K, Mann D, Nemeth B, Guiliani T. Early treatment of scoliosis with growing rods in children with severe spinal muscular atrophy: a preliminary report. J Pediatr Orthop. 2011; 31(4):450–454

[10] McElroy MJ, Shaner AC, Crawford TO, et al. Growing rods for scoliosis in spinal muscular atrophy: structural effects, complications, and hospital stays. Spine. 2011; 36(16):1305–1311

[11] McElroy MJ, Sponseller PD, Dattilo JR, et al. Growing Spine Study Group. Growing rods for the treatment of scoliosis in children with cerebral palsy: a critical assessment. Spine. 2012; 37(24):E1504–E1510

[12] Yoon WW, Sedra F, Shah S, Wallis C, Muntoni F, Noordeen H. Improvement of pulmonary function in children with early-onset scoliosis using magnetic growth rods. Spine. 2014; 39(15):1196–1202

[13] La Rosa G, Oggiano L, Ruzzin L. Magnetically controlled growing rods for the management of early onset scoliosis: a preliminary report. J Pediatr Orthop. 2017; 37(2):79–85

[14] Luque ER. Paralytic scoliosis in growing children. Clin Orthop Relat Res. 1982 (163):202–209

[15] Luque ER. The anatomic basis and development of segmental spinal instrumentation. Spine. 1982; 7(3):256–259

[16] Luque ER. Segmental spinal instrumentation for correction of scoliosis. Clin Orthop Relat Res. 1982(163):192–198

[17] McCarthy RE, Sucato D, Tuner JL, et al. Shilla growing rods in a caprine animal model: a pilot study. Clin Orthop Relat Res. 2010; 468(3):705–10

[18] McCarthy RE, McCullough F, Luhmann SJ, et al. Greater than two years follow-up Shilla growth enhancing system for the treatment of scoliosis in children. 2nd annual International Conference on Early Onset Scoliosis (ICEOS). Montreal, Canada 2008

[19] Campbell RM, Jr, Smith MD, Mayes TC, et al. The characteristics of thoracic insufficiency syndrome associated with fused ribs and congenital scoliosis. J Bone Joint Surg Am. 2003; 85-A(3):399–408

[20] Campbell RM, Jr, Hell-Vocke AK. Growth of the thoracic spine in congenital scoliosis after expansion thoracoplasty. J Bone Joint Surg Am. 2003; 85-A (3):409–420

[21] Campbell RM, Jr, Smith MD. Thoracic insufficiency syndrome and exotic scoliosis. J Bone Joint Surg Am. 2007; 89 Suppl 1:108–122

[22] Campbell RM, Jr, Smith MD, Mayes TC, et al. The effect of opening wedge thoracostomy on thoracic insufficiency syndrome associated with fused ribs and congenital scoliosis. J Bone Joint Surg Am. 2004; 86-A(8):1659–1674

[23] White KK, Song KM, Frost N, Daines BK. VEPTR™ growing rods for early-onset neuromuscular scoliosis: feasible and effective. Clin Orthop Relat Res. 2011; 469(5):1335–1341

[24] Flynn JM, Ramirez N, Emans JB, Smith JT, Mulcahey MJ, Betz RR. Is the vertebral expandable prosthetic titanium rib a surgical alternative in patients with spina bifida? Clin Orthop Relat Res. 2011; 469(5):1291–1296

[25] Smith JT. Bilateral rib-to-pelvis technique for managing early-onset scoliosis. Clin Orthop Relat Res. 2011; 469(5):1349–1355

[26] Karol LA, Johnston C, Mladenov K, Schochet P, Walters P, Browne RH. Pulmonary function following early thoracic fusion in non-neuromuscular scoliosis. J Bone Joint Surg Am. 2008; 90(6):1272–1281

[27] Tokala DP, Lam KS, Freeman BJC, Webb JK. Is there a role for selective anterior instrumentation in neuromuscular scoliosis? Eur Spine J. 2007; 16(1):91–96

[28] Basobas L, Mardjetko S, Hammerberg K, Lubicky J. Selective anterior fusion and instrumentation for the treatment of neuromuscular scoliosis. Spine. 2003; 28(20):S245–S248

[29] Dias RC, Miller F, Dabney K, Lipton G, Temple T. Surgical correction of spinal deformity using a unit rod in children with cerebral palsy. J Pediatr Orthop. 1996; 16(6) Suppl 1:734–740

[30] Dubousset J, Herring JA, Shufflebarger H. The crankshaft phenomenon. J Pediatr Orthop. 1989; 9(5):541–550

[31] Westerlund LE, Gill SS, Jarosz TS, Abel MF, Blanco JS. Posterior-only unit rod instrumentation and fusion for neuromuscular scoliosis. Spine. 2001; 26 (18):1984–1989

[32] Zebala LP, Bridwell KH, Baldus C, et al. Minimum 5-year radiographic results of long scoliosis fusion in juvenile spinal muscular atrophy patients: major curve progression after instrumented fusion. J Pediatr Orthop. 2011; 31 (5):480–488

[33] Yaszay B, Sponseller PD, Shah S, et al. Performing a definitive fusion in juvenile CP patients is a good surgical option. 2016–[Epub ahead of print]

[34] Mattila M, Jalanko T, Puisto V, Pajulo O, Helenius IJ. Hybrid versus total pedicle screw instrumentation in patients undergoing surgery for neuromuscular scoliosis: a comparative study with matched cohorts. J Bone Joint Surg Br. 2012; 94(10):1393–1398

[35] Szöke G, Lipton G, Miller F, Dabney K. Wound infection after spinal fusion in children with cerebral palsy. J Pediatr Orthop. 1998; 18(6):727–733

[36] Benson ER, Thomson JD, Smith BG, Banta JV. Results and morbidity in a consecutive series of patients undergoing spinal fusion for neuromuscular scoliosis. Spine. 1998; 23(21):2308–2317, discussion 2318

[37] Gersoff WK, Renshaw TS. The treatment of scoliosis in cerebral palsy by posterior spinal fusion with Luque-rod segmental instrumentation. J Bone Joint Surg Am. 1988; 70(1):41–44

[38] Korovessis PG, Stamatakis M, Baikousis A. Relapsing pancreatitis after combined anterior and posterior instrumentation for neuropathic scoliosis. J Spinal Disord. 1996; 9(4):347–350

[39] Leichtner AM, Banta JV, Etienne N, et al. Pancreatitis following scoliosis surgery in children and young adults. J Pediatr Orthop. 1991; 11(5):594–598

[40] Shapiro G, Green DW, Fatica NS, Boachie-Adjei O. Medical complications in scoliosis surgery. Curr Opin Pediatr. 2001; 13(1):36–41

21 Anterior Approaches to the Spine for Neuromuscular Spinal Deformity

Peter O. Newton

Abstract

Anterior exposure to the spine for the purpose of performing an anterior release has become less common as the posterior methods have become more powerful. The goals of spinal fusion in the patients with neuromuscular scoliosis cannot be forgotten, and in selected cases an anterior release (with or without instrumentation), particularly in the thoracolumbar curve pattern, is an excellent alternative to achieve pelvic obliquity correction and sitting balance. An anteroposterior approach may be safer than a posterior three-column osteotomy for the most severe cases. An approach surgeon should be utilized if the spinal deformity surgeon is not experienced with the anterior anatomy.

Keywords: anterior, neuromuscular, scoliosis, thoracoscopic, thoracotomy

21.1 Introduction

The spinal deformities of patients with neuromuscular disorders may develop at a young age and are often treated when the curves are large and rigid. Traditionally, the two main goals for an anterior procedure are the desire to prevent crankshaft, which is relatively common in these patients, and the attainment of curve flexibility. Despite the increasing popularity of posterior-only approaches for scoliosis, there remain appropriate indications for the addition of an anterior procedure in some patients with neuromuscular scoliosis.

The surgical exposure of the anterior aspect of the spine may be made by open or endoscopic methods, and the choice is determined by the intended procedure as well as the experience of the surgeon with each method. Neither of the approaches is extensile, although the standard thoracotomy can be extended into the lumbar region by dividing the diaphragm as in the thoracoabdominal approach. The thoracoscopic method is an attractive alternative to an open thoracotomy when the region of interest is between T4 and L1, allowing a less invasive alternative for performing diskectomy/release.

Additionally, there is a group of patients with specific curve features that may benefit from the addition of anterior instrumentation, generally prior to performing a longer posterior instrumented fusion procedure. The most likely candidates are those with severe/rigid thoracolumbar curves associated with marked pelvic obliquity.

The risk and benefits of adding an anterior procedure must be carefully considered in this vulnerable population. The association of medical comorbidities with many of the neuromuscular conditions should always cause one to pause when contemplating the addition of a second surgical approach. The goals of spinal deformity surgery are more likely based on functional outcomes associated with pulmonary function and comfortable sitting. Anterior procedures should be added only when the gains in achieving these goals are thought to outweigh the risks of the more invasive anterior approach. Having said that, in the myelomeningocele population, an isolated anterior approach with instrumentation may, in fact, have less risk of complications, particularly with regard to postoperative infection. As in all surgical decision making, balancing the risks and benefits is a crucial aspect of achieving success.

21.2 Open Approaches

The spinal deformity surgeon may or may not elect to utilize the skills of a general surgeon colleague for these approaches depending on his or her training and experience. In either event, an understanding of the nonskeletal anatomy (heart, lungs, great vessels, kidney, ureter, liver, bowel, etc.) is of obvious importance. With appropriate training and experience, these vital structures can be safely protected during anterior spinal surgery while enabling access to the anterior vertebral column.[1,2]

21.2.1 Standard Thoracotomy

Anterior surgical exposure of the thoracic spine is largely achieved via a lateral thoracotomy. This approach utilizes the convex side of the chest in scoliosis cases, but in some cases of severe kyphoscoliosis a concave approach may be appropriate (especially if decompression is required). Typically five or six vertebrae can be reached because the spine is exposed between two ribs that can be spread approximately 10 to 20 cm depending on the size of the patient. The level of thoracotomy must be selected proximally so that the segments of interest can be accessed. In most cases, the thoracotomy should enter via one rib above or the rib at the level of the most proximal vertebral level to be exposed.

The lateral decubitus position with an axillary roll to protect the down side arm/brachial plexus is preferred. Prominences of the greater trochanter and fibular head on the "down" leg should be padded appropriately and the "up" leg scissored and padded separately. The patient should be secured on the table with tape and or bolsters to maintain the position. The arms are positioned in 90 degrees of flexion at the shoulders and elbows. The chest wall should be prepped and draped widely from the axilla to the symphysis and beyond the midline anteriorly and posteriorly.

The skin incision generally follows a rib that may be harvested and utilized for autogenous bone graft. The subcutaneous fat and muscles of the latissimus dorsi and serratus anterior are divided in line with the incision exposing the underlying rib. Entry into the chest may be between ribs or through the rib bed itself. Subperiosteal dissection along the rib and cutting the rib at the proximal and distal extents are standard when the rib is desired for bone graft. The alternative is to divide the intercostal muscles between two ribs. The ribs are spread for access to the spine by a Finochietto chest retractor of appropriate size.

The lungs and great vessels are the relevant nonspinal anatomy within the chest. Pleural adhesions may make retraction of the lung difficult and should be expected in patients with a history of prior chest surgery or infection (fairly common in the neuromuscular population).[3] Dividing any pleural adhesions may be required to retract the lung and pack it with moist lap sponges. Selective lung ventilation is preferred by some to ease the requirement of lung retraction, but this adds complexity to the intubation (see the "Thoracoscopic Approach" section on single lung ventilation). The pleura overlying the spine is a layer that can generally be divided longitudinally in a manner that will allow closure at the end of the procedure. In the right chest, the segmental vessels are divided between the azygous vein (running longitudinally along the anterior aspect of the spine and the rib heads [posteriorly]). In the left chest, the aorta overlies more of the vertebra with shorter segmental vessels and a less developed venous hemiazygos system than in the right chest. A plane is easily developed between the vertebral column and the great vessels, thoracic duct, and esophagus once the segmental vessels are divided. Some prefer to maintain these segmental vessels; however, the circumferential exposure of the spine is limited when doing so. Utilizing the soft-tissue plane between the anterior longitudinal ligament and the great vessels allows for a safe retraction of the great vessels (▶ Fig. 21.1).

Once the spinal procedure has been addressed, the thoracotomy is closed after a chest tube is placed. In many cases, reapproximation of the pleura over the spine may be possible. This has the advantage of maintaining the position of any morselized bone graft and potentially minimizing pleural adhesions. The chest wall is closed in layers after reapproximating the ribs.

A retropleural approach to the thoracic spine is also possible. This approach avoids exposure of the lungs; however, the exposure of the spine is relatively limited compared to the transpleural thoracotomy. This is more often applicable to a tumor, an infection, or trauma, although a limited diskectomy may be approached this way.

21.2.2 Retroperitoneal Lumbar Approach

For anterior exposure limited to the lumbar spine, a retroperitoneal approach is appropriate. The potential space of the retroperitoneum, below the diaphragm, exists between the peritoneum and the abdominal wall leading to the psoas muscles and lumbar spine.[4]

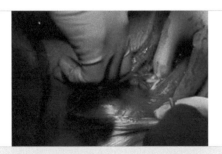

Fig. 21.1 The 12th rib cartilage tip is being split longitudinally with a scalpel. This provides a path to the retroperitoneal space. Blunt dissection deep into the cartilage and especially posteriorly opens the "potential" space posterior and lateral to the peritoneum.

The patient is placed in the lateral or three-quarter lateral (rolled slightly supine) position. The incision runs along the 11th or 12th rib and extends distally lateral to the rectus abdominis muscle. The serratus anterior and external oblique muscles overlying the 12th rib are divided along or just inferior to the rib. The cartilaginous top of the rib is sharply split, creating an interval for dissection into the retroperitoneal space (▶ Fig. 21.1). Lateral to the rectus abdominis sheath, the external oblique, internal oblique, and transverse abdominis are divided. The peritoneum is adherent to the abdominal wall musculature and must be "pushed" off the undersurface of the transverse abdominis muscle from lateral (where it is easiest to identify) to medial. The ureter should be identified (noting its peristaltic motion) and protected along with the kidney by displacing both anteriorly. Exposure of the spine is between the psoas muscle and the aorta (left side) or vena cava (right side). For full exposure at each level, the segmental vessels frequently require ligation. The segmental vein at L4 (iliolumbar vein) is quite prominent, while, more distally at the L5 level, the aorta/vena cava bifurcates into the iliac vessels. Exposure of the L5–S1 disk is often below the bifurcation.

21.2.3 Thoracoabdominal Approach

For a more extensile approach to both the thoracic and lumbar spine as is often required for release in thoracolumbar scoliosis, the thoracic and retroperitoneal approaches may be combined. Division of the diaphragm is required to connect the thoracic cavity and retroperitoneum. The thoracotomy incision (over the 9th, 10th, or 11th rib) is carried distally into the abdomen as in a retroperitoneal approach. The diaphragm is separated 1 to 2 cm from its attachment to the chest wall. Marking sutures of varying colors (e.g., black silk, white Vicryl) are placed on either side of diaphragm incision every 2 cm to aid in tissue realignment during closure (▶ Fig. 21.2). The exposure of the spinal column is as for either the thoracotomy or retroperitoneal exposures described earlier. The segmental vessels are generally divided (▶ Fig. 21.3**a**), providing circumferential exposure of the vertebral bodies and disks (▶ Fig. 21.3**b**). Closure involves an interrupted suture repair of the diaphragm and layered repair of the chest and abdominal wall (▶ Fig. 21.3**c**).

21.2.4 Thoracoscopic Approach

The thoracic cavity is particularly amenable to an endoscopic approach because with the lung deflated (with selective lung ventilation or CO_2 insufflation) a large working cavity is created.

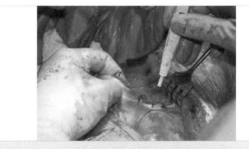

Fig. 21.2 The diaphragm is being divided with marking sutures placed to facilitate later closure of the diaphragm.

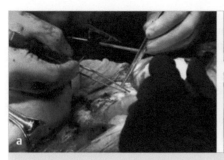
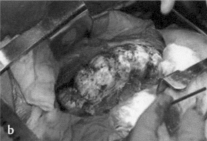
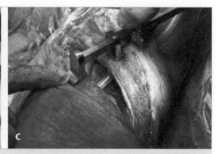

Fig. 21.3 **(a)** A thoracoabdominal exposure with division of the diaphragm provides extensile exposure to the lower thoracic and entire lumbar spine. The segmental vessels are being ligated and divided. **(b)** Circumferential exposure of the vertebral column is seen after retraction of the aorta and vena cava following segmental vessel division. This allows exposure for diskectomy, vertebrectomy, and anterior instrumentation as indicated. **(c)** The chest wall is being closed over a chest tube with the aid of a rib approximator. The chest wall is repaired in layers.

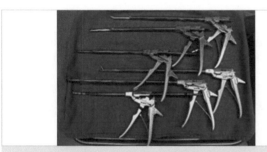

Fig. 21.4 An array of thoracoscopic instruments designed for disk removal via thoracoscopic ports (tubes 10–15 mm in diameter).

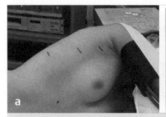
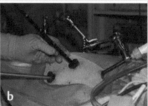

Fig. 21.5 **(a)** The markings for planned ports in an anterior release case. The incisions are planned longitudinally in the anterior axillary line. The most distal port often is more posterior to avoid placement below the diaphragm. **(b)** The three port are being utilized for a lung retractor, the endoscope, and a working tool (rongeur, ultrasonic dissector, etc.). If suction is required, an additional port may be added.

The choice of intubation may be influenced by the age of the patient, because selected intubation may be more difficult in young children. Usually, the thoracoscopy will be performed with a single lung ventilation technique using a bronchial blocker or double-lumen endotracheal tube in the lateral decubitus position. Another option is prone positioning and slight hypoventilation, creating access to the spine posterior to the lungs. Open methods have been modified to utilize 10- to 15-mm-diameter ports, telescopes, and endoscopic orthopaedic "tools" (▶ Fig. 21.4). Although this technique has advantages (smaller incisions, less pain, magnified view), there is a substantial learning curve associated with thoracoscopic anterior spinal surgery.

21.2.5 Surgical Technique

Three to four tubular ports (5–15 mm in diameter) placed between the ribs along the anterior axillary line (▶ Fig. 21.5a) provide a path to easily insert the thoracoscope and working instrument in and out of the chest (▶ Fig. 21.5b). To be certain that inferior ports are proximal to the diaphragm insertion, they should be placed under direct endoscopic visualization. The severity and location of the spinal deformity will dictate the ideal placement of the ports, but in most cases of multilevel release and fusion, the ports should be spaced widely in a single row to provide access to the greatest length of the spine.[5]

Initially, the lung will require some retraction; with time, resorptive atelectasis will shrink the lung further. The vertebral levels can be determined by counting distally from the second rib head (the first rib is palpable but not typically visible). The

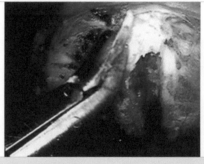

Fig. 21.6 Disk excision is done as in an open procedure. The rongeur is an efficient tool for disk removal. A 45-degree-angled scope allows visualization of the disk space. The rongeur should pass the ports that most closely aligns with the disk space.

pleura overlying the vertebrae is opened longitudinally approximately 1 cm anterior the rib heads and posterior to the azygous vein (right side) versus aorta (left side) with scissors or an ultrasonic dissector. Coagulating and dividing the segmental vessels allows a safe plane to be developed between the great vessels and the anterior longitudinal ligament. There remains a debate as to whether to divide the segmental vessels.

The anterior disk excision can be achieved with instruments that have been modified from those used for open surgery. The annulus incision is followed by diskectomy and endplate removal with thoracoscopic rongeurs, curettes, and/or elevators (▶ Fig. 21.6). The disk space is thoroughly filled with autogenous or allogeneic bone graft. Although techniques for anterior instrumentation (rod, plates, and screws) have been developed,[5,6] they are rarely indicated in neuromuscular conditions.

21.3 Mini-Open Approaches

Rivaling the truly thoracoscopic method are limited open approaches[7] (transthoracic and retroperitoneal) that may also be considered minimally invasive. Retractor systems allow one- or two-level approaches through a 3- to 7-cm incision. In the chest, a mini-open approach may be augmented with scope visualization. In the lumbar region, narrow, long blade retractors anchored in the vertebral bodies that are often secured to the operating table can be used for direct lateral exposures either anterior to the psoas or by spitting the psoas muscle.[8,9] This method is beneficial for some long neuromuscular curves that involve the thoracic and lumbar spine. The lumbar plexus is at risk in the transpsoas approaches.

21.4 Indications for Anterior Release/Diskectomy

The indications for anterior disk excision can be broadly categorized as either primarily to gain flexibility, to prevent anterior growth (crankshaft), or to decrease the risk of nonunion. There is little doubt that a circumferential release of the annulus and removal of the nucleus result in increased mobility of the motion segment. The difficulty comes in deciding when the added operative time, blood loss, and morbidity of the approach are worth the presumed gains in correction/alignment.[10,11] The principal goals for most nonambulators or

limited ambulators with neuromuscular spinal deformity are to limit progression and obtain a balanced sitting posture. Examination of the patient with forced manipulation of the torso as well as with traction/bending radiographs often provides the required information on the achievable balance by simpler posterior methods. One of the most common indications for anterior release seems to be rigid thoracolumbar scoliosis with severe pelvic obliquity. Multiple-level diskectomy may be augmented by removal of the inferior 15 to 25% of the several vertebral bodies as a means of shortening the anterior column. This is a safer alternative to performing a vertebrectomy at a single level. Rigid thoracic hyperkyphosis may also be improved by anterior thoracic disk excision.

21.5 Indications for Anterior Instrumentation

The considerations for anterior instrumentation in neuromuscular scoliosis are limited; however, specific circumstances of

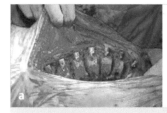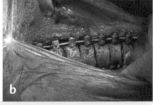

Fig. 21.7 **(a)** The appearance of the spine following anterior disk excision and vertebral body screw placement. **(b)** Following placement of an anterior rod with segmental compression, there has been substantial correction of the thoracolumbar scoliosis.

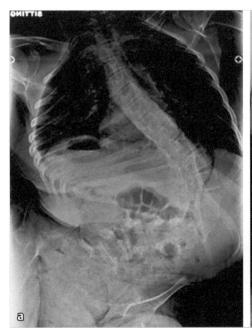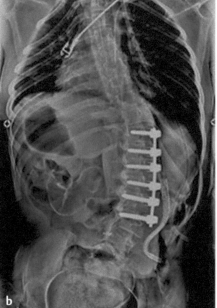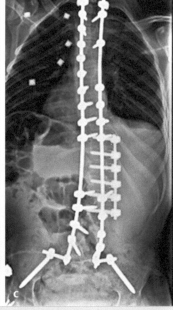

Fig. 21.8 **(a)** Preoperative posteroanterior (PA) radiograph of a patient with cerebral palsy and severe thoracolumbar scoliosis. The curvature and pelvic obliquity are creating difficulty with upright sitting. **(b)** An intraoperative PA radiograph following an anterior diskectomy and instrumentation. The majority of the deformity was corrected anteriorly. **(c)** The final correction after completing the posterior instrumentation to the pelvis. The anterior correction simplified the posterior procedure although the added morbidity of the anterior exposure was required to do so.

potential utility are highlighted. Just as in adolescent idiopathic scoliosis, anterior instrumentation with disk excision, lateral vertebral body screws, and convex compression of thoracolumbar curves provides a powerful means of deformity correction (▶ Fig. 21.7**a, b**). Given that the anterior approach is associated with less blood loss and lower rates of infection, as an isolated approach this is particularly advantageous in the patient with myelomeningocele or the ambulatory neuromuscular patient where the curve does not require fusion to the pelvis. There may also be advantages in some of the more severe thoracolumbar curves in nonambulatory patients. If an anteroposterior approach is being considered to perform an anterior release, the addition of anterior instrumentation across the apex may be considered. This is not with the goal of avoiding the posterior procedure, but it may create the majority of the deformity correction anteriorly, thus simplifying the posterior approach. Instrumenting the released levels also may allow much greater time between stages (weeks to months), optimizing physiology prior to the posterior procedure (▶ Fig. 21.8**a–c**).

References

[1] Pettiford BL, Schuchert MJ, Jeyabalan G, et al. Technical challenges and utility of anterior exposure for thoracic spine pathology. Ann Thorac Surg. 2008; 86 (6):1762–1768

[2] Tis JE, O'Brien MF, Newton PO, et al. Adolescent idiopathic scoliosis treated with open instrumented anterior spinal fusion: five-year follow-up. Spine. 2010; 35(1):64–70

[3] Lonner BS, Auerbach JD, Estreicher MB, et al. Pulmonary function changes after various anterior approaches in the treatment of adolescent idiopathic scoliosis. J Spinal Disord Tech. 2009; 22(8):551–558

[4] Gumbs AA, Bloom ND, Bitan FD, Hanan SH. Open anterior approaches for lumbar spine procedures. Am J Surg. 2007; 194(1):98–102

[5] Newton PO, Upasani VV, Lhamby J, Ugrinow VL, Pawelek JB, Bastrom TP. Surgical treatment of main thoracic scoliosis with thoracoscopic anterior instrumentation. Surgical technique. J Bone Joint Surg Am. 2009; 91 Suppl 2:233–248

[6] Hay D, Izatt MT, Adam CJ, Labrom RD, Askin GN. Radiographic outcomes over time after endoscopic anterior scoliosis correction: a prospective series of 106 patients. Spine. 2009; 34(11):1176–1184

[7] Dewald CJ, Millikan KW, Hammerberg KW, Doolas A, Dewald RL. An open, minimally invasive approach to the lumbar spine. Am Surg. 1999; 65(1):61–68

[8] Benglis DM, Vanni S, Levi AD. An anatomical study of the lumbosacral plexus as related to the minimally invasive transpsoas approach to the lumbar spine. J Neurosurg Spine. 2009; 10(2):139–144

[9] Ozgur BM, Aryan HE, Pimenta L, Taylor WR. Extreme lateral interbody fusion (XLIF): a novel surgical technique for anterior lumbar interbody fusion. Spine J. 2006; 6(4):435–443

[10] Auerbach JD, Spiegel DA, Zgonis MH, et al. The correction of pelvic obliquity in patients with cerebral palsy and neuromuscular scoliosis: is there a benefit of anterior release prior to posterior spinal arthrodesis? Spine. 2009; 34(21): E766–E774

[11] Tsirikos AI, Chang WN, Dabney KW, Miller F. Comparison of one-stage versus two-stage anteroposterior spinal fusion in pediatric patients with cerebral palsy and neuromuscular scoliosis. Spine. 2003; 28(12):1300–1305

Part IV

Postoperative Management and Complications

22 Incidence of Major Complications in Surgery for Neuromuscular Spine Deformity   150

23 Management of Early and Late Infection   155

24 Postoperative Intensive Care Unit Management   161

25 Reoperations: Instrumentation Failure, Junctional Kyphosis, and Cervical Extension   167

26 Health-Related Quality of Life in Neuromuscular Scoliosis   173

27 Baclofen Pump: Preoperative, Intraoperative, and Postoperative Management   179

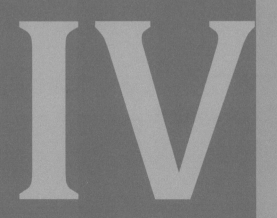

22 Incidence of Major Complications in Surgery for Neuromuscular Spine Deformity

Andrew H. Milby and Patrick J. Cahill

Abstract

Surgical correction of neuromuscular spinal deformity has been associated with higher rates of complications than correction of idiopathic spinal deformity or other spinal disorders. This disparity is the result of factors related to both the medical status of the host and the technical challenges associated with surgery in this patient population. Reported overall rates of major complications range from 17 to 63% of cases. Careful preoperative planning and optimization may help mitigate the risk of the more common complications associated with specific neuromuscular disorders.

Keywords: complications, durotomy, infection, optimization, pseudarthrosis

22.1 Introduction

Surgical correction of neuromuscular spinal deformity has historically been associated with higher rates of perioperative and postoperative complications than correction of idiopathic spinal deformity. A number of factors contribute to this disparity, including such host factors as nutritional status, continence, and bone quality, as well as structural factors related to the severity and flexibility of the curve. This combination of fragile hosts with more severe deformities demands careful preoperative planning and medical optimization to ensure the success of any surgical intervention. With a comprehensive multidisciplinary approach to perioperative care, rates of complications continue to improve over time, but additional efforts will be required in order to approach the more predictable outcomes following idiopathic deformity correction or degenerative spinal procedures.

Early reports of rates of complications associated with surgery for neuromuscular scoliosis have been as high as 63% overall[1] (▶ Table 22.1). While more recent series have demonstrated substantial improvements, certain high-risk groups have been identified. Banit et al reported a persistent 48% overall complication rate in 50 patients with myelomeningocele.[2] In a series of 110 consecutive neuromuscular deformity corrections, Duckworth et al reported a 38.5% rate in the 26 patients with muscular dystrophy.[3] Master et al in their series of 131 patients (75 with cerebral palsy [CP]) identified nonambulatory status and curve magnitude greater than 60 degrees as significant risk factors for major complications, which occurred in 28% of patients.[4] These rates are in contrast to the 16.7% overall rate for the overall Duckworth et al cohort. This latter rate is largely consistent with the 17.9% rate of overall complications observed by Reames et al in their analysis of 4,657 neuromuscular procedures in the Scoliosis Research Society's morbidity and mortality database.[5]

Perioperative complications in neuromuscular deformity correction may contribute to the relatively high in-hospital mortality rate in this patient population. An analysis of the U.S. national inpatient sample by Barsdorf et al also revealed an in-hospital mortality rate of 1.2% for 437 pediatric patients undergoing correction of neuromuscular spinal deformity as compared to 0.2% in pediatric patients with non-neuromuscular deformity.[6] A similar perioperative mortality rate of 1.0% was reported by Tsirikos et al in their series of 287 patients with CP undergoing both all-posterior and combined anteroposterior spinal deformity corrections.[7] It is important that providers, patients, and their families be aware of the rare but nontrivial risk of mortality surrounding neuromuscular deformity correction and that this information be included in the informed consent process for surgery.

We have subclassified complications by timing at presentation into (1) intraoperative, occurring during surgery, and (2) postoperative, occurring after surgery or as a consequence of decisions made during surgery. Admittedly, this classification is an oversimplification and is not meant to imply causality. For

Table 22.1 Incidence of major complications in neuromuscular spinal deformity surgery

	Incidence (range)	References
All major complications	17–63%	1–5
In-hospital mortality	1.0–1.2%	6,7
Intraoperative		
Instrumentation related	4.8%	13
Incidental durotomy	1.0%	14
Intrathecal pump dysfunction	45%	17
Blood loss > 50% estimated blood volume	65–85%	21,22
Neurologic injury	0.003–1.03%	7,26
Postoperative		
Surgical site infection	5.5–14.5%	1,5,13,32–35
Myelomeningocele	8.0–33.3%	1,2,34
Spinal cord injury	16.2%	34
Cerebral palsy	6.7–12.1%	7,32,34
Myopathies	2.7–19%	3,34
Pseudarthrosis	1.2–16%	2,7,37–39
Prominent instrumentation	2.6–15.2%	1,43,44
Medical complications		
Pulmonary dysfunction	17–50%	4,6,13,46–48
Pancreatitis in cerebral palsy	0–30.1%	39,52
Hepatotoxicity in myopathies	3.6%	3

example, surgical site infection is multifactorial and may have components in both categories, but this has been included in the postoperative category due to its typically postoperative presentation. It is likely that many complications, both intraoperative and postoperative, may be mitigated by comprehensive preoperative medical optimization to the extent that this is feasible on a case-by-case basis.

22.2 Intraoperative Complications

Complications commonly encountered intraoperatively during neuromuscular spinal deformity correction include (1) poor bone quality or instrumentation failure, (2) incidental durotomy, (3) malfunction of intrathecal medication pumps or cerebrospinal fluid shunts, when present, (4) large intraoperative blood loss (defined here as > 50% of a patient's estimated blood volume), and (5) new neurologic deficits.

A number of factors contribute to the high prevalence of osteopenia encountered in neuromuscular diseases, including nutritional deficiencies, medication side effects, and low activity level or nonambulatory status.[8,9] In particular, increasing use of corticosteroid therapy in the treatment of Duchenne muscular dystrophy, despite reducing the severity of spinal deformity and prolonging time to loss of ambulation, may result in worsening vertebral osteoporosis.[10,11,12] The potential gains in pulmonary function, time to loss of ambulatory capacity, and severity of spinal deformity must be weighed carefully against the risk of vertebral osteopenia that may increase the complexity of surgical correction. Despite the challenges inherent to instrumentation of the osteopenic spine, overall rates of reported implant-related complications with modern instrumentation remain relatively low. Sharma et al in their meta-analysis of complications in neuromuscular spinal deformity surgery found a combined rate of intraoperative and postoperative implant-related complications of 12.5%, with rates of malplacement and cutout/pullout/migration of 4.8 and 2.8%, respectively.[13] While there is little literature specifically reporting intraoperative rates of screw malposition, pedicle fracture, or cutout during deformity correction, such reports are likely to underestimate the true incidence as corrective measures may be taken when these occurrences are recognized intraoperatively.

While uncommon, incidental durotomy remains an undesirable complication in this group of patients at high risk for infection and often with preexisting disturbances in cerebrospinal fluid circulation. In their analysis of the Scoliosis Research Society morbidity and mortality database, Williams et al reported 5,191 neuromuscular deformity cases with a 1% rate of incidental durotomy.[14] This compares favorably to the 1.6% overall rate and the 2.2% rate seen in degenerative spinal deformity correction. While the overall incidence is relatively low, there are a number of patient-specific factors that may increase the risk of incidental durotomy in patients with neuromuscular scoliosis. Preoperative imaging must be carefully reviewed for the presence of dural ectasia that may contribute to the risk of inadvertent dural injury. Patients with myelomeningocele present additional challenges as disturbances in cerebrospinal fluid flow and even neurologic deterioration have been reported in the setting of deformity correction.[15] Untethering of the cord has been advocated prior to deformity correction to minimize

these risks, though one recent series suggests that this may not be required in otherwise asymptomatic patients.[16] In addition, the presence of laminotomies for intrathecal pump placement may increase the potential for inadvertent canal penetration, and dislodgement of the pump catheter itself may also result in persistent cerebrospinal fluid leakage.[17]

Many patients with spastic CP have intrathecal catheters in place. The local delivery of intrathecal baclofen reduces the dose required to decrease spasticity compared to oral baclofen, thus decreasing undesirable side effects.[18] Gerszten et al reported on the effect of baclofen in reducing the occurrence and postoperative recurrence of lower extremity contractures.[19] However, these catheters are frequently associated with scar tissue formation and are at risk of being damaged or dislodged during surgery. Caird et al reported a matched series of patients with spastic CP with and without baclofen pumps.[17] Nine of 20 patients (45%) experienced complications related to their pumps, including 3 patients who had their catheters inadvertently damaged or pulled out intraoperatively. More recently, Yaszay et al have reported equivalent surgical time, blood loss, curve correction, and rates of wound complications in groups with and without baclofen pumps in place preoperatively.[20] It is possible that greater awareness and familiarity with the perioperative management of such pumps over time may reduce the complications associated with their use.

Neuromuscular spinal deformity correction has been associated with greater overall estimated blood loss than idiopathic deformity correction. While not necessarily a complication when accompanied by appropriate resuscitation, increasing blood loss may increase the likelihood of developing life-threatening coagulopathy.[4] Edler et al performed a retrospective comparison of 18 patients with neuromuscular spinal deformity to 145 patients with non-neuromuscular (congenital or idiopathic) deformity.[21] The authors found that over 65% of the neuromuscular patients experienced a total blood loss of greater than 50% of their estimated blood volume (EBV). After statistically adjusting for total number of levels fused, neuromuscular patients had an almost seven times higher risk (adjusted odds ratio of 6.9; $p < 0.05$) of losing greater than 50% of their EBV when compared to patients with non-neuromuscular scoliosis. Modi et al, in their series of 27 patients undergoing all-posterior corrections of flaccid myopathic spinal deformities, reported a mean estimated blood loss of 123% of the EBV, with 85% of patients experiencing blood loss of greater than 50% of their EBV.[22] Several factors may contribute to the predisposition toward increased blood loss seen in the neuromuscular population, including nutritional status, smaller body habitus,[23] and disease-specific factors such as inherent clotting dysfunction observed in CP.[24] In addition, certain antiseizure medications, especially valproic acid, have been associated with increased blood loss despite otherwise normal coagulation testing.[25] Consideration should be given to bridging with alternative antiepileptic medications perioperatively, whenever feasible per the patient's neurologist.

Neurologic injury is a potentially devastating complication in an already impaired host. Loss of bladder control and protective sensation can compound the risk of decubiti in nonambulatory patients. Fortunately, neurologic injury is relatively rare and is becoming even more rare with the development of better neuromonitoring techniques and the trend away from implants that occupy the spinal canal such as sublaminar wires and laminar hooks. Tsirikos et al reported only one possible neurologic injury in their series of 287 patients with CP.[7] In their analysis of the Scoliosis Research Society's morbidity and mortality database, Hamilton et al found a 1.03% rate of new neurologic deficit following 5,147 cases of neuromuscular deformity correction in adult and pediatric patients.[26] These rates are similar to the 1.0% overall rate for all reported spinal procedures, and compare favorably to the 2.49% rate seen with adult degenerative deformity correction. With the exception of patients with complete spinal cord injuries, intraoperative neurophysiologic monitoring is often feasible. Ashkenaze et al reported that they were able to obtain somatosensory evoked potential (SSEP) signals reliably in 72% of their neuromuscular patients.[27] Subsequent series have confirmed the feasibility and utility of SSEP monitoring in the neuromuscular population.[28,29] Some surgeons consider motor evoked potential (MEP) monitoring to be contraindicated in patients with shunts and/or a history of seizures. However, Schwartz et al reported no difficulties or complications in a series of 30 patients with neuromuscular scoliosis undergoing fusion who had a seizure history and intraoperative MEP monitoring.[30]

Cerebrospinal fluid shunts are common in patients with CP and myelomeningocele. As these shunts are often gravity dependent, prolonged periods of time intraoperatively and postoperatively in a prone or supine position may lead to shunt malfunction. Preoperative evaluation by the patient's neurosurgeon is advised. In rare cases, it may be necessary to perform intraoperative intracranial pressure monitoring and periodic intraoperative decompression via removal of cerebrospinal fluid through the cranial shunt portal. While rates of shunt failure have not been examined in large series, this complication has been reported in the literature and requires vigilance on the part of the surgical and anesthesia teams.[31]

22.3 Postoperative Complications

The most frequently encountered postoperative complications following neuromuscular spinal deformity correction include (1) surgical site infection, (2) pseudarthrosis, (3) prominent or symptomatic instrumentation, and (4) medical complications related to the stress of surgery and underlying neurologic diagnoses.

Infection after scoliosis surgery is a devastating complication that has been difficult to eradicate in the neuromuscular population despite continued progress in the idiopathic and degenerative populations. Szöke et al reported an 8.7% infection rate in spastic CP, with all infections occurring in patients who were nonambulatory and had severe neurologic involvement.[32] Sponseller et al subsequently reported a rate of 11.9% in a series of patients with both CP and myelomeningocele.[33] In their 30-year experience, the Shriners Hospital of Philadelphia group reported an infection rate of 13.3% in a series of 323 neuromuscular deformity corrections.[34] The authors identified the patient's age at surgery as being inversely related to the risk of infection and also noted significant disparities in infection rates by diagnosis, with a 17.9% rate in myelomeningocele, a 16.2% rate in spinal cord injury, a 12.1% rate in CP, and a 2.7% rate in myopathies. These stand in contrast to the 0.5% rate following idiopathic deformity correction at the same institution. Values

from other multicenter series have shown considerable variability. Reames et al reported a 5.5% overall infection rate (1.7% superficial, 3.8% deep) for pediatric neuromuscular cases in the Scoliosis Research Society morbidity and mortality database.[5] Contrary to the Shriners experience, the analysis of the adult data from the same database by Smith et al yielded a higher (8.9%) rate for adult neuromuscular deformity patients.[35] One meta-analysis from Sharma et al included studies with infection rates ranging from 0 to 62%, with a pooled overall estimate of 10.9%.[13] Certainly there is significant variability within the neuromuscular population, and an individual patient's infection risk is likely due to a combination of multiple factors. Patients lacking protective sensation are at risk for the development of decubiti, which can lead to infection by either direct contamination or hematologic spread. These risks are compounded by incontinence of urine and/or feces. Patients with frequent urinary tract infections may also seed implanted instrumentation and a surgical wound via Batson's venous plexus.[36]

Patients with neuromuscular spinal deformity also remain at increased risk of pseudarthrosis postoperatively. Poor bone mineral density may contribute to loss of fixation with repetitive loading prior to the onset of bony fusion. In addition, patients with myelomeningocele may have missing or dysplastic posterior elements yielding a greatly decreased surface area of bone for fusion. Boachie-Adjei et al noted a 6.5% rate of pseudarthrosis and Gau et al a 10% rate in their series of patients with mixed diagnoses treated with Luque segmental instrumentation.[37,38] Lonstein et al reported a similar 7.5% rate with use of the Luque–Galveston technique in 93 patients with CP or static encephalopathy.[39] Pseudarthrosis rates as high as 16% have been reported in patients with myelomeningocele undergoing all-posterior fusion with segmental instrumentation.[2] Sharma et al meta-analytically demonstrated pooled estimates of loosening and implant breakage of 2.4 and 4.6%, respectively.[13] More recent series examining the use of hook-based, hybrid, or all pedicle-screw instrumentation have reported lower pseudarthrosis rates[40,41]; however, it remains uncertain to what extent instrumentation techniques are responsible for improvements in pseudarthrosis rates over time. Indeed, Tsirikos et al reported on 242 patients with CP who underwent all-posterior fusion using unit rod instrumentation with a 1.2% rate of pseudarthrosis[7] and subsequently no detectable pseudarthroses using all-pedicle screw instrumentation in both posterior and combined approaches.[42] Additional high-quality evidence is needed to clarify the indications for segmental wiring versus hook-/screw-based instrumentation strategies, as well as all-posterior versus combined approaches.

Implant prominence is frequent in patients with neuromuscular spinal deformity, especially in the setting of impaired nutrition. Historically, the rate of revision surgery for prominent iliac instrumentation with the unit rod technique has been approximately 10%.[1,43] When including proximal prominence, symptomatic instrumentation has been reported in up to 15.2% of patients undergoing unit rod fixation; this was reduced to 2.6% with the use of modular custom bent rods.[44] One promising technique that may further reduce the prominence of iliac fixation is a trans-sacral iliac screw trajectory. As described by Sponseller et al, this screw takes a trajectory starting on the dorsal sacrum at S2, traverses through the sacroiliac joint, and rests just superior to the sciatic notch within the ilium.[45] As described further in Chapter 17, this technique results in a much lower profile implant and also provides inline fixation, thus obviating the need for offset connectors. In a series of 32 consecutive patients in whom this sacropelvic fixation technique was used, the authors reported equivalent radiographic outcomes with no pelvic instrumentation prominence, skin breakdown, or deep infections.

While the spine surgeon is often focused on the technical considerations regarding correction of the spinal deformity, it is important to retain a wide perspective on the patient's underlying disease process. In particular, neuromuscular disorders have far-ranging impacts on other organ systems beyond the more visible musculoskeletal manifestations. As such, careful consideration must be given to potential medical complications in the perioperative period. Perhaps the most commonly described and most morbid of these are pulmonary complications, including respiratory failure, aspiration, pneumonia, pneumothorax, or pleural effusion. Such complications have been reported in 17 to 50% of patients,[4,6,13,46,47,48] with preexisting pulmonary dysfunction, worsening Cobb angle, and increasing age associated with increased risk.[46,47,48] Identification of preexisting pulmonary compromise is essential for perioperative management and does not necessarily represent a contraindication to surgery.[49,50] Other gastrointestinal complications, including ileus and superior mesenteric artery syndrome,[51] may also occur in a manner similar to that seen in idiopathic deformity correction. Neuromuscular disease-specific complications include postoperative pancreatitis and hepatotoxicity. Pancreatitis has been observed in up to 30% of patients with CP following deformity correction, with feeding intolerance and the presence of a gastrostomy tube being risk factors.[52] Hepatotoxicity has also been observed in up to 3.6% of patients with muscular dystrophy following deformity correction.[3] Awareness of these patterns on the part of the surgical team is essential to the multidisciplinary treatment approach required to optimize outcomes in this patient population.

22.4 Conclusion

Surgical correction of neuromuscular spinal deformity has been associated with significant perioperative complications and represents an especially challenging patient population for the spine surgeon. Careful consideration of the patient's underlying disease process and specific risk factors is essential to the ultimate success of any planned surgical procedure. With ongoing study and a multidisciplinary treatment approach, neuromuscular spinal deformity correction will continue to progress toward the safety and predictability of other spinal procedures.

References

[1] Stevens DB, Beard C. Segmental spinal instrumentation for neuromuscular spinal deformity. Clin Orthop Relat Res. 1989(242):164–168

[2] Banit DM, Iwinski HJ, Jr, Talwalkar V, Johnson M. Posterior spinal fusion in paralytic scoliosis and myelomeningocele. J Pediatr Orthop. 2001; 21(1):117–125

[3] Duckworth AD, Mitchell MJ, Tsirikos AI. Incidence and risk factors for postoperative complications after scoliosis surgery in patients with Duchenne muscular dystrophy : a comparison with other neuromuscular conditions. Bone Joint J. 2014; 96-B(7):943–949

[4] Master DL, Son-Hing JP, Poe-Kochert C, Armstrong DG, Thompson GH. Risk factors for major complications after surgery for neuromuscular scoliosis. Spine. 2011; 36(7):564–571

[5] Reames DL, Smith JS, Fu KM, et al. Scoliosis Research Society Morbidity and Mortality Committee. Complications in the surgical treatment of 19,360 cases of pediatric scoliosis: a review of the Scoliosis Research Society Morbidity and Mortality database. Spine. 2011; 36(18):1484–1491

[6] Barsdorf AI, Sproule DM, Kaufmann P. Scoliosis surgery in children with neuromuscular disease: findings from the US National Inpatient Sample, 1997 to 2003. Arch Neurol. 2010; 67(2):231–235

[7] Tsirikos AI, Lipton G, Chang WN, Dabney KW, Miller F. Surgical correction of scoliosis in pediatric patients with cerebral palsy using the unit rod instrumentation. Spine. 2008; 33(10):1133–1140

[8] Söderpalm AC, Magnusson P, Ahlander AC, et al. Low bone mineral density and decreased bone turnover in Duchenne muscular dystrophy. Neuromuscul Disord. 2007; 17(11–12):919–928

[9] Joyce NC, Hache LP, Clemens PR. Bone health and associated metabolic complications in neuromuscular diseases. Phys Med Rehabil Clin N Am. 2012; 23(4):773–799

[10] King WM, Ruttencutter R, Nagaraja HN, et al. Orthopedic outcomes of long-term daily corticosteroid treatment in Duchenne muscular dystrophy. Neurology. 2007; 68(19):1607–1613

[11] Houde S, Filiatrault M, Fournier A, et al. Deflazacort use in Duchenne muscular dystrophy: an 8-year follow-up. Pediatr Neurol. 2008; 38(3):200–206

[12] Lebel DE, Corston JA, McAdam LC, Biggar WD, Alman BA. Glucocorticoid treatment for the prevention of scoliosis in children with Duchenne muscular dystrophy: long-term follow-up. J Bone Joint Surg Am. 2013; 95(12):1057–1061

[13] Sharma S, Wu C, Andersen T, Wang Y, Hansen ES, Bünger CE. Prevalence of complications in neuromuscular scoliosis surgery: a literature meta-analysis from the past 15 years. Eur Spine J. 2013; 22(6):1230–1249

[14] Williams BJ, Sansur CA, Smith JS, et al. Incidence of unintended durotomy in spine surgery based on 108,478 cases. Neurosurgery. 2011; 68(1):117–123

[15] Geiger F, Parsch D, Carstens C. Complications of scoliosis surgery in children with myelomeningocele. Eur Spine J. 1999; 8(1):22–26

[16] Samdani AF, Fine AL, Sagoo SS, et al. A patient with myelomeningocele: is untethering necessary prior to scoliosis correction? Neurosurg Focus. 2010; 29(1):E8

[17] Caird MS, Palanca AA, Garton H, et al. Outcomes of posterior spinal fusion and instrumentation in patients with continuous intrathecal baclofen infusion pumps. Spine. 2008; 33(4):E94–E99

[18] Albright AL, Barron WB, Fasick MP, Polinko P, Janosky J. Continuous intrathecal baclofen infusion for spasticity of cerebral origin. JAMA. 1993; 270(20):2475–2477

[19] Gerszten PC, Albright AL, Johnstone GF. Intrathecal baclofen infusion and subsequent orthopedic surgery in patients with spastic cerebral palsy. J Neurosurg. 1998; 88(6):1009–1013

[20] Yaszay B, Scannell BP, Bomar JD, et al. Harms Study Group. Although inconvenient, baclofen pumps do not complicate scoliosis surgery in patients with cerebral palsy. Spine. 2015; 40(8):E504–E509

[21] Edler A, Murray DJ, Forbes RB. Blood loss during posterior spinal fusion surgery in patients with neuromuscular disease: is there an increased risk? Paediatr Anaesth. 2003; 13(9):818–822

[22] Modi HN, Suh SW, Hong JY, Cho JW, Park JH, Yang JH. Treatment and complications in flaccid neuromuscular scoliosis (Duchenne muscular dystrophy and spinal muscular atrophy) with posterior-only pedicle screw instrumentation. Eur Spine J. 2010; 19(3):384–393

[23] Jain A, Njoku DB, Sponseller PD. Does patient diagnosis predict blood loss during posterior spinal fusion in children? Spine. 2012; 37(19):1683–1687

[24] Brenn BR, Theroux MC, Dabney KW, Miller F. Clotting parameters and thromboelastography in children with neuromuscular and idiopathic scoliosis undergoing posterior spinal fusion. Spine. 2004; 29(15):E310–E314

[25] Chambers HG, Weinstein CH, Mubarak SJ, Wenger DR, Silva PD. The effect of valproic acid on blood loss in patients with cerebral palsy. J Pediatr Orthop. 1999; 19(6):792–795

[26] Hamilton DK, Smith JS, Sansur CA, et al. Scoliosis Research Society Morbidity and Mortality Committee. Rates of new neurological deficit associated with spine surgery based on 108,419 procedures: a report of the Scoliosis Research Society Morbidity and Mortality Committee. Spine. 2011; 36(15):1218–1228

[27] Ashkenaze D, Mudiyam R, Boachie-Adjei O, Gilbert C. Efficacy of spinal cord monitoring in neuromuscular scoliosis. Spine. 1993; 18(12):1627–1633

[28] Ecker ML, Dormans JP, Schwartz DM, Drummond DS, Bulman WA. Efficacy of spinal cord monitoring in scoliosis surgery in patients with cerebral palsy. J Spinal Disord. 1996; 9(2):159–164

[29] Fehlings MG, Kelleher MO. Intraoperative monitoring during spinal surgery for neuromuscular scoliosis. Nat Clin Pract Neurol. 2007; 3(6):318–319

[30] Schwartz DM, Sestokas AK, Dormans JP, et al. Transcranial electric motor evoked potential monitoring during spine surgery: is it safe? Spine. 2011; 36 (13):1046–1049

[31] Samdani A, Cahill P, Garg H, Bonet H, Betz RR. Acute intraoperative shunt failure in a child with myelomeningocele: case report. JBJS Case Connect. 2012; 2(1:e5)

[32] Szöke G, Lipton G, Miller F, Dabney K. Wound infection after spinal fusion in children with cerebral palsy. J Pediatr Orthop. 1998; 18(6):727–733

[33] Sponseller PD, LaPorte DM, Hungerford MW, Eck K, Bridwell KH, Lenke LG. Deep wound infections after neuromuscular scoliosis surgery: a multicenter study of risk factors and treatment outcomes. Spine. 2000; 25(19):2461–2466

[34] Cahill PJ, Warnick DE, Lee MJ, et al. Infection after spinal fusion for pediatric spinal deformity: thirty years of experience at a single institution. Spine. 2010; 35(12):1211–1217

[35] Smith JS, Shaffrey CI, Sansur CA, et al. Scoliosis Research Society Morbidity and Mortality Committee. Rates of infection after spine surgery based on 108,419 procedures: a report from the Scoliosis Research Society Morbidity and Mortality Committee. Spine. 2011; 36(7):556–563

[36] Batson OV. The function of the vertebral veins and their role in the spread of metastases. Ann Surg. 1940; 112(1):138–149

[37] Boachie-Adjei O, Lonstein JE, Winter RB, Koop S, vanden Brink K, Denis F. Management of neuromuscular spinal deformities with Luque segmental instrumentation. J Bone Joint Surg Am. 1989; 71(4):548–562

[38] Gau YL, Lonstein JE, Winter RB, Koop S, Denis F. Luque-Galveston procedure for correction and stabilization of neuromuscular scoliosis and pelvic obliquity: a review of 68 patients. J Spinal Disord. 1991; 4(4):399–410

[39] Lonstein JE, Koop SE, Novachek TF, Perra JH. Results and complications after spinal fusion for neuromuscular scoliosis in cerebral palsy and static encephalopathy using Luque Galveston instrumentation: experience in 93 patients. Spine. 2012; 37(7):583–591

[40] Teli M, Elsebaie H, Biant L, Noordeen H. Neuromuscular scoliosis treated by segmental third-generation instrumented spinal fusion. J Spinal Disord Tech. 2005; 18(5):430–438

[41] Piazzolla A, Solarino G, De Giorgi S, Mori CM, Moretti L, De Giorgi G. Cotrel-Dubousset instrumentation in neuromuscular scoliosis. Eur Spine J. 2011; 20 Suppl 1:S75–S84

[42] Tsirikos AI, Mains E. Surgical correction of spinal deformity in patients with cerebral palsy using pedicle screw instrumentation. J Spinal Disord Tech. 2012; 25(7):401–408

[43] Peelle MW, Lenke LG, Bridwell KH, Sides B. Comparison of pelvic fixation techniques in neuromuscular spinal deformity correction: Galveston rod versus iliac and lumbosacral screws. Spine. 2006; 31(20):2392–2398, discussion 2399

[44] Sponseller PD, Shah SA, Abel MF, et al. Harms Study Group. Scoliosis surgery in cerebral palsy: differences between unit rod and custom rods. Spine. 2009; 34(8):840–844

[45] Sponseller PD, Zimmerman RM, Ko PS, et al. Low profile pelvic fixation with the sacral alar iliac technique in the pediatric population improves results at two-year minimum follow-up. Spine. 2010; 35(20):1887–1892

[46] Padman R, McNamara R. Postoperative pulmonary complications in children with neuromuscular scoliosis who underwent posterior spinal fusion. Del Med J. 1990; 62(5):999–1003

[47] Miller F, Moseley CF, Koreska J. Spinal fusion in Duchenne muscular dystrophy. Dev Med Child Neurol. 1992; 34(9):775–786

[48] Kang GR, Suh SW, Lee IO. Preoperative predictors of postoperative pulmonary complications in neuromuscular scoliosis. J Orthop Sci. 2011; 16(2):139–147

[49] Wazeka AN, DiMaio MF, Boachie-Adjei O. Outcome of pediatric patients with severe restrictive lung disease following reconstructive spine surgery. Spine. 2004; 29(5):528–534, discussion 535

[50] Modi HN, Suh SW, Hong JY, Park YH, Yang JH. Surgical correction of paralytic neuromuscular scoliosis with poor pulmonary functions. J Spinal Disord Tech. 2011; 24(5):325–333

[51] Tsirikos AI, Jeans LA. Superior mesenteric artery syndrome in children and adolescents with spine deformities undergoing corrective surgery. J Spinal Disord Tech. 2005; 18(3):263–271

[52] Borkhuu B, Nagaraju D, Miller F, et al. Prevalence and risk factors in postoperative pancreatitis after spine fusion in patients with cerebral palsy. J Pediatr Orthop. 2009; 29(3):256–262

23 Management of Early and Late Infection

Mark Shasti, Paul D. Sponseller, and Stefan Parent

Abstract

Early or late deep wound infection after scoliosis surgery in pediatric patients is a devastating complication. Differentiating between early and late infection is important for treatment purposes. Empirical treatment of these infections should include both gram-negative and gram-positive antibiotics because of their polymicrobial nature. The treatment algorithm for early infections includes aggressive surgical irrigation and debridement followed by long-term parenteral antibiotics. Late infections require explantation of instrumentation and sometimes staged instrumentation once the infection is cleared. Late infections may be treated with oral antibiotics. In this chapter, risk factors, preventative measures, and treatment protocols for these infections are discussed in detail, along with the most recent scientific evidence.

Keywords: early infection, explants, irrigation and debridement, late infection, neuromuscular scoliosis

23.1 Introduction and Background

According to the Centers for Disease Control and Prevention, deep surgical site infection (SSI) is an "infection that appears to be related to the operative procedure and involves deep soft tissue (e.g., fascial and muscle layers of the incision)."[1] In addition, it must have at least one characteristic listed in ▶ Table 23.1. According to Aleissa et al,[2] deep wound infection after spinal surgery is defined as "infection in which there is a direct communication between the infected materials and the spinal instrumentation and bone graft/fusion mass." Deep SSI after spinal deformity surgery can be further classified as early or late infection. The definition of "late" SSI after spinal fusion is unclear. Two large studies of deep SSI after pediatric spinal deformity surgery defined early SSI as occurring less than 3 months after surgery and late SSI as occurring 3 months or more after surgery.[3,4] As discussed later in this chapter, we used 3 months postoperatively as the cutoff between early and late infections.

Deep wound infection after pediatric scoliosis surgery is a devastating complication that typically requires prolonged surgical and medical management. These infections can compromise the outcome of deformity correction, especially in patients who require subsequent removal of implants. The other comorbidities and potentially life-threatening complications associated with spinal deep SSI include sepsis, vertebral osteomyelitis, neurologic compromise, and clinically important soft-tissue defects.[5] Deep SSIs also add substantial costs to treating patients.[6]

The incidence of SSI after pediatric spinal deformity surgery varies by patient diagnosis.[7] The term "neuromuscular scoliosis" covers a wide variety of conditions, each with its own rate of infection associated with spinal deformity surgery. It is well established that infection rates are higher in patients with neuromuscular scoliosis compared with patients with adolescent idiopathic scoliosis. ▶ Table 23.2[5,8,9,10,11,12,13,14,15,16,17,18,19] summarizes the rate of deep SSI after pediatric scoliosis spinal surgery.

23.2 Risk Factors for Infection and Microbiological Data

Risk factors and microbiological data for patients with neuromuscular scoliosis who have developed deep SSI after spinal surgery are critical to understand, not only for prevention but also for formulating treatment plans. Surgical scoliosis correction is a major intervention in patients who typically have limited ability to adapt to imposed stress. Some of the factors that may account for the higher deep SSI rate in patients with neuromuscular scoliosis may be related to diminished or absent sensation in the lower body, lack of bowel or bladder control, previous spine surgery (e.g., myelomeningocele closure after birth), and altered soft-tissue coverage. Patients without sensation in the lower body are more prone to develop pressure sores and decubiti, which can lead to infection by either direct contamination or hematologic spread. Patients who lack bowel and bladder control are at risk of seeding a wound with feces or urine. Furthermore, these patients develop frequent urinary tract infections, which can spread to implanted instrumentation or a surgical wound.[3]

Several studies have identified risk factors and bacteria associated with deep SSI after neuromuscular scoliosis corrective surgery. In a multicenter retrospective case control study, the degree of cognitive impairment was identified as a significant risk factor for deep SSI after scoliosis surgery in patients with cerebral palsy and myelodysplasia.[20] Other risk factors identified in this study are listed in ▶ Table 23.3.[20] In the same study, 52% of the infections were polymicrobial. The most common organisms were coagulase-negative *Staphylococcus*, *Enterobacter*,

Table 23.1 Deep surgical site infection characteristics

Purulent discharge
Positive cultures
Evidence of infection on physical examination (tenderness, swelling, redness, or heat)
Wound dehiscence
Abscess discovery upon reoperation
Evidence of infection on histopathologic or radiologic examination

Table 23.2 Rates of deep surgical site infection after pediatric scoliosis spinal surgery

Diagnosis	Rate of infection (%)
Adolescent idiopathic scoliosis[8,9,10]	0.9–3
Cerebral palsy[5,17,18,19]	6.1–8.7
Myelomeningocele[11,12,13,14,15,16]	8–24

Table 23.3 Predictive values for risk factors

Parameter	p-value
Previous spine surgery	0.129
Posterior versus anterior/posterior	0.382
Preoperative urinary tract infection	0.171
Estimated blood loss	0.216
Allograft versus autograft	0.010[a]
Operating time	0.586
Cognitive impairment	<0.01[a]

Source: Adapted from Sponseller et al.[20]
[a]Represents a significant difference.

Enterococcus, and *Escherichia coli*.[20] In a multicenter study, Mackenzie et al[7] showed that nearly half of SSIs after scoliosis surgery contained at least one gram-negative organism. Significantly higher rates of gram-negative infections were found in patients with nonidiopathic scoliosis. In this study, *Pseudomonas* was the third most common organism after *S. aureus* and *S. epidermidis*. Aleissa et al[2] reported that more virulent enteric and gram-negative organisms were more commonly isolated from early deep SSIs (e.g., *Pseudomonas*, *Enterococcus*), whereas low-virulence cutaneous organisms were more commonly cultured from late infections (e.g., *Propionibacterium acnes*, *S. epidermidis*). This is an important finding, especially when choosing antibiotic treatment for these infections.

Preoperative nutritional status and a positive urine culture have been evaluated as risk factors for deep SSI in patients with neuromuscular scoliosis.[20,21,22] It was previously reported that malnutrition may be associated with an increased rate of postoperative complications.[21,22] In a multicenter study, Sponseller et al[20] found that markers such as a preoperative albumin level below 3.5 mg/dL, a total lymphocyte count below 1,500 cells/mm[3], and a hematocrit level of 33 g/L or less were not statistically correlated with increased risk of infection.[20] Hatlen et al[22] showed that a positive preoperative urine culture was a significant independent risk factor for SSI after spinal fusion in patients with myelodysplasia.

The risk of deep SSI varies according to surgical approach and instrumentation type. It is higher after posterior spinal fusion, whereas infection after anterior spinal fusion is rare.[2] Use of allograft bone has been identified as a significant risk factor for deep SSI after scoliosis surgery, particularly in patients with neuromuscular conditions.[2,20] Sponseller et al[23] found a significantly higher risk of SSI after scoliosis surgery in patients with cerebral palsy who had undergone instrumentation with unit rods (15%) versus custom bent rods (5%). Furthermore, although stainless steel implants have not been studied in patients with neuromuscular scoliosis, their use in patients with adolescent idiopathic scoliosis has been associated with a higher risk of late deep SSI compared with titanium implants.[24,25]

23.3 Prevention

Various approaches have been proposed to prevent deep SSIs in pediatric spine surgery, supported by different levels of

Table 23.4 Final best-practice guidelines: consensus recommendations to prevent surgical site infections in high-risk pediatric spine surgery

Guideline	Consensus (%)		
	Total		Agree
Patients should have a chlorhexidine skin wash at home the night before surgery[a]	91	61	30
Patients should have preoperative urine cultures obtained and treated if positive[a]	91	26	65
Patients should receive a preoperative Patient Education Sheet[a]	91	48	43
Patients should have a preoperative nutritional assessment[a]	96	57	39
If removing hair, clipping is preferred to shaving[b]	100	61	39
Patients should receive perioperative intravenous cefazolin[a]	91	65	26
Patients should receive perioperative intravenous prophylaxis for gram-negative bacilli[a]	95	65	30
Adherence to perioperative antimicrobial regimens should be monitored (i.e., agent, timing, dosing, redosing, cessation)[a]	96	61	35
Operating room access should be limited during scoliosis surgery whenever practical[a]	96	61	35
Ultraviolet lights need not be used in the operating room[a]	87	48	39
Patients should have intraoperative wound irrigation[a]	100	83	17
Vancomycin powder should be used in the bone graft and/or the surgical site[b]	91	48	43
Impervious dressings are preferred postoperatively[b]	91	56	35
Postoperative dressing changes should be minimized before discharge to the extent possible[b]	91	52	39

Source: Adapted from Vitale et al.[26]
[a]Consensus reached after the first round of voting.
[b]Consensus reached after the second round of voting.

scientific evidence. In 2013, a group of 20 pediatric spine surgeons and 3 infectious disease specialists from North America gathered to establish best-practice guidelines for SSI prevention in high-risk pediatric spine surgery. The objective of this initiative was to decrease the extensive variability in SSI prevention strategies, improve patient outcomes, and reduce health care costs. Using available evidence in the literature and expert opinion, this initiative resulted in consensus regarding 14 "best practices" in high-risk pediatric spine surgery.[26] ▶ Table 23.4 summarizes the final best-practice guidelines consensus recommendations.

23.4 Treatment of Early Postoperative Infection

There is no consensus on preferred medical and surgical treatment strategies, particularly for early postoperative infections. The goal is to eradicate infection and achieve a pain-free, stable spine. The main concern with early postoperative infection is lack of stable fusion mass formation. Therefore, removal of spinal implants at an early postoperative stage is avoided because implant removal may compromise fusion and curve correction, leading to deformity progression. For infections in the acute postoperative period, aggressive irrigation and debridement, wound closure over drains, retention of instrumentation, and long-term parenteral and oral antibiotics are recommended by many experts.[4,20] One-stage irrigation and closure is recommended when there is no deep purulence and the wound edges are clean, pink, and viable. If tissue quality or patient health status is poor and multiple debridements are needed, the wound may be left open to granulate over.[5] This is a reliable method, as long as the implants are well below the surrounding muscle surface.

Recently, the use of the vacuum-assisted closure (VAC) system has gained popularity. The VAC promotes formation of granulation tissue, and when changing the VAC, necrotic tissue is debrided. Canavese et al[27] described application of a VAC sponge at the time of initial surgical debridement in 14 patients who developed acute deep SSI after spinal fusion. Twelve of the wounds healed by secondary intention with the use of VAC. No instrumentation was removed in any patient, and there were no recurrent infections. Van Rhee et al[28] published similar findings in six patients who developed acute deep SSI after posterior spinal fusion. All patients in both studies received long-term parenteral and oral antibiotics.

Rohmiller et al[29] described a closed suction irrigation system placed at the time of initial debridement for deep SSI in 28 patients. They placed a proximal inflow catheter deep into the fascia and two to three distal outflow catheters superficial and deep into the fascia. The wounds were irrigated with normal saline for approximately 3 days. The catheters were removed sequentially as the drainage became clearer and decreased in volume. Two-thirds of early SSIs were treated successfully with this method. One-third of patients developed a recurrent infection, which resolved after a second course of closed suction irrigation. Removal of instrumentation was not required in any patient. ▶ Fig. 23.1 provides an algorithm for treatment of early postoperative deep SSI based on current literature.

23.5 Treatment of Late Postoperative Infection

Treatment of late infections (3 months or more after surgery[3,4]) in patients with spinal deformity requires a different approach. Whereas the external and systemic signs are more indolent, the deep extent of granulation tissue and osteolysis is much more extensive and usually involves the entire surgical field. Debridement without implant removal does not work because of retained areas of infected tissue under the instrumentation. Therefore, consensus among most authors is that implant removal is necessary for the complete debridement and effective treatment of delayed deep SSIs after spinal deformity

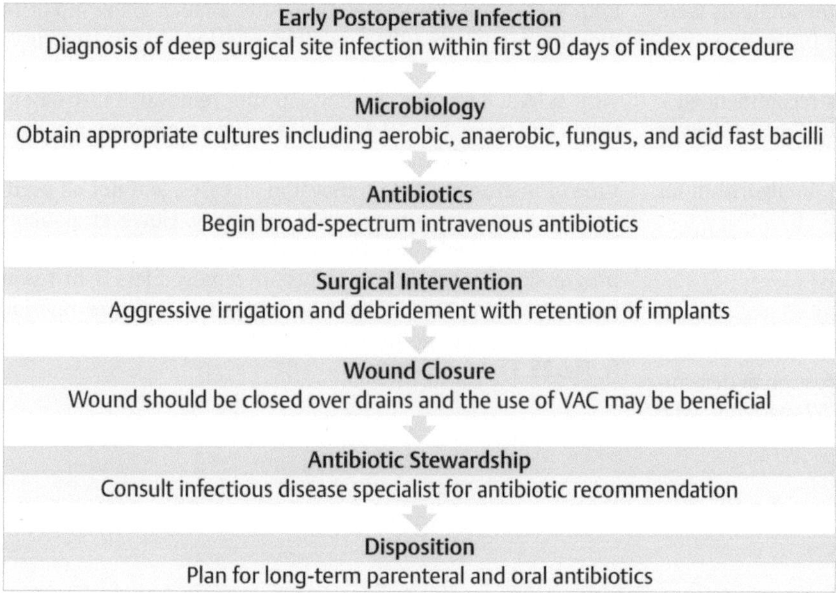

Early Postoperative Infection
Diagnosis of deep surgical site infection within first 90 days of index procedure

Microbiology
Obtain appropriate cultures including aerobic, anaerobic, fungus, and acid fast bacilli

Antibiotics
Begin broad-spectrum intravenous antibiotics

Surgical Intervention
Aggressive irrigation and debridement with retention of implants

Wound Closure
Wound should be closed over drains and the use of VAC may be beneficial

Antibiotic Stewardship
Consult infectious disease specialist for antibiotic recommendation

Disposition
Plan for long-term parenteral and oral antibiotics

Fig. 23.1 Early postoperative infection management algorithm.

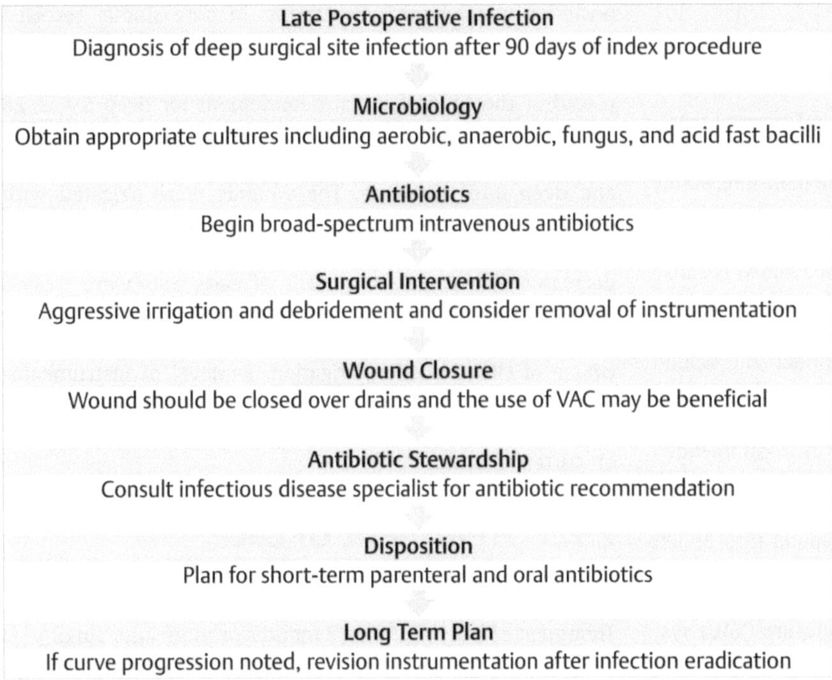

Late Postoperative Infection
Diagnosis of deep surgical site infection after 90 days of index procedure

Microbiology
Obtain appropriate cultures including aerobic, anaerobic, fungus, and acid fast bacilli

Antibiotics
Begin broad-spectrum intravenous antibiotics

Surgical Intervention
Aggressive irrigation and debridement and consider removal of instrumentation

Wound Closure
Wound should be closed over drains and the use of VAC may be beneficial

Antibiotic Stewardship
Consult infectious disease specialist for antibiotic recommendation

Disposition
Plan for short-term parenteral and oral antibiotics

Long Term Plan
If curve progression noted, revision instrumentation after infection eradication

Fig. 23.2 Late postoperative infection management algorithm.

surgery.[3,4,20,30] Hedequist et al[4] retrospectively reviewed 26 patients who developed late SSI after spinal fusion. They found that patients who retained their instrumentation always returned with recurrent infection and required further debridement until the implants were removed. In most cases, no repeat surgeries were necessary after instrumentation removal.

Two studies reported that deep SSIs after spinal fusion are soft-tissue infections and not osteomyelitis.[31,32] In these studies, when the soft tissues and bone surrounding the implants were examined, there was no sequestrum, and the fusion mass was viable. This explains why short-term antibiotics are adequate after instrumentation removal. These studies recommended 2 to 5 days of parenteral antibiotics, followed by 7 to 14 days of oral antibiotics. Several authors have reported success with this treatment protocol.[4,20,30] ▶ Fig. 23.2 provides an algorithm for treatment of late postoperative deep SSI.

23.6 Effect on Outcomes

Implant removal is associated with certain risks. Implant removal prior to bony fusion can lead to progression of deformity. Cahill et al[3] retrospectively reviewed 57 patients who developed SSI after scoliosis surgery. Instrumentation was removed in 51% of patients. Forty-four percent of these patients developed greater than 10 degrees of curve progression. Notably, the patients whose implants were removed within 1 year of their initial surgery had a mean of 30 degrees of progression, compared with 20 degrees for those who underwent removal more than 1 year after initial surgery. Hedequist et al[4] reported on a series of 26 patients who were treated for late infection with removal of instrumentation. After a mean follow-up of 14 months, 6 patients (23%) required revision surgery for curve progression. Similarly, Ho et al[30] reported that 6 of 10 patients with at least 4 months of follow-up after removal of instrumentation had more than 10 degrees of curve progression in at least one plane. Furthermore, pseudarthrosis is not evident at the time of instrumentation removal in all cases, and not all pseudarthrosis results in progressive deformity. However, patients and families should be counseled about the possibility of curve progression, especially if implants are removed less than 1 year postoperatively. They should be advised that future revision surgery may be necessary once the infection has cleared (▶ Fig. 23.3).

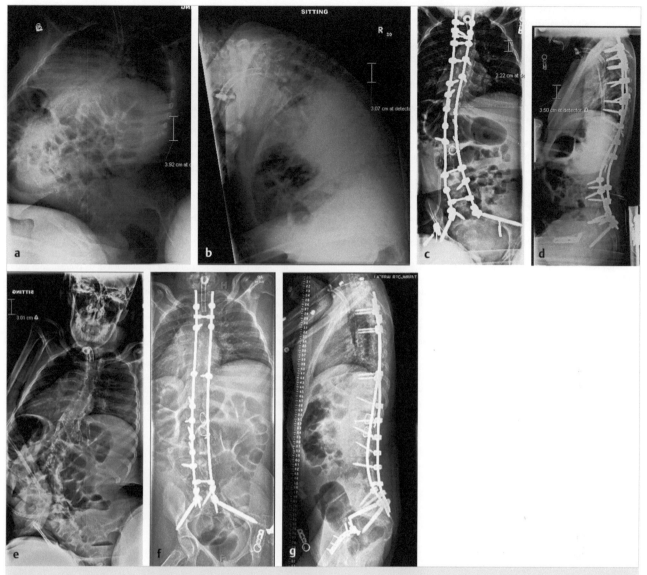

Fig. 23.3 Radiographs of a 20-year-old woman with cerebral palsy who underwent surgery to correct neuromuscular scoliosis. She was diagnosed with late postoperative infection and underwent explantation of instrumentation, debridement, and treatment with antibiotics. One year later, her curve had progressed and initial curve correction was lost. Ultimately, she underwent revision scoliosis surgery. Preoperative (a) anteroposterior and (b) lateral views; postoperative index procedure (c) anteroposterior and (d) lateral views; (e) 1 year after instrumentation removal; postoperative final procedure (f) anteroposterior and (g) lateral views.

References

[1] Horan TC, Gaynes RP, Martone WJ, Jarvis WR, Emori TG. CDC definitions of nosocomial surgical site infections, 1992: a modification of CDC definitions of surgical wound infections. Infect Control Hosp Epidemiol. 1992; 13(10):606–608

[2] Aleissa S, Parsons D, Grant J, Harder J, Howard J. Deep wound infection following pediatric scoliosis surgery: incidence and analysis of risk factors. Can J Surg. 2011; 54(4):263–269

[3] Cahill PJ, Warnick DE, Lee MJ, et al. Infection after spinal fusion for pediatric spinal deformity: thirty years of experience at a single institution. Spine. 2010; 35(12):1211–1217

[4] Hedequist D, Haugen A, Hresko T, Emans J. Failure of attempted implant retention in spinal deformity delayed surgical site infections. Spine. 2009; 34(1):60–64

[5] Szöke G, Lipton G, Miller F, Dabney K. Wound infection after spinal fusion in children with cerebral palsy. J Pediatr Orthop. 1998; 18(6):727–733

[6] Sparling KW, Ryckman FC, Schoettker PJ, et al. Financial impact of failing to prevent surgical site infections. Qual Manag Health Care. 2007; 16(3):219–225

[7] Mackenzie WGS, Matsumoto H, Williams BA, et al. Surgical site infection following spinal instrumentation for scoliosis: a multicenter analysis of rates, risk factors, and pathogens. J Bone Joint Surg Am. 2013; 95(9):800–806, S1–S2

[8] Buchowski JM, Lenke LG, Kuhns CA, et al. Infections following spinal deformity surgery. A twenty-year assessment of 2876 patients [paper #34]. Presented at the Scoliosis Research Society 41st Annual Meeting, Monterey, CA, September 13–16; 2006

[9] Coe JD, Arlet V, Donaldson W, et al. Complications in spinal fusion for adolescent idiopathic scoliosis in the new millennium. A report of the Scoliosis Research Society Morbidity and Mortality Committee. Spine. 2006; 31(3):345–349

[10] Rihn JA, Lee JY, Ward WT. Infection after the surgical treatment of adolescent idiopathic scoliosis: evaluation of the diagnosis, treatment, and impact on clinical outcomes. Spine. 2008; 33(3):289–294

[11] Banit DM, Iwinski HJ, Jr, Talwalkar V, Johnson M. Posterior spinal fusion in paralytic scoliosis and myelomeningocele. J Pediatr Orthop. 2001; 21(1):117–125

[12] Benson ER, Thomson JD, Smith BG, Banta JV. Results and morbidity in a consecutive series of patients undergoing spinal fusion for neuromuscular scoliosis. Spine. 1998; 23(21):2308–2317

[13] Geiger F, Parsch D, Carstens C. Complications of scoliosis surgery in children with myelomeningocele. Eur Spine J. 1999; 8(1):22–26

[14] McMaster MJ. Anterior and posterior instrumentation and fusion of thoracolumbar scoliosis due to myelomeningocele. J Bone Joint Surg Br. 1987; 69 (1):20–25

[15] Osebold WR, Mayfield JK, Winter RB, Moe JH. Surgical treatment of paralytic scoliosis associated with myelomeningocele. J Bone Joint Surg Am. 1982; 64 (6):841–856

[16] Stella G, Ascani E, Cervellati S, et al. Surgical treatment of scoliosis associated with myelomeningocele. Eur J Pediatr Surg. 1998; 8 Suppl 1:22–25

[17] Dias RC, Miller F, Dabney K, Lipton G, Temple T. Surgical correction of spinal deformity using a unit rod in children with cerebral palsy. J Pediatr Orthop. 1996; 16(6):734–740

[18] Teli MGA, Cinnella P, Vincitorio F, Lovi A, Grava G, Brayda-Bruno M. Spinal fusion with Cotrel-Dubousset instrumentation for neuropathic scoliosis in patients with cerebral palsy. Spine. 2006; 31(14):E441–E447

[19] Tsirikos AI, Lipton G, Chang WN, Dabney KW, Miller F. Surgical correction of scoliosis in pediatric patients with cerebral palsy using the unit rod instrumentation. Spine. 2008; 33(10):1133–1140

[20] Sponseller PD, LaPorte DM, Hungerford MW, Eck K, Bridwell KH, Lenke LG. Deep wound infections after neuromuscular scoliosis surgery: a multicenter study of risk factors and treatment outcomes. Spine. 2000; 25(19):2461–2466

[21] Jevsevar DS, Karlin LI. The relationship between preoperative nutritional status and complications after an operation for scoliosis in patients who have cerebral palsy. J Bone Joint Surg Am. 1993; 75(6):880–884

[22] Hatlen T, Song K, Shurtleff D, Duguay S. Contributory factors to postoperative spinal fusion complications for children with myelomeningocele. Spine. 2010; 35(13):1294–1299

[23] Sponseller PD, Shah SA, Abel MF, Newton PO, Letko L, Marks M. Infection rate after spine surgery in cerebral palsy is high and impairs results: multicenter analysis of risk factors and treatment. Clin Orthop Relat Res. 2010; 468 (3):711–716

[24] Di Silvestre M, Bakaloudis G, Lolli F, Giacomini S. Late-developing infection following posterior fusion for adolescent idiopathic scoliosis. Eur Spine J. 2011; 20 Suppl 1:S121–S127

[25] Soultanis KC, Pyrovolou N, Zahos KA, et al. Late postoperative infection following spinal instrumentation: stainless steel versus titanium implants. J Surg Orthop Adv. 2008; 17(3):193–199

[26] Vitale MG, Riedel MD, Glotzbecker MP, et al. Building consensus: development of a Best Practice Guideline (BPG) for surgical site infection (SSI) prevention in high-risk pediatric spine surgery. J Pediatr Orthop. 2013; 33 (5):471–478

[27] Canavese F, Gupta S, Krajbich JI, Emara KM. Vacuum-assisted closure for deep infection after spinal instrumentation for scoliosis. J Bone Joint Surg Br. 2008; 90(3):377–381

[28] van Rhee MA, de Klerk LW, Verhaar JA. Vacuum-assisted wound closure of deep infections after instrumented spinal fusion in six children with neuromuscular scoliosis. Spine J. 2007; 7(5):596–600

[29] Rohmiller MT, Akbarnia BA, Raiszadeh K, Raiszadeh K, Canale S. Closed suction irrigation for the treatment of postoperative wound infections following posterior spinal fusion and instrumentation. Spine. 2010; 35(6):642–646

[30] Ho C, Skaggs DL, Weiss JM, Tolo VT. Management of infection after instrumented posterior spine fusion in pediatric scoliosis. Spine. 2007; 32 (24):2739–2744

[31] Clark CE, Shufflebarger HL. Late-developing infection in instrumented idiopathic scoliosis. Spine. 1999; 24(18):1909–1912

[32] Richards BR, Emara KM. Delayed infections after posterior TSRH spinal instrumentation for idiopathic scoliosis: revisited. Spine. 2001; 26(18):1990–1996

24 Postoperative Intensive Care Unit Management

Sandeep Khanna and Kathleen Gorenc

Abstract

The postoperative period after scoliosis repair requires a multidisciplinary approach with coordination of multiple services including intensive care, the pain service, nutrition, rehabilitation, and social services. This chapter focuses on components of postsurgical care including intraoperative concerns, initial assessment of the patient after arrival to the intensive care unit, physiologic principles of optimal function of different organs, multiorgan dysfunction following surgery, and complications encountered in the postoperative period.

Keywords: blood loss, coagulopathy, electrolytes, hypovolemia, infection intubation, monitoring, nutrition, pain control, scoliosis

24.1 Introduction

Postoperative care of the patient following scoliosis surgery begins by obtaining the information pertaining to the cardiopulmonary status of the patient, as well as other pertinent medical history. History of seizures, nutritional status, mobility, and home medications are all crucial to obtain preoperatively, and will allow optimal care to be provided intraoperatively and postoperatively. History of pulmonary or cardiac disease is essential to elicit. Patients may require a preoperative ECHO (or echocardiogram) or pulmonary function tests (PFTs). The anesthesiologist and the surgeon accomplish a smooth transfer to the intensive care unit (ICU) by providing a detailed verbal report describing preoperative and intraoperative events (▶ Table 24.1).

During this transfer of care, invasive and noninvasive monitoring, including electrocardiogram (ECG), blood pressure, heart rate, ventilation, and oxygenation, is maintained. A rapid assessment of the cardiopulmonary status of the patient, with special attention to ventilation, oxygenation, perfusion, and urine output, is then made. A chest radiograph is obtained immediately upon arrival at the ICU to assess the lung fields, position of tubes and lines, as well as the new spinal implant (▶ Table 24.2).

Recovery following spinal fusion may be classified as either normal or abnormal. A normal recovery is expected based upon the preoperative state of the patient and intraoperative course. Prolonged recovery may occur as a result of unexpected complications of the surgical correction and/or complication effecting organ systems either directly as a result of surgery or in the form of a secondary complication such as sepsis or pneumonia.

24.1.1 Mechanical Ventilation and Pulmonary Support

Patients with idiopathic scoliosis are often healthy preoperatively, and therefore experience a complication-free surgery. As

Table 24.1 Information passed between anesthesiologist and ICU (intensive care unit) team following surgery (the hand-off)

Preoperative history	Etiology of scoliosis Past medical illnesses Comorbidities Pulmonary function tests ECHO Medications Allergies Previous surgeries Nutritional status
Intraoperative considerations	Airway (difficult intubation?) Respiratory parameters, ventilator settings Anesthetic agents Hemodynamic parameters Vasoactive agents Blood loss and blood products Fluids and electrolytes Levels of vertebra involved Correction Neurophysiologic monitoring

Table 24.2 Immediate postoperative assessment performed by ICU (intensive care unit) team

Pulmonary	Breath sounds Endotracheal tube size position leak Chest expansion Facial edema and airway edema from positioning
Cardiovascular	Heart rate Blood pressure invasive and noninvasive Cardiac output Capillary refill Peripheral perfusion color Filling pressures
CNS	Pupils Wakefulness Motor and sensory assessment
Abdomen	Distention Ileus
Labs	CBC, electrolytes, ABG, coagulation chest X-ray
ECG	Ischemia Arrhythmia
Temperature	Cardiac output Hypothermia
BP invasive and noninvasive	Hypotension or hypertension
Pulse oximeter	Saturations peripheral perfusion
Urine	Cardiac output, fluid status
End-tidal CO_2	Dead space, compliance, ventilation
CVP	Fluid status

Abbreviations: ABG, arterial blood gas; BP, blood pressure; CBC, complete blood count; CNS, central nervous system; CVP, central venous pressure; ECG, electrocardiogram.

a result, they commonly tolerate extubation immediately postoperatively or on the same day of surgery. For those patients with neuromuscular scoliosis, comorbidities including cerebral palsy, seizure disorder, congenital anomalies, cardiac anomalies such as Fontan patients, myopathies, and muscular dystrophies such as Duchenne muscular dystrophy increase the likelihood that they will require respiratory support postoperatively in the ICU.

Mechanical ventilation in the postoperative period may be required for a variety of reasons including airway control, inappropriate oxygen delivery, abnormal lung function, inadequate cardiac output and fluid overload, significant abdominal distension, residual anesthesia, and neurologic complications. It has been shown that scoliosis surgery produces immediate and transient decrease of up to 40% in vital capacity (VC) in almost all patients undergoing surgery.[1] The reasons for this decline are many, including the duration of the operation, patient positioning, and surgical trauma to various muscle groups (especially with thoracotomy). Given that the VC is usually much lower than normal before surgery, any further reduction can easily lead to respiratory failure. This risk is significantly higher in patients with neuromuscular scoliosis.

An early goal of ICU care is to proceed with a safe and expedited wean from mechanical ventilation. A systematic review of the criteria for extubation is performed (▶ Table 24.3). Chest radiographs, blood gas sampling, pulse oximetry, end tidal carbon dioxide, lung mechanics, and physical examination are the parameters used to determine the weaning from mechanical ventilation and pulmonary adequacy. Dexamethasone is sometimes initiated to prevent airway edema, while diuretics may be started to achieve a negative fluid balance prior to extubation.

After weaning from mechanical ventilation, aggressive pulmonary toilet should be initiated to prevent atelectasis, which is more commonly seen in patients with neuromuscular scoliosis or myopathies. Patients at risk for postextubation atelectasis are weaned to noninvasive ventilation (bilevel positive airway pressure [BiPAP], nasal continuous positive airway pressure [NCPAP]), frequent chest percussion treatments and postural drainage are provided, and routine chest radiographs are performed to assess lung expansion. The efficacy of noninvasive ventilation in prevention of tracheal intubation due to respiratory failure is well supported.[2,3] Patients who require noninvasive ventilation at home should be placed on noninvasive ventilation via BiPAP or NCPAP immediately following extubation. Over the course of a few days, the noninvasive ventilation can be weaned as patient strength improves and pain is reduced.

Pleural effusions may develop in response to the fluids administered in the operating room. A chest tube may be placed in the operating room or a thoracentesis may need to be performed prior to extubation for resolution of the pleural effusion and optimization of functional residual capacity. Postsurgical thoracotomy complications including air leak, hemothorax, and persistent chest pain[4] are commonly observed, whereas chylothorax has been noted much less frequently and is most often associated with an anterior surgical approach.[4]

Halo placement and cervical fusion pose unique challenges to the anesthesiologists and intensivists while securing an airway. Fixed position, limited access to the face, and immobilization of neck due to halo and cervical fusion make it difficult to visualize the larynx, thus increasing the level of difficulty for successful tracheal intubation, as well as increasing the upper airway obstruction following tracheal extubation. Patients placed in a halo vest sometimes experience a decrease in VC that may reduce their pulmonary reserve and ability to tolerate any pulmonary insult.[5]

Prior to tracheal extubation, patients must be able to maintain their airway, demonstrate adequate gag reflex and cough, and be able to manage secretions, as well as demonstrate adequate strength to support spontaneous respirations. The intubation and anesthetic record should be reviewed prior to extubation. For patients with pre-existing pulmonary disease or airway control issues, preoperative PFTs, chest X-rays, and medications should be reviewed. Prolonged mechanical ventilation can be necessary in patients with severe restrictive lung disease prior to scoliosis repair. Based on these considerations, if it has been determined safe, experienced personnel (intensivists, anesthesiologists, ear nose throat specialists if difficult airway) should be readily available at the time of extubation. If there is concern that the patient's trachea may need to be re-intubated due to weakness, excessive secretions, or known future procedures such as staged repair, extubation should be postponed. It should be noted that one should have a low threshold for re-intubating these patients under more controlled and elective circumstances. In these situations, a fiberoptic bronchoscope, glidescope, or laryngeal mask airway may be helpful.

24.1.2 Cardiac Support

Support of the cardiovascular system is directed at optimizing cardiac output and oxygen delivery. This is achieved by optimization of preload, afterload, and inotropy, and is guided by invasive, noninvasive, and laboratory monitoring.

Requirement for cardiac support in patients with no associated heart diseases, such as cardiomyopathy, is minimal. Hypovolemia is the most commonly recognized complication following scoliosis surgery and results from inadequate replacement of intraoperative fluid losses, as well as from fluid third spacing. Unless there are complications associated with loss of motor evoked potential (MEP) and somatosensory evoked potential (SSEP) in the operating room, patients do not routinely require vasopressor support.

For patients who experienced loss of MEP and SSEP during scoliosis surgery, support of blood pressure is achieved using vasopressors and fluid replacement to optimize nerve and spinal cord perfusion. SSEP and MEP are particularly sensitive to

---

Table 24.3 Criteria for extubation

Oxygen saturations adequate with minimal ventilator support on $FiO_2 < 50\%$

Spontaneous breathing with good tidal volumes of 4–7 mL/kg

Resolution of airway and facial swelling

Airway protective reflexes intact

Need for tracheal suctioning and quality and quantity of secretions

Good cardiac output and hemodynamics

Adequate urine output and no evidence of fluid overload

Heart rate normal

Chest X-ray shows good expansion and clear lung fields

Adequate pain control

blood pressure changes and can be used quite effectively to titrate the degree of hypotensive state that the spinal cord will withstand.[6] At the time of transfer to the pediatric intensive care unit (PICU), anesthesiologists will report the use of vasopressor support intraoperatively, and will note the mean arterial pressure utilized to preserve evoked potentials during surgery. In these patients, the mean arterial blood pressure is usually maintained at a slightly higher-than-normal value by administering intravenous fluids, intravenous calcium, and vasopressor therapy. Dopamine is commonly used; however, epinephrine and norepinephrine can be added if there is a need to increase systemic vascular resistance.

Patients with pre-existing heart disease, such as Duchenne muscular dystrophy, are maintained on their preoperative medications. It is pertinent to review the preoperative echocardiogram and utilize invasive and noninvasive monitoring to follow hemodynamics. Prior to induction of anesthesia, every effort should be made to obtain a baseline echocardiogram so that baseline cardiac function may be well understood and to determine what cardiac support the patient will need in the perioperative period.

24.2 Fluids, Electrolytes, and Renal Function

Postoperative fluid management is immensely influenced by heart rate, blood pressure, perfusion, and urine output. The anesthesiologist communicates optimal right atrial pressure, along with blood pressure upon arrival at the ICU. The optimum right atrial pressure, blood pressure, and urine output is then maintained by administering colloid and/or crystalloid intravenous fluids and blood products.

Maintenance intravenous fluids are administered during the first postoperative day, followed by either enteral feeds or hyperalimentation on subsequent days depending on the patient's ability to tolerate enteral feeds.

Syndrome of inappropriate antidiuretic hormone (SIADH) has been reported in patients after spinal surgery. The incidence of SIADH varies from 5 to 30%.[7,8,9] SIADH is defined as the retention of water, loss of sodium, and inappropriately concentrated urine, in normovolemic and hypervolemic patients in whom renal and adrenal functions are normal. In these patients, the loss of sodium and water retention has been attributed to sustained endogenous production and release of antidiuretic hormone (ADH) or ADH-like substances without any physiologic and pharmacological stimuli to ADH release. Postoperative SIADH has been attributed to invasion of dura mater and traction on the neural pathways[9] and to stress after surgery.[10] SIADH resolves spontaneously and in the immediate postoperative period is treated with diuresis and replacement of sodium with normal saline, hypertonic saline, or fluid restriction.

Hypokalemia occurs infrequently, but when seen is often due to the use of diuretics in the postoperative period. Hyperkalemia rarely occurs and is a consequence of renal dysfunction. This is rarely seen in this patient population unless the patient develops prerenal failure due to inadequate fluid administration in the perioperative period, thus leading to low cardiac output and renal perfusion.

Hypomagnesemia and hypophosphatemia are very common in the postoperative period following spinal surgery. These electrolyte imbalances result from the administration of fluids and intracellular shifts, thus causing a dilution effect. Hypophosphatemia is especially important as it can lead to impaired oxygen delivery, myocardial depression, and respiratory insufficiency.[11,12,13]

Another common electrolyte disturbance commonly seen following spine surgery is hypocalcemia. Factors contributing to hypocalcemia are citrate in packed red blood cells which binds free calcium, diuretic therapy, and the use of albumin to expand intravascular volume. Albumin decreases the proportion of ionized calcium available for cellular interaction by binding calcium.

Surgical stress and exogenous glucose administration associated with surgical repair can affect blood glucose levels and can result in hyperglycemia. Hyperglycemia, in turn, can result in osmotic diuresis and intravascular dehydration. High levels of hyperglycemia are treated with continuous insulin infusions.

Renal function is mostly well preserved and diuretics are frequently utilized in the case of total body fluid overload secondary to fluid replacement therapy. Renal failure after scoliosis surgery may be related to inadequate fluid administration intraoperatively, subsequent development of sepsis, or infection.

24.2.1 Infection

The child who undergoes scoliosis surgery is at an increased risk for postoperative infection related to surgery duration, requirement for number and duration of intravascular catheters, bladder catheterization, malnutrition, multiple stages of scoliosis surgeries, etc. Surgery alone can add to the risk of infection because of surgical trauma, immunologic depression, and possible surgical entry of organisms. Patients with neuromuscular causes of scoliosis have a much higher incidence of postoperative infection, ranging from 4 to 14% in some studies. Impaired immune status, poor personal hygiene, degree of cognitive impairment, use of allograft, and contamination of the wound contribute to the higher incidence of infection in patients with neuromuscular disorders.[14,15,16,17]

Antibiotic prophylaxis is recommended, consisting of a first-generation cephalosporin 20 to 30 minutes prior to the initiation of surgery, during intraoperative period, and then postoperatively for at least 24 to 48 hours. First-generation cephalosporins are recommended as first-line therapy, since they provide coverage against staphylococcus aureus, a frequently identified organism isolated following scoliosis surgery. Cefazolin is one example of a first-generation cephalosporin that is commonly used.[18] In the case that the patient has an allergy to cephalosporins, Vancomycin is frequently recommended for antibiotic prophylaxis after surgery. Patients who are incontinent of bladder or bowel are at increased risk of infection with gram-negative organisms. Coverage for these organisms, such as aminoglycosides, is recommended in these patients. Broad-spectrum antibiotics are not recommended due to concerns of emergence of resistant bacteria and opportunistic infections.

Systemic signs of infection include fever, leukocytosis, elevated erythrocyte sedimentation rate and C-reactive protein, chest infiltrates, and hemodynamic instability due to sepsis. However, temperature elevations are also common in the first 4 days after surgery due to metabolic changes, so a fever workup is often not appropriate for an isolated fever during this time. If systemic signs of infection are present, antibiotics therapy may be broadened and blood, tracheal, urinary, and wound cultures should be sent. The antibiotic spectrum is narrowed once the culture results and organism sensitivities and susceptibility are available. Urinary tract infections are usually secondary to a Foley catheter–associated infection. Treatment for postoperative urinary tract infections consists of removal of the contaminated catheter and administration of the appropriate antibiotic for the organism identified. Blood and urine cultures should be collected daily until all cultures result as negative for growth. Deep central lines can be a common source of bacteremia and sepsis. If blood cultures remain positive for bacteria despite appropriate antibiotic therapy, then deep intravenous catheters should be removed or exchanged. Infectious disease consultants should be involved to help direct therapy and provide recommendations for further care. All invasive lines and tubes should be removed as soon as clinically acceptable to decrease the risk of catheter-associated infections.

Deep wound infection after surgery for scoliosis correction is considered a significant complication that requires prolonged medical and surgical management. Infection can occur early or late. Wound infections are aggressively treated both medically and surgically, which can involve debridement and removal of infected material, instrumentation or tissue. The critical care team is involved only when deep wound infections are severe, associated with severe sepsis, systemic inflammatory response syndrome, or renal and cardiopulmonary complications.

24.2.2 Neurological Complications

After arrival in the ICU, the initiation of sedation and analgesia is postponed until the patient is awake. Once the patient is awake, a rapid neurologic examination is performed to document any signs of sensory or motor deficits and the level of consciousness. This should be compared against the patient's baseline, which is relayed during the hand-off (▶ Table 24.1). If the patient is ready for tracheal extubation at that time, mechanical ventilation is weaned and the patient is extubated. If factors preclude tracheal extubation, sedation and analgesia are resumed and hourly neurological exams are performed.

Any neurological abnormality recognized in the intraoperative period is aggressively treated. Reversal of paraplegia or normalization of SSEP and MEP occur with restoration of normal to higher mean arterial pressure, correction of anemia, and release of distraction in the operating room.[19] Mean arterial pressure should be maintained above normal as needed to prevent or, in severe cases, to improve the spinal cord ischemia. This can be achieved by fluid administration, vasopressor therapy, or a combination of both. Mild hyperosmolar therapy with hypertonic saline and mannitol is also initiated to improve the potential spinal cord injury, which may have resulted from direct trauma. Hyperosmolar therapy also improves rheology and has been found to improve spinal cord perfusion. Methylprednisolone is controversial but, if used, starts at a dose of 30 mg/kg administered, followed by a continuous infusion of 5.4 mg/kg/h

for a total of 24 hours in line with accepted spinal injury protocols after discussion with orthopaedic surgery.[20]

Postoperative pain control is achieved with narcotics, which include fentanyl or morphine infusions with or without patient-controlled analgesia, and anxiolysis with benzodiazepines. NSAIDs (nonsteroidal anti-inflammatory drugs) such as Ketorolac may be utilized for four to six doses in the postoperative period and have been found to offer good pain control. Diazepam is also useful in the postoperative period to alleviate pain or discomfort that may result from muscle spasm. Effective pain control and active rehabilitation following scoliosis correction require a multimodal regimen of pain management.[21] The pain service is often actively involved in the management of pain in the postoperative period.

24.3 Gastrointestinal

It is important to optimize the nutritional status of the patient before and after surgery. There is considerable variability among patients in tolerating nasogastric feeds postoperatively, and close examination during advancement of feeds is essential. Transpyloric feeding is frequently employed in postoperative, ventilated patients after scoliosis surgery to achieve targeted calorie intake rapidly. A nutritional plan should be developed on arrival.

Paralytic ileus, stress ulcers, pancreatitis, and superior mesenteric artery syndrome are postoperative complications seen in the ICU after scoliosis surgery.

Postoperative ileus is frequently present after scoliosis surgery. Distraction mechanisms that are performed during surgery that causes a mechanism of traction affect the peritoneum and, in combination with opioid use for pain control, can result in an ileus. Placement of the nasogastric tube to low intermittent wall suction for 12 to 24 hours can treat or prevent postoperative ileus. Slow feeds are started in these patients, and use of narcotics is reduced for pain control. Scoliosis patients after surgery also develop severe constipation due to decreased physical activity level and opioid use. Stool softeners should be initiated early to prevent this complication.

As in all major surgical procedures, stress ulcers can occur. Antacids such as ranitidine and omeprazole are routinely administered to reduce stress ulcers. Early initiation of enteral feeds has also been found to prevent stress ulceration.

Pancreatitis appears as a postoperative complication of scoliosis surgery in children and adults. Gastroesophageal reflux disease, reactive airway disease, patient position, anemia and blood loss, anesthetic agents, metabolic factors, and autonomic nervous system abnormalities are implicated in the pathogenesis of pancreatitis after scoliosis surgery.[22],[23],[24] It should be suspected with the appearance of vomiting, abdominal distension, and abdominal pain. Abdominal ultrasound and laboratory tests, which include serum amylase and lipase, are done for confirmation. Pancreatitis resolves with resting the bowel and by replacing enteral nutrition with parenteral nutrition.

Superior mesenteric artery (SMA) syndrome is an uncommon but well-recognized clinical entity characterized by compression of the third or transverse portion of the duodenum between the aorta and the SMA. The syndrome is attributed to excessive stretching of the spine or extrinsic compression with corrective casts. The syndrome usually develops 6 to 10 days after scoliosis surgery and is rarely encountered in the ICU but should be considered in the differential for any gastrointestinal disturbance.

The symptoms of SMA syndrome are nonspecific. These patients may present with postoperative nausea, permanent bilious vomiting, pain, and bloating. Diagnosis is made by abdominal radiography showing dilation of gastric and first portions of the duodenum. Obstruction of the duodenum, with proximal dilation, can be identified with a barium swallow series.[25] Doppler ultrasonography and angiography are also used to evaluate the aortomesenteric angle. Using oral and intravenous contrast-enhanced abdominal tomography and angiography, duodenum and the vascular structures can be evaluated simultaneously.[26] Medical treatment with fluid therapy, parenteral nutrition, and nasogastric tube usually results in improvement.[25] In extreme cases, surgery is the only option and a duodenojejunostomy should be undertaken.

24.4 Hematology

Hematological stability is one of the most important postoperative considerations following a surgical correction of scoliosis. Significant blood loss and coagulopathy are common in the operative and postoperative period. It is not uncommon for a patient to lose 50% or greater of their total blood volume. Much of the blood volume loss is associated with the length of the procedure and number of segments fused during the correction; an ongoing blood loss in the postoperative period can account for approximately 30% of the total blood loss. Some studies have found a direct correlation between milliliters of blood loss for every segment fused.[27]

Close monitoring with serial CBCs (complete blood counts) as well as activated partial thromboplastin time (APTT), partial thromboplastin time (PT), and thrombin time is crucial. Blood loss during surgical correction of scoliosis should be discussed preoperatively, and replacement of blood products should be anticipated throughout the perioperative period. Depending on the degree of blood loss, it is common for patients to require multiple transfusions of varying blood products including packed red blood cells, fresh frozen plasma, platelets, and cryoprecipitate.

In addition to blood loss, patients can develop coagulopathy following surgical correction of scoliosis. Similar to the blood loss, the degree of coagulopathy can be directly related to the number of segments fused and length of the procedure. Severe coagulopathy is more often observed in patients with neuromuscular scoliosis due to longer operative periods, more segments fused, and a history of osteopenia that is associated with more bleeding and longer operative times. Patients undergoing surgical correction of idiopathic scoliosis are less likely to have other underlying conditions such as pre-existing coagulation abnormalities or anemia, thus experiencing less severe blood loss and or coagulopathies.

Intravenous (IV) access with large bore IVs, central-line catheters, or arterial catheters are often placed and utilized during the operative period. These catheters are often left in place for the first 24 to 48 hours postoperatively to continue close monitoring and to carefully assess blood loss. CVP (central venous pressure) monitoring may help indicate fluid status of the patient. Close hemodynamic monitoring and blood sampling is necessary to closely monitor blood loss and coagulopathies so that adequate replacement can occur in a timely manner.

24.5 Skin

Skin integrity should be taken into consideration throughout the perioperative course of surgical scoliosis repair. All patients undergoing surgical correction should undergo a thorough skin examination prior to surgical repair, in the immediate postoperative period, and throughout the duration of their hospital stay.

Multiple aspects of the surgical correction impact skin integrity, beginning with the preoperative status of the patients. Any patient undergoing surgical correction of scoliosis is at significant risk for altered skin integrity, but children suffering from neuromuscular scoliosis are especially at risk for potential skin breakdown. Neuromuscular scoliosis is often associated with significant comorbidities, which increase the risk of skin breakdown and altered skin integrity. Neuromuscular scoliosis negatively affects skin integrity as the degree of developmental delay significantly interferes with the ability to perform activities of daily living independently, thus requiring help with positioning during elimination, bathing, and feeding. As a result, skin integrity may be altered prior to surgical correction.

During the operative period, it is pertinent that proper precautions are taken to reduce or eliminate new or further skin breakdown. Surgical correction of scoliosis can be a lengthy operation. Often, the patient is required to be in a prone position and can develop pressure ulcers during this period of time alone if the necessary precautions are not taken. Therefore, it is crucial that upon completion of the surgical correction, in the immediate postoperative assessment, a thorough skin exam is completed to assess for old, new, and potential areas of concern, as well as to evaluate new surgical sites.

The surgical incision should be assessed immediately postoperatively, and any drainage should be noted and documented. Significant saturation of any surgical dressing can lead to further skin breakdown, and dressing changes should be made accordingly at the discretion of the surgical team. Surgical dressings shall also remain occlusive to prevent possible infection of the surgical site. Drain sites should also be closely monitored following discontinuity of the drains for fluid accumulation or leaking at the site of insertion.

Pain can often limit the patient's ability to be mobile and can potentiate further skin breakdown. Therefore, adequate pain management will facilitate proper position changes, ambulation, and spontaneous movement, preventing or reducing the risk of skin breakdown. Adequate nutrition is another important factor in maintaining skin integrity in the postoperative period. Early initiation of optimal nutrition will promote wound healing and assist in maintaining the integrity of the skin, thus aiding in preventing skin breakdown. Finally, patients are often sedated or unable to ambulate to the restroom. Incontinence, dependence on diaper, or inability to ambulate to void may lead to further skin breakdown. Proper positioning and frequent position changes are extremely important for this patient population. Positioning can be painful and patients may be hesitant or resistant to move. Logrolling the patient in the initial post-operative period every 2 hours is optimal for maintaining proper alignment following the surgical repair as well as preventing pressure ulcers or skin breakdown.

References

[1] Koumbourlis AC. Scoliosis and the respiratory system. Paediatr Respir Rev. 2006; 7(2):152–160

[2] Doherty MJ, Millner PA, Latham M, Dickson RA, Elliott MW. Non-invasive ventilation in the treatment of ventilatory failure following corrective spinal surgery. Anaesthesia. 2001; 56(3):235–238

[3] Kindgen-Milles D, Müller E, Buhl R, et al. Nasal-continuous positive airway pressure reduces pulmonary morbidity and length of hospital stay following thoracoabdominal aortic surgery. Chest. 2005; 128(2):821–828

[4] Grossfeld S, Winter RB, Lonstein JE, Denis F, Leonard A, Johnson L. Complications of anterior spinal surgery in children. J Pediatr Orthop. 1997; 17(1):89–95

[5] Lind B, Bake B, Lundqvist C, Nordwall A. Influence of halo vest treatment on vital capacity. Spine. 1987; 12(5):449–452

[6] Schwartz DM, Auerbach JD, Dormans JP, et al. Neurophysiological detection of impending spinal cord injury during scoliosis surgery. J Bone Joint Surg Am. 2007; 89(11):2440–2449

[7] Callewart CC, Minchew JT, Kanim LE, et al. Hyponatremia and syndrome of inappropriate antidiuretic hormone secretion in adult spinal surgery. Spine. 1994; 19(15):1674–1679

[8] Elster AD. Hyponatremia after spinal fusion caused by inappropriate secretion of antidiuretic hormone (SIADH). Clin Orthop Relat Res. 1985(194):136–141

[9] Lieh-Lai MW, Stanitski DF, Sarnaik AP, et al. Syndrome of inappropriate antidiuretic hormone secretion in children following spinal fusion. Crit Care Med. 1999; 27(3):622–627

[10] Philbin DM, Coggins CH. Plasma antidiuretic hormone levels in cardiac surgical patients during morphine and halothane anesthesia. Anesthesiology. 1978; 49(2):95–98

[11] Knochel JP. The pathophysiology and clinical characteristics of severe hypophosphatemia. Arch Intern Med. 1977; 137(2):203–220

[12] Newman JH, Neff TA, Ziporin P. Acute respiratory failure associated with hypophosphatemia. N Engl J Med. 1977; 296(19):1101–1103

[13] O'Connor LR, Wheeler WS, Bethune JE. Effect of hypophosphatemia on myocardial performance in man. N Engl J Med. 1977; 297(17):901–903

[14] Szöke G, Lipton G, Miller F, Dabney K. Wound infection after spinal fusion in children with cerebral palsy. J Pediatr Orthop. 1998; 18(6):727–733

[15] Lonstein J, Winter R, Moe J, Gaines D. Wound infection with Harrington instrumentation and spine fusion for scoliosis. Clin Orthop Relat Res. 1973 (96):222–233

[16] Sponseller PD, LaPorte DM, Hungerford MW, Eck K, Bridwell KH, Lenke LG. Deep wound infections after neuromuscular scoliosis surgery: a multicenter study of risk factors and treatment outcomes. Spine. 2000; 25(19):2461–2466

[17] Smith JS, Shaffrey CI, Sansur CA, et al. Scoliosis Research Society Morbidity and Mortality Committee. Rates of infection after spine surgery based on 108,419 procedures: a report from the Scoliosis Research Society Morbidity and Mortality Committee. Spine. 2011; 36(7):556–563

[18] Barker FG, II. Efficacy of prophylactic antibiotic therapy in spinal surgery: a meta-analysis. Neurosurgery. 2002; 51(2):391–400

[19] Winter RB. Neurologic safety in spinal deformity surgery. Spine. 1997; 22 (13):1527–1533

[20] Mooney JF, III, Bernstein R, Hennrikus WL, Jr, MacEwen GD. Neurologic risk management in scoliosis surgery. J Pediatr Orthop. 2002; 22(5):683–689

[21] Kehlet H, Dahl JB. The value of "multimodal" or "balanced analgesia" in postoperative pain treatment. Anesth Analg. 1993; 77(5):1048–1056

[22] Leichtner AM, Banta JV, Etienne N, et al. Pancreatitis following scoliosis surgery in children and young adults. J Pediatr Orthop. 1991; 11(5):594–598

[23] Borkhuu B, Nagaraju D, Miller F, et al. Prevalence and risk factors in postoperative pancreatitis after spine fusion in patients with cerebral palsy. J Pediatr Orthop. 2009; 29(3):256–262

[24] Laplaza FJ, Widmann RF, Fealy S, et al. Pancreatitis after surgery in adolescent idiopathic scoliosis: incidence and risk factors. J Pediatr Orthop. 2002; 22 (1):80–83

[25] Biank V, Werlin S. Superior mesenteric artery syndrome in children: a 20-year experience. J Pediatr Gastroenterol Nutr. 2006; 42(5):522–525

[26] Applegate GR, Cohen AJ. Dynamic CT in superior mesenteric artery syndrome. J Comput Assist Tomogr. 1988; 12(6):976–980

[27] Murray DJ, Forbes RB, Titone MB, Weinstein SL. Transfusion management in pediatric and adolescent scoliosis surgery. Efficacy of autologous blood. Spine. 1997; 22(23):2735–2740

25 Reoperations: Instrumentation Failure, Junctional Kyphosis, and Cervical Extension

Vidyadhar V. Upasani, Corey B. Fuller, and Munish Gupta

Abstract

Surgical correction of neuromuscular scoliosis is associated with a higher complication rate compared to idiopathic scoliosis.[1,2] Most of the published outcomes and complication data are in patients with cerebral palsy; however, a number of large studies have been published in patients with myelodysplasia and muscular dystrophy. There are many reasons for failures after surgery for neuromuscular spinal deformity, which include pseudarthrosis, rod failure, adding-on, junctional deformity, and recurrence of deformity due to crankshaft. The most common complications in these patient populations are related to infection, pseudarthrosis, and implant failure, as well as pulmonary and neurologic compromise. The primary indication for reoperation after spinal deformity correction is pain. Although the etiology of postoperative pain may be multifactorial, this chapter will focus on reoperations related to instrumentation failure, junctional kyphosis, and cervical extension.

Keywords: cervical extension, crankshaft, instrumentation failure, junctional kyphosis, neuromuscular scoliosis, revision surgery

25.1 Instrumentation Failure

The instrumentation used to correct neuromuscular scoliosis has evolved over the last 60 years. The Luque–Galveston technique, with dual rods or the unit rod, has traditionally been the most common posterior instrumentation used.[3,4] More recently, segmental fixation with all-pedicle screws or hybrid constructs has increased in popularity to improve deformity correction and lower rates of pseudarthrosis and implant failure.[5] Spinal instrumentation complications can be classified as biologic failures due to infection or pseudarthrosis or biomechanical failures resulting in implant breakage. A recent meta-analysis of complications in neuromuscular spinal deformity surgery included 7,612 patients and found an overall implant complication rate of 12.5%.[6] It is important to note, however, that implant failure does not always necessitate revision surgery. A study of 74 neuromuscular patients who underwent spinal fusion reported 6 cases of broken rods, yet 4 were asymptomatic and did not require revision surgery.[7] It is not infrequent to see loosening around the iliac screws, which do not need to be revised. Revision surgery for implant failure in the patient with neuromuscular scoliosis should be reserved for pain or significant loss of correction (▸ Fig. 25.1).

25.1.1 Pseudarthrosis

Biologic pseudarthrosis in the spine is a lack of bony fusion with formation of a false joint. A pseudarthrosis can result from several causes including insufficient stability or infection and often presents in the form of pain, deformity progression, or failed instrumentation. If there is no evidence of implant failure or

obvious lucency in the fusion mass, workup often proceeds to computed tomography (CT) scan for more definitive diagnosis. Magnetic resonance imaging (MRI) can be helpful to assess the central canal and neuroforamina.

Unfortunately, a pseudarthrosis can occur in these patients even after a technically well-performed spinal surgery. The lever arm is often long in the neuromuscular patient and places a tremendous amount of stress at the end of fusion, especially at the lumbosacral junction. Prevention lies in being meticulous in surgery with facetectomies, use of robust bone graft, and stable fixation. Overall incidence of pseudarthrosis after spinal deformity surgery in the neuromuscular population is 1.88% with higher rates in myelomeningocele (12.63%) compared to cerebral palsy (0.05%) and Duchenne muscular dystrophy (2.97%).[6] In cerebral palsy, the incidence has declined over the last 50 years with the advancement of spinal implants. Pseudarthrosis rates from 11 to 40% were reported with use of Harrington rods and improved to 13% with Luque instrumentation. More recently Tsirikos et al reported on 45 consecutive patients with cerebral palsy who underwent posterior spinal fusion with a pedicle screw construct and reported no cases of pseudarthrosis.[8]

Despite its relatively low incidence, pseudarthrosis is the most common reason for revision surgery in the neuromuscular population outside the immediate postoperative period.[9] Although not all pseudarthroses necessitate revision surgery, in the setting of pain or implant failure with loss of correction, surgical revision may be required. Infection should be ruled out as the cause of the pseudarthrosis prior to planning reoperation. Revision surgery for pseudarthrosis typically involves assessment and debridement of the pseudarthrosis with deformity correction and rigid stabilization of the segment.

Fortunately, if appropriately managed, pseudarthrosis can be treated successfully. Dias et al reported on four children with cerebral palsy who underwent revision spine surgery at their intuition for symptomatic pseudarthrosis with progressive deformity and implant failure.[10] Resolution of symptoms and correction of deformity were successfully achieved in three patients. The fourth child underwent revision with takedown and bone grafting of the pseudarthrosis without instrumentation, resulting in persistent and symptomatic pseudarthrosis. They concluded that rigid instrumentation combined with pseudarthrosis debridement and bone grafting is imperative for successful deformity correction and resolution of symptoms.

Yagi et al had similar findings on 50 cases of pediatric revision spine surgeries, of which 13 involved neuromuscular scoliosis.[11] Nine of 13 patients (69%) underwent revision for pain or progressive deformity from pseudarthrosis. Eight patients had resolution of symptoms after undergoing revision and one patient had residual symptoms with recurrent pseudarthrosis, which was treated successfully with a second revision. This is consistent with previous reports in that pseudarthrosis is the most common postoperative complication requiring revision in the neuromuscular scoliosis population, and with clear

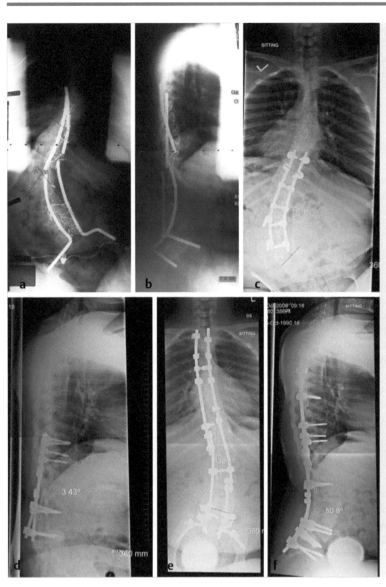

Fig. 25.1 (a–f) A patient with broken instrumentation and pseudarthrosis that was revised. The patient had failure again and then underwent another revision.

indications, bone grafting, osteotomies if necessary, and appropriate instrumentation, the risk of pseudarthrosis recurrence is minimized and successful outcome is likely.

25.1.2 Biomechanical Failure

Other sources of increased stress on the bone–implant interface and potential biomechanical failure beside pseudarthrosis include obesity, poor bone quality, and significant preoperative spinal deformity, especially in the sagittal plane and at the lumbopelvic junction. The larger the curve, the stiffer the curve, and the softer the bone, the more important the bone–implant interface. Sink et al found a high rate of proximal and distal instrumentation pullout and failure in the management of cerebral palsy spinal deformity using the Luque–Galveston instrumentation and identified hyperkyphosis as a significant risk factor for implant failure.[12] With a 54% failure rate, they concluded that the Luque–Galveston instrumentation was not ideal given the significant deforming forces in hyperkyphotic spinal deformities.

Although once the most popular instrumentation for neuromuscular spinal deformities, the Luque–Galveston instrumentation has fallen out of favor in recent years due to biomechanical advantages of newer screw-based constructs.[13] This is especially true in treating the significant pelvic obliquity often found in neuromuscular scoliosis. Options have expanded significantly including iliosacral screw fixation, iliac screw fixation, and sacral–alar–iliac (SAI) screw fixation. Although these new techniques have been shown to be powerful in the correction and maintenance of pelvic obliquity, they also have introduced new modes of failure.

Iliac screws became popular with proponents citing diminished implant failure and lower pseudarthrosis rates; however, complications related to rod disengagement from screws and connectors were reported.[14,15] More recently, S2-iliac screw fixation has been gaining popularity as a powerful technique to control pelvic obliquity; however, the course of S2-iliac screws crosses the sacroiliac joint in the majority of cases and the long-term clinical significance of this is unknown.[16,17]

Although uncommon, revision for failed pelvic fixation in neuromuscular scoliosis is generally reserved for symptoms or significant loss of deformity correction. In the case of implant failure in Galveston rods, revision to modern screw-based constructs is commonly used if fusion is not present. Revision of screw-based constructs commonly consists of additional or longer screw placement with deformity correction and debridement and bone grafting of pseudarthrosis, if present. Longer screws have been shown to improve implant stability if they reach anterior to the caudal extension of the middle osteoligamentous column.[18]

Sponseller et al compared 32 patients who underwent S2-iliac fixation to 27 patients who had traditional sacral or iliac screws in patients with significant pelvic obliquity from cerebral palsy.[16] Revision rates were comparable as each group had one revision for implant failure. One patient in the S2-alar group required revision for sacral joint pain, which improved with longer screw placement, and one patient in the traditional group required revision for failure of fixation and pain at implant site.

Myung et al retrospectively looked at 41 patients with neuromuscular scoliosis who underwent posterior spinal fusion to the pelvis with iliac screws in 31 patients and S2-iliac screws in 10 patients.[19] They reported an overall implant complication rate of 29% with 9 occurring in the iliac screw group and 1 in the S2-iliac screw group. Despite this, only 2 patients required revision surgery, both in the iliac screw group for failed pelvic anchors. They noted that no failure occurred in patients in whom there were 6 or more screws in L5 and below. They concluded that more robust distal pelvic anchorage was protective against implant failure and this was easier to achieve with S2-iliac screws.

In neuromuscular spinal deformity, there are considerable forces the implant must withstand to prevent complications and achieve a successfully outcome. Each technique has cited advantages and disadvantages, and understanding several is necessary to manage a revision surgery for failed spinal or sacropelvic instrumentation.

25.2 Junctional Kyphosis

Junctional kyphosis is a postoperative phenomenon seen after spinal fusion in scoliosis and kyphosis deformities in which a focal kyphosis develops adjacent to the end of the fusion. This phenomenon has been described extensively in adolescent idiopathic scoliosis (AIS) and Scheuermann's kyphosis and can occur above or below the fusion. There are various definitions of junctional kyphosis with no clear consensus; however, the most commonly used in the literature is a greater than 10-degree difference in the Cobb angle in the sagittal plane between the lower endplate of the upper instrumented vertebra (UIV) and the upper endplate of the vertebrae two levels above and at least 10 degrees greater than the preoperative measurement.[20]

There are several different mechanisms that are thought to cause junctional kyphosis after fusion for spinal deformity that have mainly been described in patients with adolescent and adult idiopathic scoliosis. Violation of the posterior tension soft-tissue band near the end of the fusion level and thoracoplasty are both thought to destabilize the spine, leading to junctional kyphosis. Preoperative hyperkyphoses greater than 50-degree and greater than 10-degree intraoperative reduction of thoracic kyphosis have both been identified as a risk factor for junctional kyphosis as significant intraoperative correction of kyphosis can concentrate this stress at the ends of the fusion. Also a more rigid construct using all pedicle screws, especially at the transition between instrumented and uninstrumented vertebrae, has been found to have a higher incidence of junctional kyphosis compared to less rigid constructs using all-hook or hybrid fixation.[12,21,22,23,24]

Although junctional kyphosis does occur after spinal fusion in neuromuscular scoliosis, it more commonly occurs at the proximal end of the fusion in the upper thoracic region, as many fusions are extended to the pelvis in this patient population (▶ Fig. 25.2). The incidence of junctional kyphosis in cerebral palsy is less (< 2–5%) compared to published incidence of 17 to 46% in AIS.[9,25,26] Despite its occurrence, the clinical significance of junctional kyphosis is not clear. In the AIS group, several studies have not found a clinical difference between patients who develop junctional kyphosis and those who do not.[27] The clinical significance of junctional kyphosis has not been analyzed as closely in the neuromuscular population, and although there are certainly cases of junctional kyphosis that develop symptoms that require treatment, most do not.[9]

Despite the controversy, preventing junctional kyphosis is recommended and strategies directed at the risk factors. Minimizing soft-tissue dissection and preserving the facet joints, interspinous, and supraspinous ligaments near the ends of the construct are commonly recommended to preserve the posterior tension band near transitions.[27] Some surgeons will place transverse process hooks at the superior level of the fusion in order to preserve soft tissue and decrease the rigidity at the UIV in an effort to ease the stress at the end of the fusion. In spinal deformity in thepatients with cerebral palsy, ending the proximal instrumentation high in the thoracic spine around T2 is recommended to decrease the incidence of proximal junctional kyphosis (PJK) and proximal failure.[28]

Although symptomatic PJK is relatively rare in neuromuscular scoliosis, symptomatic progression does occur and may warrant surgical correction. Management strategies of symptomatic PJK in the neuromuscular patient generally involve extension of the posterior fusion to include the involved segments, with or without osteotomies. An anterior approach is generally unnecessary as the kyphosis can be managed posteriorly. If there is associated neuroforaminal or central stenosis, decompression may be a necessary addition as well.

Osteotomies are sometimes a necessary addition for correction of the junctional deformity along with proximal extension of the fusion. As the deformity in junctional kyphosis is often focal and rigid, occurring at only one or two levels above the previous UIVs, posteriorly based osteotomies such as pedicle subtraction and vertebral column resection are particularly well suited to correct focal deformities. However, the goal in revision surgery for junctional kyphosis should be a moderate correction. If too much correction is attempted, the kyphotic deforming forces can be translated into the new end vertebra and a compensatory curve can even develop.[29]

Often in revision surgery for junctional kyphosis, it is possible to perform the revision through a much smaller incision than the initial surgery. Sponseller describes a technique to

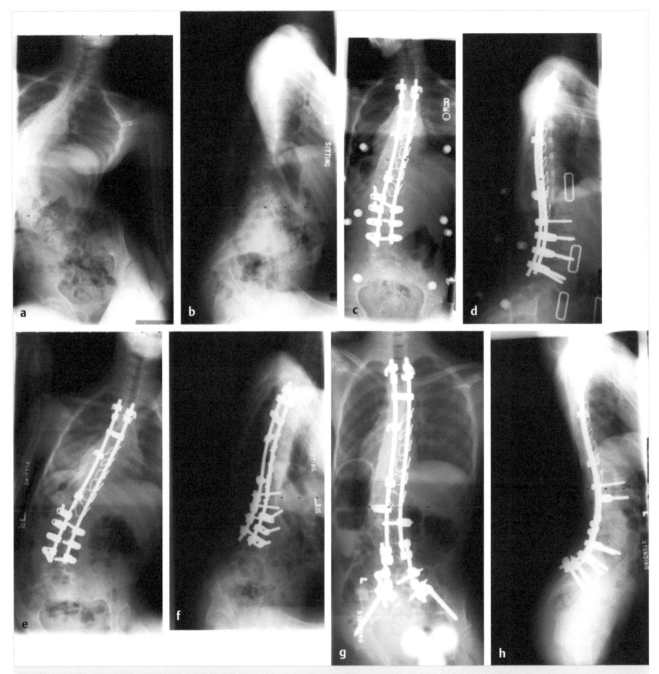

Fig. 25.2 (a–h) Patient with cerebral palsy had a fusion to the distal lumbar spine. Patient had to undergo a revision due to decompensation in the coronal and sagittal plane.

extend the fusion superiorly and recommends using enough anchors (usually two to three pairs) in order to withstand the stress of the deformity correction. The technique includes locking the new rods to all of the anchors superior to the previous UIV first, then compressing toward the existing fusion using cantilevering mechanism to correct the deformity. Once corrected, rod-to-rod connectors are used to attach the new rods to the existing ones.[30]

There is little literature on revisions in the neuromuscular population for PJK. In a recent study of 93 patients with neuromuscular scoliosis with posterior spine fusion, 2 patients underwent revision for PJK. Both of these were successfully treated by extending the posterior fusion several levels superiorly.[9] A recent case report details an adolescent with cerebral palsy who developed PJK with significant neurological deficits and inability to walk several months postoperatively after T2–L4 posterior spinal fusion.[31] He underwent cervical extension to C6 with hybrid pedicle screw and hook fixation and regained ambulation without assistive device by 6 months postoperatively. Although revisions are uncommon, both of these studies highlight the fact that revision spine surgery for junctional kyphosis in the neuromuscular patient is technically demanding, but successful outcomes are possible with careful planning.

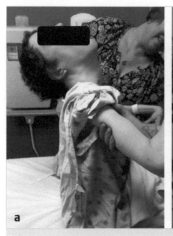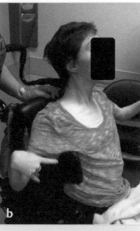

Fig. 25.3 (a) This 26-year-old with athetoid cerebral palsy developed severe neck extension 10 years after spinal fusion. It impaired swallowing and communication. (b) After anterior diskectomies and posterior extension of the fusion from T2 to C2, she had significant improvement in her position.

25.3 Cervical Extension

Compared to thoracolumbar spinal deformity in neuromuscular patients, significant cervical involvement is rare but can occur in patients with underlying myopathies. Cervical hyperextension deformity has been described in Duchenne muscular dystrophy as well as many of the congenital muscular dystrophies and is characterized by weak neck flexors and subsequent contractures of the neck extensors (▶ Fig. 25.3). This muscle imbalance, especially in the setting of remaining growth, leads to poor head control in extension and often to progressive cervical lordosis and fixed hyperextension contractures. This can be debilitating as loss of control in extension results in falling backward with torso extension, and fixed hyperextension makes basic tasks difficult, requiring the patient to bend forward through their trunk or even their hips and knees just to maintain level gaze (see ▶ Fig. 25.3a, b).

Addressing the cervical spine deformity when present with the thoracolumbar curve can significantly improve these patients' quality of life. Giannini et al described a technique to address cervical spine hyperextension that has been successfully applied to patients with various underlying myopathies.[32] A posterior approach to the cervical spine is performed and the posterior spinal ligaments and facet joints are released from C2 to C7. Next the interspinous spaces are freed using a rongeur, as they are typically very narrow, and then the neck is then forward flexed, correcting the deformity. Finally, wedge-shaped autograft bone without instrumentation is placed between the spinous processes posteriorly to maintain the correction and facilitate arthrodesis.

This technique was applied to seven patients with Duchenne muscular dystrophy with rigid neck hyperextension or poor head control in extension in addition to a significant thoracolumbar spinal deformity. Both deformities were corrected in the same operative setting with the cervical extension deformity addressed by the Giannini technique after posterior fusion from T1 to sacrum was complete. All of the patients achieved significant deformity correction, improved posture, and head control postoperatively. Six of these patients maintained correction through final follow-up at 7.6 years; however, one patient developed a cervical extension and rotational deformity through the occiput to C2 at 3 years postoperative. The authors concluded that cervical deformity correction should be offered to patients with Duchenne muscular dystrophy with significant neck deformities at the same time as undergoing thoracolumbar curve correction as these patients are vulnerable to repeat anesthesia and surgery.[32]

Giannini et al also had success with this technique using similar indications in seven patients with underlying myopathies such as both merosin-positive and merosin-negative congenital muscular dystrophy, Emery–Dreifuss muscular dystrophy, and rigid spine syndrome.[33] None of these patients had significant associated thoracolumbar deformity and underwent isolated cervical deformity correction. They achieved significant correction without significant complication. All patients had stable arthrodesis with significant clinical improvement in posture and were able to maintain horizontal gaze compensatory postures through 10.4 years. Although the technique of Giannini does not typically use instrumentation, posteriorly based instrumentation and extension to the occiput has been described with success in addition to posterior releases and bone graft in the treatment of these rare and challenging deformities.[34]

References

[1] Sarwark J, Sarwahi V. New strategies and decision making in the management of neuromuscular scoliosis. Orthop Clin North Am. 2007; 38(4):485–496, v

[2] McDonnell MF, Glassman SD, Dimar JR, II, Puno RM, Johnson JR. Perioperative complications of anterior procedures on the spine. J Bone Joint Surg Am. 1996; 78(6):839–847

[3] Luque ER. Segmental spinal instrumentation for correction of scoliosis. Clin Orthop Relat Res. 1982(163):192–198

[4] Allen BL, Jr, Ferguson RL. A 1988 perspective on the Galveston technique of pelvic fixation. Orthop Clin North Am. 1988; 19(2):409–418

[5] Imrie MN, Yaszay B. Management of spinal deformity in cerebral palsy. Orthop Clin North Am. 2010; 41(4):531–547

[6] Sharma S, Wu C, Andersen T, Wang Y, Hansen ES, Bünger CE. Prevalence of complications in neuromuscular scoliosis surgery: a literature meta-analysis from the past 15 years. Eur Spine J. 2013; 22(6):1230–1249

[7] Broom MJ, Banta JV, Renshaw TS. Spinal fusion augmented by Luque-rod segmental instrumentation for neuromuscular scoliosis. J Bone Joint Surg Am. 1989; 71(1):32–44

[8] Tsirikos AI, Mains E. Surgical correction of spinal deformity in patients with cerebral palsy using pedicle screw instrumentation. J Spinal Disord Tech. 2012; 25(7):401–408

[9] Lonstein JE, Koop SE, Novachek TF, Perra JH. Results and complications after spinal fusion for neuromuscular scoliosis in cerebral palsy and static encephalopathy using Luque Galveston instrumentation: experience in 93 patients. Spine. 2012; 37(7):583–591

[10] Dias RC, Miller F, Dabney K, Lipton GE. Revision spine surgery in children with cerebral palsy. J Spinal Disord. 1997; 10(2):132–144

[11] Yagi M, King AB, Kim HJ, Cunningham ME, Boachie-Adjei O. Outcome of revision surgery in pediatric spine deformity patients. Spine Deform. 2013; 1 (1):59–67

[12] Sink EL, Newton PO, Mubarak SJ, Wenger DR. Maintenance of sagittal plane alignment after surgical correction of spinal deformity in patients with cerebral palsy. Spine. 2003; 28(13):1396–1403

[13] Jones-Quaidoo SM, Yang S, Arlet V. Surgical management of spinal deformities in cerebral palsy. A review. J Neurosurg Spine. 2010; 13(6):672–685

[14] Gitelman A, Joseph SA, Jr, Carrion W, Stephen M. Results and morbidity in a consecutive series of patients undergoing spinal fusion with iliac screws for neuromuscular scoliosis. Orthopedics. 2008; 31(12):31

[15] Phillips JH, Gutheil JP, Knapp DR, Jr. Iliac screw fixation in neuromuscular scoliosis. Spine. 2007; 32(14):1566–1570

[16] Sponseller PD, Zimmerman RM, Ko PS, et al. Low profile pelvic fixation with the sacral alar iliac technique in the pediatric population improves results at two-year minimum follow-up. Spine. 2010; 35(20):1887–1892

[17] O'Brien JR, Yu WD, Bhatnagar R, Sponseller P, Kebaish KM. An anatomic study of the S2 iliac technique for lumbopelvic screw placement. Spine. 2009; 34 (12):E439–E442

[18] McCord DH, Cunningham BW, Shono Y, Myers JJ, McAfee PC. Biomechanical analysis of lumbosacral fixation. Spine. 1992; 17(8) Suppl:S235–S243

[19] Myung KS, Lee C, Skaggs DL. Early pelvic fixation failure in neuromuscular scoliosis. J Pediatr Orthop. 2015; 35(3):258–265

[20] Glattes RC, Bridwell KH, Lenke LG, Kim YJ, Rinella A, Edwards C, II. Proximal junctional kyphosis in adult spinal deformity following long instrumented posterior spinal fusion: incidence, outcomes, and risk factor analysis. Spine. 2005; 30(14):1643–1649

[21] Helgeson MD, Shah SA, Newton PO, et al. Harms Study Group. Evaluation of proximal junctional kyphosis in adolescent idiopathic scoliosis following pedicle screw, hook, or hybrid instrumentation. Spine. 2010; 35(2):177–181

[22] Kim YJ, Lenke LG, Bridwell KH, et al. Proximal junctional kyphosis in adolescent idiopathic scoliosis after 3 different types of posterior segmental spinal instrumentation and fusions: incidence and risk factor analysis of 410 cases. Spine. 2007; 32(24):2731–2738

[23] Kim YJ, Bridwell KH, Lenke LG, Kim J, Cho SK. Proximal junctional kyphosis in adolescent idiopathic scoliosis following segmental posterior spinal instrumentation and fusion: minimum 5-year follow-up. Spine. 2005; 30 (18):2045–2050

[24] Wang J, Zhao Y, Shen B, Wang C, Li M. Risk factor analysis of proximal junctional kyphosis after posterior fusion in patients with idiopathic scoliosis. Injury. 2010; 41(4):415–420

[25] Nectoux E, Giacomelli MC, Karger C, Herbaux B, Clavert JM. Complications of the Luque-Galveston scoliosis correction technique in paediatric cerebral palsy. Orthop Traumatol Surg Res. 2010; 96(4):354–361

[26] Cho SK, Kim YJ, Lenke LG. Proximal junctional kyphosis following spinal deformity surgery in the pediatric patient. J Am Acad Orthop Surg. 2015; 23 (7):408–414

[27] Yagi M, King AB, Boachie-Adjei O. Incidence, risk factors, and natural course of proximal junctional kyphosis: surgical outcomes review of adult idiopathic scoliosis. Minimum 5 years of follow-up. Spine. 2012; 37(17):1479–1489

[28] Sanders JO, Evert M, Stanley EA, Sanders AE. Mechanisms of curve progression following sublaminar (Luque) spinal instrumentation. Spine. 1992; 17 (7):781–789

[29] Sponseller PD, Jain A, Lenke LG, et al. Vertebral column resection in children with neuromuscular spine deformity. Spine. 2012; 37(11):E655–E661

[30] Sponseller PD. Pediatric revision spinal deformity surgery: issues and complications. Spine. 2010; 35(25):2205–2210

[31] Cruz D, Mendoza-Lattes S, Weinstein SL. Nontraumatic proximal junctional kyphosis with catastrophic neurologic deficits after instrumented arthrodesis in an adolescent with cerebral palsy: case report and review of the literature. JBJS Case Connect. 2014; 3:e:58

[32] Giannini S, Faldini C, Pagkrati S, Grandi G, Romagnoli M, Merlini L. Surgical treatment of neck hyperextension in Duchenne muscular dystrophy by posterior interspinous fusion. Spine. 2006; 31(16):1805–1809

[33] Giannini S, Ceccarelli F, Faldini C, Pagkrati S, Merlini L. Surgical treatment of neck hyperextension in myopathies. Clin Orthop Relat Res. 2005(434):151–156

[34] Arkader A, Hosalkar H, Dormans JP. Scoliosis correction in an adolescent with a rigid spine syndrome: case report. Spine. 2005; 30(20):E623–E628

26 Health-Related Quality of Life in Neuromuscular Scoliosis

James H. Stephen, Eve Hoffman, Unni G. Narayanan, Paul D. Sponseller, and Amer F. Samdani

Abstract

This chapter provides an overview of health-related quality of life (HRQoL) in patients with neuromuscular scoliosis including cerebral palsy (CP), myelomeningocele, spinal cord injury (SCI), and flaccid neuromuscular disease. In CP an increasing curvature and pelvic obliquity has been implicated in worsening sitting tolerance, impaired mobility, decreased pulmonary function, gastroesophageal reflux, and feeding difficulty. The Child Health Index of Life with Disabilities (CPCHILD) is a validated proxy for health status in children with CP and was used in multiple studies to show improvement following spinal fusion. In patients with myelomeningocele the Spina Bifida Spine Questionnaire (SBSQ) was validated to assess physical disability related to scoliosis. The SBSQ was shown to have no significant relationship between the magnitude of the spinal deformity and self-perception or overall physical function; however, increased coronal imbalance was associated with worse sitting balance. There are not yet any validated condition-specific instruments for measuring HRQoL in patients with SCI-related scoliosis. Shriners Hospitals for Children has developed the Shriners Pediatric Instrument for Neuromuscular Scoliosis (SPINS) with the future aim of validating the instrument and eventually to compare the impact of bracing versus surgery on HRQoL. The Pediatric Quality of Life Inventory (PedsQL) is the most commonly used scale in flaccid neuromuscular disease; however, it has not been used to investigate the effects of spinal deformity in this population. The development of validated disease-specific metrics for neuromuscular scoliosis and their use in prospective studies will further help guide decision-making to maximize patient quality of life.

Keywords: cerebral palsy, Duchenne muscular dystrophy, flaccid neuromuscular disease, health-related quality of life, myelomeningocele, neuromuscular scoliosis, spinal cord injury, spinal muscular atrophy.

26.1 Introduction

Surgical deformity correction in patients with neuromuscular scoliosis is fraught with challenges. Given the high complication rates and the underlying baseline neurological and medical comorbidities of the patients, there is debate about the impact that surgical correction has on patient health-related quality of life (HRQoL). This chapter will provide an overview of HRQoL in the neuromuscular population, including the challenges and available outcome metrics for the specific patient populations of cerebral palsy (CP), myelomeningocele, spinal cord injury (SCI), and flaccid neuromuscular disease.

26.2 Cerebral Palsy

CP is a heterogeneous disorder caused by a static injury in the developing fetal or infant nervous system. This nonprogressive insult results in permanent disorders of movement and coordination. However, such motor disorders are often accompanied by disturbances of sensation, perception, cognition, and communication. Despite the static nature of the original insult, patients may also go on to develop secondary musculoskeletal problems, which may be progressive throughout life.[1]

The musculoskeletal consequences of CP, secondary to imbalances of strength and tone, include muscle contractures as well as deformities of the appendicular and axial skeleton.

26.2.1 Natural History

Children with CP are at increased risk for developing spinal deformity when compared to the general pediatric population. There is large variation in the estimated prevalence of scoliosis in CP, ranging from 20 to 77%.[2,3,4,5,6,7] This variation may be explained by the heterogeneity of CP and the fact that the risk of deformity increases with the severity of CP. For example, scoliosis is more common in children with tetraplegia, when compared with paraplegia or hemiplegia, and is more common in spastic CP.[8] Severity of CP as measured by the Gross Motor Function Classification System (GMFCS) is the most important risk factor of scoliosis, with a strong association between increasing GMFCS level and scoliosis.[8] Nonambulatory children (GMFCS levels IV and V) have a 50% probability of acquiring a moderate or severe scoliosis by 18 years, whereas for ambulatory children who do not need walking aids (GMFCS levels I and II) the risk of developing scoliosis is not significantly different from the general population.[3] Scoliosis tends to progress most rapidly before skeletal maturity but routinely continues beyond skeletal maturity, particularly in nonambulatory patients with a curve of greater than 40 degrees by 12 years of age.[9,10] Skeletal maturity may also be delayed in these patients, which also contributes to a prolonged period of increased risk of curve progression.

26.2.2 Comorbidities

The secondary musculoskeletal consequences of CP, including scoliosis, get progressively worse with increasing age. These consequences include the development of contractures of the upper and lower extremities that can interfere with the child's care and comfort. Patients are at increased risk for progressive hip displacement, and this risk is also strongly related to the GMFCS levels.[6] Therefore, a thorough evaluation of the hips for the presence of contractures or dislocation is necessary in the evaluation of spinal deformity. Hip displacement usually precedes the onset of scoliosis, but this is not always the case. These musculoskeletal effects of CP can result in children relying on wheelchairs for their mobility. This immobility and lack of load bearing can lead to osteoporosis. Children are dependent on their caregivers for much of their care and activities of daily living.

Patients with CP who are at greatest risk for developing a spinal deformity are also those most likely to have significant nonmusculoskeletal comorbidities. These comorbidities may include seizure disorder, hydrocephalus, bowel and bladder incontinence, urinary tract infection, gastroesophageal reflux, malnutrition, constipation, aspiration pneumonia, and cardiopulmonary issues.[4,5] Their neurological impairment can lead to swallowing difficulties, which cause an increased risk for developing aspiration pneumonias. They also experience distressing gastroesophageal reflux, which can be exacerbated in certain positions. Gastric tube feeding is often necessary both to overcome the malnutrition associated with feeding difficulties and to protect against aspiration. Tracheostomy is also common in patients with severe CP, again to protect against aspiration. Most of these patients are incontinent of bowel and bladder. Children may develop pressure sores as their spinal deformity worsens, especially if they are thin.

26.2.3 Spinal Deformity and Comorbidities: Impact on QoL

These comorbidities collectively have a significant impact on the longevity and HRQoL in these severely involved children with CP and scoliosis. An increasing curvature has been implicated in worsening sitting tolerance and impaired mobility. Sitting upright is an important aspect of these children's lives, given the lack of ambulation. The presence of a significant spinal deformity (specifically, the presence of pelvic obliquity) has the potential to impact sitting balance, comfort, and endurance. The inability to sit upright might compound the impact of patients' baseline visual impairments and thus affect their ability to process visual information. Furthermore, progressive scoliosis might directly or indirectly exacerbate some of the medical comorbidities. Worsening scoliosis is implicated in decreased pulmonary function, gastroesophageal reflux, and feeding difficulties. The location and magnitude of the curve might negatively impact pulmonary function. Cardiopulmonary function declines with age as a function of the underlying disease, but this deterioration correlates better with GMFCS level than curve magnitude. It can be difficult to test pulmonary function directly in patients with CP due to their inability to participate, particularly those at GMFCS levels IV and V. However, studies have shown no difference between oxygen saturation and heart rate in patients with mild or no scoliosis as compared to those with curves greater than 45 degrees[11,12] Other factors such as presence of a tracheostomy,[9] pelvic obliquity, and hip dislocation[13,14,15,16] have been shown to be associated with worsening scoliosis in CP. The relationship between scoliosis and all these factors remains unclear and worsening cardiopulmonary comorbidities may be related to underlying disease severity rather than a causal relationship with scoliosis. What is clear is that this population has significant comorbidities, and these comorbidities lead to challenges in the treatment of the scoliosis.

In the presence of multiple comorbidities, the additional negative impact of scoliosis on HRQoL of these children has been difficult to quantify. It is a challenge to measure patient-reported HRQoL in patients who are unable to communicate their quality of life due to cognitive and/or communication impairments. Consequently, there is some controversy about the benefit and indications for the surgical treatment of scoliosis in this population. These are major interventions with significant complication rates and high costs associated with surgery and rehabilitation.[7,9] Surgical outcomes have been typically reported based on radiographic measures, fusion rates, early and late complications, and mortality from uncontrolled case series. More important HRQoL outcomes are infrequently reported, mostly using unvalidated measures. There is an imperative for prospective, comparative studies using validated HRQoL measures to address the uncertainty about the true benefits of surgery.

26.2.4 Interventions

The problems associated with increasing spinal deformity in patients with CP might be effectively managed using nonoperative means or by definitive surgical correction. Any intervention should progress from a clear understanding of the natural history of the disease. It should modify the disease in such a way that the patient's general state of health is improved in some way and the intervention is tolerable. Traditionally, in patients with CP and spinal deformity, radiographic measures or morbidity and mortality data were primarily used to follow the observed natural history and the response to treatments. Validated HRQoL outcomes comparing bracing, observation, or surgery are not currently available in the literature.

26.2.5 Satisfaction and HRQoL Studies

CP is a chronic disease, with no cure. As such, outcome studies should reflect subtle changes in functional status and general well-being, distinguishing the results of an intervention with the natural history. Over the past 20 years, there has been growing interest and understanding of the importance of parent and patient satisfaction following spinal surgery for CP. Given the high rates of complications in this challenging population, the effect of correction and complications on functional outcomes has been examined. Sponseller et al[17]suggested that deep infection rates were comparatively higher in CP spinal deformity correction population and that such infections may be associated with worse pain outcomes. Posterior-only pedicle screw constructs produce satisfactory radiographic coronal and sagittal correction, without higher complication rates. They are associated with functional improvements (using a modified Rancho Los Amigos Hospital system criteria score).[18] Another study has suggested that there was no correlation between the occurrence of complications and changes in HRQoL. Furthermore, extension of spinal fusion to the pelvis to manage pelvic obliquity had no impact on the occurrence of complications in these patients.[19]

Several studies report high retrospective parental/caregiver satisfaction with their decision to undergo surgical correction of spinal deformity[17,20,21,22,23,24,25,26] though these studies did not use validated outcome instruments for children with severe CP. Comstock et al[27] in a series of 79 patients with a median follow-up of 4 years reported a late progression of scoliosis greater than 10 degrees, worsening pelvic obliquity, and decompensation greater than 4 cm in more than 30% of patients following surgery, noting that the majority of patients who progressed underwent surgery while skeletally immature. Despite this, the study reported an 85% satisfaction rate from parents or caregivers following surgery and noted a beneficial impact on physical appearance, comfort, ease of care, and sitting ability. A longitudinal study of parental perceptions following spinal surgery using the POSNA (Pediatric Orthopaedic Society of North America) outcomes questionnaire reported no difference between preoperative and postoperative physical functions, comorbidities, and parental health. Patient pain and happiness as well as parental satisfaction were significantly improved by 1 year.[28,29] The lack of perceived functional improvements in this study may have underestimated the potential functional benefit of surgery secondary to a ceiling effect of this instrument in children with severe CP. In a retrospective study of 84 patients with spastic CP, Watanabe et al[30] reported 85% satisfaction with surgery. Most improvement was felt to be related to posture and sitting balance as well as cosmetic appearance. Interestingly, the least improved scores postoperatively concerned walking ability, use of arms and hands, ability to eat, sleeping patterns, perineal care, number of pressure sores, ability to dress, and pain.[20] Given the lack of validated questionnaires with unknown responsiveness, it is difficult to ascertain the true effects of surgery in children with scoliosis and severe CP. There is a need for a validated measure of quality of life in this population to elucidate which radiographic or clinical outcomes may lead to improved quality of life.

26.2.6 Developing Appropriate HRQoL Instruments for Children with CP

There has been a general move within medicine toward HRQoL measures to assess the global impact of disease and interventions. Ideally, a single instrument could be used across all diseases, allowing standardized data collection and interpretation. In children, the Child Health Questionnaire (CHQ) and Pediatric Outcomes Data Collection Instrument (PODCI) were developed and have been used in both healthy children and those with chronic disease. The PODCI has been used to study ambulatory children with CP; however, its usefulness in children with GMFCS levels IV and V is limited, exhibiting ceiling and floor effects, which renders it poorly responsive. It is this group of patients who are most likely to develop significant scoliosis. When looking at the responsiveness of an outcome instrument —the ability to accurately reflect a change following an intervention—the tool must be sensitive enough to discriminate subtle changes in a population with preexisting functional limitations.

To develop a useful HRQoL construct for CP interventions, we must first identify what is important to patients and caregivers. However, the perceptions of health and function to the general public, health care professionals, and caregivers may be substantially different than those of patients with CP. Ideally it would be the patient who tells us the important functions and goals we should be measuring, but in this population, their neurological impairment may prevent such communication. In developing a list of areas to study (construct), we have to be confident that the content is important (content validity), that it examines whether an instrument appears to be measuring what it intends to measure (face validity), and that the metrics used are sensitive enough to identify subtle changes following an intervention (responsiveness). Construct validity is generally used when dealing with abstract variables, such as quality of life, and is the most rigorous test of validity. The proposed or hypothetical underlying factors are referred to as constructs.

Construct validity examines the logical relations that should exist between a measure and characteristics of patients and patient groups. This test tries to address the question of whether or not the scores of the questionnaire correlate with other related constructs in the anticipated manner. Construct validation is an ongoing process of learning more about the construct, making new predictions, and then testing them. Given that a proxy is required to give this information, the tool must be proven to be accurate between different people and at different times (reliable).

Sources of Bias

Proxies (parents/caregivers) may be prone to overestimating disability prior to an intervention (in order to justify making a decision on a major intervention) or overestimating postoperative improvement for the same reason. This is particularly the case with retrospective studies but may also be seen prospectively when the study is carried out around the time of a major decision/intervention. Such biases may be minimized by performing not only prospective studies, but also longitudinal studies that capture prospective data long before and after a specific intervention is undertaken.

Caregiver Priorities and Child Health Index of Life with Disabilities Project

The Child Health Index of Life with Disabilities (CPCHILD) questionnaire was devised to address the lack of an instrument specific to interventions in children with severe CP. Acknowledging it as a proxy measure for functional and health status, extensive development of the construct was performed. Parents, caregivers, and health care workers were involved in formulating questions, and assigning relative importance of each. Face, content, and construct validation as well as its reliability and responsiveness to change were rigorously assessed by the developers.[21,31] A separate study to assess the validity and reliability of CPCHILD (Dutch version) found it to be sufficiently reliable and valid as a proxy for health status and well-being in nonambulatory patents with CP.[22]

The CPCHILD consists of 37 items distributed over six sections representing the following domains:
- Activities of daily living/personal care (nine items).
- Positioning, transferring, and mobility (eight items).
- Comfort and emotions (nine items).
- Communication and social interaction (seven items).
- Health (three items).
- Overall quality of life (one item).

A higher score reflects a better quality of life, and is transformed to a scale of 0 to 100.

Using the CPCHILD tool to assess outcomes following spinal fusion surgery, Bohtz et al[29] retrospectively studied a series of 50 consecutive patients undergoing spinal fusion with a minimum 2-year follow-up. They noted no correlation between complications and HRQoL or satisfaction following surgery. They observed an improvement in HRQoL and a high satisfaction rate following surgery but noted it did not significantly correlate with objective radiographic changes. In a similar-style retrospective review of 33 patients, Sewell et al[32] compared the radiographs and the CPCHILD score of patients with scoliosis who underwent observational treatment and compared them to those undergoing surgery. They found that in the observation group scoliosis worsened on radiographic parameters and that there was a slight worsening of the overall CPCHILD scores. In the operative group, radiographic parameters improved, and the overall CPCHILD score also significantly improved. In both groups, a change in pain was the most significant factor affecting quality of life. Neither group showed a difference in mobility, GMFCS level, feeding, or communication before and after treatment. This suggests that the presence of pain is an important factor when considering the potential benefit of surgery.

26.2.7 Future Directions

Further study is required to assess the long-term outcomes of surgery in patients with CP to see if these benefits are long-lasting and have any impact on patient quality of life. Large cohorts of patients across multiple centers are required to study the effects of confounding factors such as disease heterogeneity or surgical variation. Elucidation of variables that effect changes in quality of life will be important in determining which patients benefit the most from surgery and which are most at risk. The expansion of the Harms Study Group to include spinal deformity in patients with CP promises to yield useful data. This prospectively collected, multicenter database records CPCHILD scores at preoperative, operative, and postoperative visits. Current analysis of these data with 2-year follow-up will yield results about impact on quality of life utilizing a reliable, valid outcome measure, CPCHILD. In tandem, research to demonstrate the responsiveness of CPCHILD to detecting quality-of-life changes with interventions in this population is also underway. Additionally, 5-year results from the Harms Study Group database will be instrumental in examining longer term quality-of-life outcomes.

26.3 Myelomeningocele

Most patients with myelomeningocele and scoliosis who undergo deformity correction surgery are full-time sitters, and the goals of surgery are to correct sitting balance and improve self-reported outcome measures including physical function and self-perception.[33] Historically, Mazur et al[34] reported on functional outcomes following correction of scoliosis deformity in 49 patients with myelomeningocele. The best sitting balance was obtained with a combined anterior and posterior fusion, where improvement in sitting balance occurred in 70% of the patients. When investigating the outcomes of the subset of ambulatory patients in this series, none of the patients had improvement in their ambulatory status postoperatively, and 67% had decreased walking ability following anterior and posterior spinal fusion. While their series and others[35,36] have focused on clinician-driven outcome measures such as sitting balance and ambulation, more recent research has focused on patient- and caregiver-reported quality-of-life measures.

Wai et al[37] have published their work developing and validating the Spina Bifida Spine Questionnaire (SBSQ) to assess physical disability related to scoliosis. The SBSQ is a 25-item questionnaire designed to incorporate quality-of-life measurements from the viewpoint of the patients and caregivers. The same group of researchers then used the SBSQ to investigate the relationship of spinal deformity with physical function.[33] They administered the SBSQ questionnaire to 80 children with myelomeningocele, including 24 who had undergone surgical stabilization, and found that after adjusting for neurological level, there was no significant relationship between the magnitude of the spinal deformity and self-perception or overall physical function. In the subgroup of 24 patients who had undergone surgical stabilization, increased coronal imbalance was associated with a worse outcome in sitting balance.

Sibinski et al[38] investigated long-term outcomes of patients with myelomeningocele treated nonoperatively for scoliosis. They performed a prospective study of 19 skeletally mature patients. Patients were divided into groups based on neurologic motor level, ambulation status, and sitting stability. They then filled out several questionnaires in order to assess different aspects of physical function and quality of life including the SBSQ. Their results showed that while the severity of the scoliosis deformity decreases quality-of-life outcomes, it had no correlation with physical function, self-perception, or self-motivation. They hypothesized that the decrease in quality-of-life scores may be related to other aspects of the condition, for instance, the ability to walk, rather than the scoliosis itself.

26.4 Spinal Cord Injury

Data on the HRQoL outcomes in children and adolescents with SCI have been sparse. There are currently no validated condition-specific instruments for measuring HRQoL in SCI-related scoliosis. In other forms of neuromuscular scoliosis, higher level of neurologic injury and disability is related to lower HRQoL outcomes;[39] however, Vogel et al[40] followed 46 adult patients who sustained SCI as children and found that life satisfaction was not significantly associated with level of injury, age at injury, or duration of injury. Instead, they found that satisfaction was related to education level and employment. Similarly, there were no differences between HRQoL in children with tetraplegia and those with paraplegia when a generic pediatric quality-of-life measurement was administered to children with SCI and to their parents.[41]

Research done at Shriners Hospitals for Children has laid the groundwork for a disease-specific HRQoL instrument to be used in pediatric neuromuscular scoliosis related to SCI. Hunter et al[42] developed the Shriners Pediatric Instrument for Neuromuscular Scoliosis (SPINS) and tested the instrument on 14 children with SCI, demonstrating comprehensibility in that group. Following validity testing, the aim of SPINS is to allow for measurement of the impact of bracing versus surgery on the HRQoL of children with SCI and neuromuscular scoliosis.

26.5 Duchenne Muscular Dystrophy/Spinal Muscular Atrophy

Instruments used to measure HRQoL in progressive, flaccid neuromuscular disorders are varied. A recent literature review identified 21 articles using 15 different quality-of-life scales applied to patients with muscular dystrophy.[43] In the pediatric and adolescent groups, the most commonly used scale included the generic Pediatric Quality of Life Inventory (PedsQL) or one of two disease-specific subsets of this scale: the PedsQL Duchenne Module or the PedsQL Neuromuscular Module. The PedsQL Duchenne Module has been validated by comparing the results of a group of 117 boys with Duchenne muscular dystrophy (DMD) with those of matched healthy children.[44] This study showed that mean scores were significantly lower for boys with DMD in the physical and psychosocial domains. The PedsQL Neuromuscular Module was validated by comparing the results of a group of 167 children with spinal muscular atrophy (SMA) to a healthy control group.[45] Similarly, children with SMA and their parents report significantly lower HRQoL than the healthy children. However, neither of these disease-specific instruments has been used to investigate spinal deformity in this population or the effects of treatment on HRQoL.

To address HRQoL specifically related to scoliosis in this patient population, Bridwell et al[46] devised and validated a questionnaire that was administered to 55 patients with DMD or SMA who had previously undergone spinal fusion. The questionnaire assessed patient function, pain, cosmesis, self-image, and quality of life at the most recent follow-up examination. They showed that 81% of the patients had overall improvement in their quality of life compared to preoperatively, and 96% of the patients had an improvement in sitting balance. Despite the overwhelming positive quality-of-life scores, 5 patients (10%) who were able to feed themselves prior to surgery were no longer able to feed themselves following fusion because their spine was taller and they could no longer get their hands to their mouth. A study similar to Bridwell's using the PedsQL generic and disease-specific modules has not yet been published but will contribute more objective data regarding the effect of scoliosis treatment in this patient population.

26.6 Conclusion

Patients with neuromuscular scoliosis remain a challenging population for spinal deformity surgeons. Collecting and evaluating HRQoL data to assess for response to intervention also represents a challenge. Available data are often sparse, flawed, or conflicted when examining the effects of surgical deformity correction on HRQoL outcomes in these patients. However, the development of validated disease-specific metrics and prospectively collected data comparing the effects of interventions may provide answers and guide decision-making to maximize patient quality of life.

References

[1] Rosenbaum P, Paneth N, Leviton A, et al. A report: the definition and classification of cerebral palsy April 2006. Dev Med Child Neurol Suppl. 2007; 109:8–14

[2] Madigan RR, Wallace SL. Scoliosis in the institutionalized cerebral palsy population. Spine. 1981; 6(6):583–590

[3] Persson-Bunke M, Hägglund G, Lauge-Pedersen H, Wagner P, Westbom L. Scoliosis in a total population of children with cerebral palsy. Spine. 2012; 37 (12):E708–E713

[4] Himmelmann K, Beckung E, Hagberg G, Uvebrant P. Gross and fine motor function and accompanying impairments in cerebral palsy. Dev Med Child Neurol. 2006; 48(6):417–423

[5] Shevell MI, Dagenais L, Hall N, REPACQ Consortium. Comorbidities in cerebral palsy and their relationship to neurologic subtype and GMFCS level. Neurology. 2009; 72(24):2090–2096

[6] Soo B, Howard JJ, Boyd RN, et al. Hip displacement in cerebral palsy. J Bone Joint Surg Am. 2006; 88(1):121–129

[7] Mercado E, Alman B, Wright JG. Does spinal fusion influence quality of life in neuromuscular scoliosis? Spine. 2007; 32(19) Suppl:S120–S125

[8] Palisano R, Rosenbaum P, Walter S, Russell D, Wood E, Galuppi B. Development and reliability of a system to classify gross motor function in children with cerebral palsy. Dev Med Child Neurol. 1997; 39(4):214–223

[9] Whitaker AT, Sharkey M, Diab M. Spinal fusion for scoliosis in patients with globally involved cerebral palsy: an ethical assessment. J Bone Joint Surg Am. 2015; 97(9):782–787

[10] Koop SE. Scoliosis in cerebral palsy. Dev Med Child Neurol. 2009; 51 Suppl 4:92–98

[11] Balmer GA, MacEwen GD. The incidence and treatment of scoliosis in cerebral palsy. J Bone Joint Surg Br. 1970; 52(1):134–137

[12] Edebol-Tysk K. Epidemiology of spastic tetraplegic cerebral palsy in Sweden. I. Impairments and disabilities. Neuropediatrics. 1989; 20(1):41–45

[13] Pritchett JW. The untreated unstable hip in severe cerebral palsy. Clin Orthop Relat Res. 1983; 173(173):169–172

[14] Porter D, Michael S, Kirkwood C. Patterns of postural deformity in non-ambulant people with cerebral palsy: what is the relationship between the direction of scoliosis, direction of pelvic obliquity, direction of windswept hip deformity and side of hip dislocation? Clin Rehabil. 2007; 21(12):1087–1096

[15] Rosenthal RK, Levine DB, McCarver CL. The occurrence of scoliosis in cerebral palsy. Dev Med Child Neurol. 1974; 16(5):664–667

[16] Saito N, Ebara S, Ohotsuka K, Kumeta H, Takaoka K. Natural history of scoliosis in spastic cerebral palsy. Lancet. 1998; 351(9117):1687–1692

[17] Sponseller PD, Shah SA, Abel MF, Newton PO, Letko L, Marks M. Infection rate after spine surgery in cerebral palsy is high and impairs results: multicenter analysis of risk factors and treatment. Clin Orthop Relat Res. 2010; 468 (3):711–716

[18] Terjesen T, Lange JE, Steen H. Treatment of scoliosis with spinal bracing in quadriplegic cerebral palsy. Dev Med Child Neurol. 2000; 42(7):448–454

[19] Tsirikos AI, Chang WN, Dabney KW, Miller F. Comparison of one-stage versus two-stage anteroposterior spinal fusion in pediatric patients with cerebral palsy and neuromuscular scoliosis. Spine. 2003; 28(12):1300–1305

[20] Cassidy C, Craig CL, Perry A, Karlin LI, Goldberg MJ. A reassessment of spinal stabilization in severe cerebral palsy. J Pediatr Orthop. 1994; 14(6):731–739

[21] Tsirikos AI, Chang W-N, Dabney KW, Miller F. Comparison of parents' and caregivers' satisfaction after spinal fusion in children with cerebral palsy. J Pediatr Orthop. 2004; 24(1):54–58

[22] Dias RC, Miller F, Dabney K, Lipton G, Temple T. Surgical correction of spinal deformity using a unit rod in children with cerebral palsy. J Pediatr Orthop. 1996; 16(6):734–740

[23] Lonstein JE, Akbarnia A. Operative treatment of spinal deformities in patients with cerebral palsy or mental retardation. An analysis of one hundred and seven cases. J Bone Joint Surg Am. 1983; 65(1):43–55

[24] Lipton GE, Letonoff EJ, Dabney KW, Miller F, McCarthy HC. Correction of sagittal plane spinal deformities with unit rod instrumentation in children with cerebral palsy. J Bone Joint Surg Am. 2003; 85-A(12):2349–2357

[25] Lipton GE, Miller F, Dabney KW, Altiok H, Bachrach SJ. Factors predicting postoperative complications following spinal fusions in children with cerebral palsy. J Spinal Disord. 1999; 12(3):197–205

[26] Tsirikos AI, Lipton G, Chang WN, Dabney KW, Miller F. Surgical correction of scoliosis in pediatric patients with cerebral palsy using the unit rod instrumentation. Spine. 2008; 33(10):1133–1140

[27] Comstock CP, Leach J, Wenger DR. Scoliosis in total-body-involvement cerebral palsy. Analysis of surgical treatment and patient and caregiver satisfaction. Spine. 1998; 23(12):1412–1424, discussion 1424–1425

[28] Jones KB, Sponseller PD, Shindle MK, McCarthy ML. Longitudinal parental perceptions of spinal fusion for neuromuscular spine deformity in patients with totally involved cerebral palsy. J Pediatr Orthop. 2003; 23(2):143–149

[29] Bohtz C, Meyer-Heim A, Min K. Changes in health-related quality of life after spinal fusion and scoliosis correction in patients with cerebral palsy. J Pediatr Orthop. 2011; 31(6):668–673

[30] Watanabe K, Lenke LG, Daubs MD, et al. Is spine deformity surgery in patients with spastic cerebral palsy truly beneficial?: a patient/parent evaluation. Spine. 2009; 34(20):2222–2232

[31] Narayanan UG, Fehlings D, Weir S, Knights S, Kiran S, Campbell K. Initial development and validation of the Caregiver Priorities and Child Health Index of Life with Disabilities (CPCHILD). Dev Med Child Neurol. 2006; 48 (10):804–812

[32] Sewell MD, Malagelada F, Wallace C, et al. A preliminary study to assess whether spinal fusion for scoliosis improves carer-assessed quality of life for

children with GMFCS level IV or V cerebral palsy. J Pediatr Orthop. 2016; 36 (3):299–304

[33] Wai EK, Young NL, Feldman BM, Badley EM, Wright JG. The relationship between function, self-perception, and spinal deformity: implications for treatment of scoliosis in children with spina bifida. J Pediatr Orthop. 2005; 25 (1):64–69

[34] Mazur J, Menelaus MB, Dickens DRV, Doig WG. Efficacy of surgical management for scoliosis in myelomeningocele: correction of deformity and alteration of functional status. J Pediatr Orthop. 1986; 6(5):568–575

[35] Müller EB, Nordwall A, von Wendt L. Influence of surgical treatment of scoliosis in children with spina bifida on ambulation and motoric skills. Acta Paediatr. 1992; 81(2):173–176

[36] Osebold WR, Mayfield JK, Winter RB, Moe JH. Surgical treatment of paralytic scoliosis associated with myelomeningocele. J Bone Joint Surg Am. 1982; 64 (6):841–856

[37] Wai EK, Owen J, Fehlings D, Wright JG. Assessing physical disability in children with spina bifida and scoliosis. J Pediatr Orthop. 2000; 20(6):765–770

[38] Sibinski M, Synder M, Higgs ZC, Kujawa J, Grzegorzewski A. Quality of life and functional disability in skeletally mature patients with myelomeningocele-related spinal deformity. J Pediatr Orthop B. 2013; 22(2):106–109

[39] Varni JW, Burwinkle TM, Sherman SA, et al. Health-related quality of life of children and adolescents with cerebral palsy: hearing the voices of the children. Dev Med Child Neurol. 2005; 47(9):592–597

[40] Vogel LC, Klaas SJ, Lubicky JP, Anderson CJ. Long-term outcomes and life satisfaction of adults who had pediatric spinal cord injuries. Arch Phys Med Rehabil. 1998; 79(12):1496–1503

[41] Oladeji O, Johnston TE, Smith BT, Mulcahey MJ, Betz RR, Lauer RT. Quality of life in children with spinal cord injury. Pediatr Phys Ther. 2007; 19(4):296–300

[42] Hunter L, Molitor F, Chafetz RS, et al. Development and pilot test of the Shriners Pediatric Instrument for Neuromuscular Scoliosis (SPINS): a quality of life questionnaire for children with spinal cord injuries. J Spinal Cord Med. 2007; 30 Suppl 1:S150–S157

[43] Bann CM, Abresch RT, Biesecker B, et al. Measuring quality of life in muscular dystrophy. Neurology. 2015; 84(10):1034–1042

[44] Uzark K, King E, Cripe L, et al. Health-related quality of life in children and adolescents with Duchenne muscular dystrophy. Pediatrics. 2012; 130(6): e1559–e1566

[45] Iannaccone ST, Hynan LS, Morton A, Buchanan R, Limbers CA, Varni JW, AmSMART Group. The PedsQL in pediatric patients with Spinal Muscular Atrophy: feasibility, reliability, and validity of the Pediatric Quality of Life Inventory Generic Core Scales and Neuromuscular Module. Neuromuscul Disord. 2009; 19(12):805–812

[46] Bridwell KH, Baldus C, Iffrig TM, Lenke LG, Blanke K. Process measures and patient/parent evaluation of surgical management of spinal deformities in patients with progressive flaccid neuromuscular scoliosis (Duchenne's muscular dystrophy and spinal muscular atrophy). Spine. 1999; 24(13):1300–1309

27 Baclofen Pump: Preoperative, Intraoperative, and Postoperative Management

Brian P. Scannell and Burt Yaszay

Abstract

Spasticity and dystonia can be managed operatively with the placement of an intrathecal baclofen pump. This therapy has been shown to improve spasticity, range of motion, ease of care, and patient/caregiver satisfaction. Preoperatively, it is important to determine indications for implantation of the baclofen pump and identify treatment goals. Test dosing can be performed prior to implantation to ensure appropriate therapeutic response. Many patients who are candidates for intrathecal baclofen also are candidates for spinal fusion. Timing of pump implantation is controversial, but based on the available literature, it appears to be safe for implantation before, during, or after spinal fusion. There is no conclusive evidence that baclofen pumps increase the risk of scoliosis requiring surgery. We describe various surgical techniques for implantation based on this timing. Postoperatively, the surgeon and multidisciplinary team managing these patients need to be aware of potential medical and surgical complications related to intrathecal baclofen pumps.

Keywords: baclofen, spasticity, neuromuscular scoliosis, spinal fusion, intrathecal baclofen

27.1 Preoperative Management

27.1.1 Tone Management

Hypertonia can manifest itself secondary to a number of different etiologies. Neuromuscular disorders such as cerebral palsy (CP) are the most common, but many other disorders such as traumatic/acquired brain injury, metabolic disorders, leukodystrophies, hydrocephalus, and spinal cord injuries are also associated with hypertonia.[1] Hypertonia can cause impairments in quality of life and lead to problems with rehabilitation.[2] It can present as spasticity, dystonia, rigidity, or a mixed combination. Spasticity is the most frequently observed form. It is an increased muscle tone as a result of an externally imposed muscle movement.[3] Dystonia is a less common but more complicated form of hypertonia.[1] It consists of abnormal involuntary contractions in muscle groups causing abnormal posturing of the neck, torso, or extremities.[3] Both spasticity and dystonia can lead to rigidity or simultaneous contracture of muscle agonists and antagonists.[3] Often, there is a mixture of spasticity and dystonia in children with various tone disorders.

Management of hypertonia can involve both nonoperative and operative approaches. Nonoperative approaches include physical/occupational therapy, orthoses, casting, chemodenervation with botulinum toxin, and enteral medications such as benzodiazepines. One enteral medication that is frequently used is baclofen. Baclofen binds to $GABA_B$ receptors (metabotropic transmembrane receptors for gamma-aminobutyric acid) and inhibits the release of excitatory neurotransmitters and substance P, which results in decreased spasticity.[4] The enteral form of baclofen can work very well but can also cause significant sedation, fatigue, and hypotonia.[1] Sedation is reported to occur in 7 to 70% of patients on enteral baclofen.[2]

Operative management of hypertonia consists of various orthopaedic surgeries (soft tissue and bony), dorsal rhizotomy, intrathecal baclofen, deep brain stimulation, and other methods.[1] Intrathecal baclofen delivered by an implanted pump was first approved by the Food and Drug Administration in 1996 for the treatment of hypertonia. Intrathecal baclofen is approved for treatment of spasticity related to a number of disorders including CP.[5] Evidence for its efficacy in spastic and dystonic CP was first published by Butler et al[6] in 2000. It results in fewer systemic side effects than enteral baclofen and has a higher efficacy rate.[7] Due to systemic absorption of enteral baclofen, only small concentrations reach the spinal cord and cerebrospinal fluid (CSF) despite high doses. Intrathecal delivery of baclofen allows for high concentrations to diffuse into the superficial layers of the spinal cord dorsal horn, often avoiding the cerebral side effects.[8]

27.1.2 Indications/Treatment Goals for Intrathecal Baclofen Pump

The indications for implantation of intrathecal baclofen pumps are primarily for intractable spasticity or spasticity not optimally managed by physical therapies, oral baclofen, or other medications including botulinum toxin injections.[9,10] Additionally, patients with intolerable side effects to enteral baclofen may be good candidates.[9] Patients and their family members need to have the ability and motivation to attend regular follow-ups and monitoring.[10]

The treatment goals and benefits of intrathecal baclofen are well documented in the neuromuscular population. Penn and Kroin[11] first reported its use for severe spasticity with immediate reduction of muscle tone to near normal levels, and others have demonstrated the efficacy of intrathecal baclofen in children with CP.[12] Multiple studies have shown benefits in patients with CP. Gooch et al[13] demonstrated improved satisfaction of care providers, ease of care, and decreased pain. Other studies have also found improved ease of care[14] as well as improved gait in ambulatory patients.[15] Additionally, Gerszten et al[15] demonstrated a decreased need for subsequent orthopaedic surgery for lower extremity spasticity. In summary, intrathecal baclofen pumps have the ability to improve spasticity, range of motion, ease of care, pain, caregiver satisfaction, hygiene, and gait.[9,10]

27.1.3 Timing of Intrathecal Baclofen Implantation

Many patients who are candidates for intrathecal baclofen pumps are also at risk for the development of scoliosis. Thus, the timing for intrathecal baclofen pump and catheter placement is often discussed in reference to the timing of spinal fusion: before, during, or after scoliosis surgery. Although there is extensive literature discussing this timing, significant controversy remains as to whether insertion of an intrathecal baclofen pump causes progression of scoliosis.[16,17,18,19,20,21,22,23,24] There is also concern and debate as to whether prior placement of an intrathecal baclofen pump can further complicate CP scoliosis surgery and increase the risk for wound complications.[23,24,25] Specifically, there is concern that the intrathecal baclofen catheter can prevent complete closure of the fascia, result in a CSF leak, or interfere with placement of instrumentation.

Numerous studies have evaluated progression of scoliosis after placement of a baclofen pump. Two small series of patients reported accelerated scoliosis progression after baclofen pump placement.[17,18] Segal et al,[17] in their series of five patients with a rapid curve progression, found a mean progression of 44 degrees over 11 months leading to spinal fusion in all patients. Burn et al[20] found an annual progression of Cobb angle of 19 degrees in 32 patients after intrathecal baclofen pump placement. This study also found that the Cobb progression was higher in patients who were skeletally immature. Another study found an increase in scoliosis progression from 1.8 degrees per year prior to implantation to 10.9 degrees per year after implantation.[16]

Despite these studies suggesting curve progression, two studies that compared matched cohorts of CP patients with and without a baclofen pump found no difference in the rate of scoliosis progression.[21,22] Senaran et al[21] compared 25 matched patients with quadriplegic CP who had scoliosis (controls) who did not receive an intrathecal baclofen pump to 26 patients who did receive the pump. The average curve progression for the baclofen pump group after implantation was 16.3 degrees per year compared to 16.1 degrees per year in the control group. Shilt et al[22] also found that patients receiving an intrathecal baclofen pump experience a natural progression of scoliosis similar to that of patients without this therapy.

Timing of baclofen pump placement and spinal fusion has also been studied. Controversy exists as to whether the presence of a baclofen pump complicates posterior spinal fusion. Caird et al[23] and Borowski et al[24] both report single center experiences evaluating complications associated with intrathecal baclofen pump placement and spinal fusion. Caird et al[23] compared 20 patients with spastic quadriplegic CP with baclofen who underwent posterior spinal fusion to 20 matched patients without a baclofen pump. They found increased reoperation and rehospitalization and a higher infection rate in the baclofen pump group (20 vs. 0%, $p = 0.063$). However, in this series, two patients who developed wound infection had a history of decubitus ulcers prior to the spinal fusion, and four patients who were readmitted postoperatively for complications had been previously hospitalized for pulmonary problems.

Borowski et al[24] compared four groups of patients with CP. The four groups included: (1) posterior spinal fusion prior to baclofen pump placement ($n = 26$); (2) posterior spinal fusion and baclofen pump placement concurrently ($n = 11$); (3) posterior spinal fusion after baclofen pump placement ($n = 25$); and (4) baclofen pump placement only ($n = 103$). In all four groups, they found an infection rate of 8 to 9% with no differences between groups. There was also no difference in device or catheter complications between groups. They concluded that

baclofen pumps can be implanted and managed without any increase in complication rate before, during, or after spinal fusion.

A recent multicenter study by Yaszay et al[25] is the largest study to date comparing patients undergoing posterior spinal fusion with ($N = 32$) and without ($N = 155$) previously placed intrathecal baclofen pumps. This study found no difference between groups in OR (operating room) time or intraoperative EBL (estimated blood loss), and an overall wound complication rate was not significant between the baclofen pump group (16%) and the nonbaclofen pump group (15%). The deep infection rate was 6.3% in the baclofen pump group and 5.8% in the nonbaclofen pump group. Both of these complication rates compare favorably to that of Caird et al.[23]

Based on the studies by Borowski et al[24] and Yaszay et al,[25] while it may be inconvenient for the surgeon, baclofen pumps do not appear to increase the complexity of surgery or the risk for wound complications. Yaszay et al[25] states that when counseling patients and their caregivers on the timing of pump placement, it does not appear to compromise the care of the patient if the baclofen pump is placed first.

27.1.4 Test Dose for Intrathecal Baclofen Implantation

Commonly a trial test dose is given prior to proceeding with placement of an intrathecal baclofen pump. This can be performed on an inpatient or outpatient basis and will vary from center to center. The goal is to determine whether the patient responds to the treatment rather than to determine long-term functional improvements.[10] Typically, the test dose of baclofen is administered via lumbar puncture or a temporary catheter into the CSF. The amount for the test dose is typically between 10 and 50 µg in children and 25 and 100 µg in adults. The largest effect of a test dose in cerebral spasticity is between 2 and 8 hours with a maximum effect seen typically around 4 hours after injection.[26]

After administration of the test dose, it is important to have the resources in place to fully assess the effect of the medication. Trained medical personnel typically perform this assessment. Assessments should be at multiple time points after injection and include spasticity assessments with scales such as the modified Ashworth scale and should also include patient/caregiver subjective assessment.[2] Based on the response, it may be recommended to proceed with intrathecal baclofen pump implantation.

Some centers no longer perform test dosing for children with spasticity as nearly all have a good response to the therapy. However, the majority of children who "do not respond" to bolus doses have dystonia, and therefore, a trial is strongly recommended in these patients prior to implantation.[27]

27.2 Intraoperative Management

27.2.1 Surgical Placement of Intrathecal Baclofen Pump

There are two components to the intrathecal baclofen pump infusion systems: pump and catheter. The pump commonly is implanted subcutaneously below the fascia on the abdominal wall and the catheter is implanted and travels from the pump to the CSF. The pump commonly holds enough drug for 4 to 6 months of therapy and should be replaced at the end of its battery life at approximately 5 to 7 years.[2] Because of its subcutaneous location, it can be refilled with a subcutaneous injection into the pump.

As many of these patients undergo spinal fusion, the surgical approach for intrathecal baclofen pump placement may vary depending on whether it is being done before, during, or after the scoliosis surgery. Intrathecal baclofen pumps placed prior to spinal fusion are technically less demanding than after spinal fusion. Under general anesthesia, patients can be positioned prone or in a lateral decubitus position. A midline incision is placed at approximately L2/L3 or L3/L4. A 14-gauge Tuohy needle is placed into the dural sac. The catheter is then advanced to the desired level. Most pumps are placed on the right side to avoid current or future gastrostomy tubes. A separate incision is made in this location, and a subcutaneous or subfascial pocket is developed in order to place the pump. The catheter is then tunneled from the spine to the pump and is tested to ensure backflow of CSF.[9]

Borowski et al[24] describe their technique when placing the intrathecal baclofen pump after a spinal fusion. Patients are typically positioned in a lateral decubitus position and a 5-cm incision is made through the previous midline scar. Subperiosteal exposure of the fusion mass is performed. Fluoroscopy is used to locate the implants, and then a burr is then used to open a hole in the fusion mass at L2–L3 or L3–L4. The Tuohy needle is then used to penetrate the dural sac and the remaining procedure is similar to that described earlier.

Other authors describe a different technique via a cervical approach when inserting an intrathecal baclofen pump after a spinal fusion.[28,29] A 5-cm incision is made midline at the superior aspect of the fusion mass. A limited laminectomy in the cervical spine can expose the dura. A purse-string suture is then inserted into the dura, which is then opened with a no. 11 blade. The catheter is then advanced to the appropriate level. Implantation via a cervical approach has been shown to be safe and feasible with low complications.[29]

Concurrent spinal fusion and intrathecal baclofen pump placement has also been described by Borowski et al.[24] The spinal fusion is completed in the standard fashion with the surgical drapes brought more lateral toward the flank. Prior to wound closure, the Tuohy needle is inserted at the levels discussed previously. The catheter is then inserted and anchored to the spinous process nearest the puncture site with a strain-relief fastener. The catheter is then pulled through the paraspinal muscles and tunneled into the subcutaneous tissue and anchored to the fascia laterally. CSF flow is confirmed and the spinal incision is closed. The patient is then turned supine and re-prepped. The subfascial pump pocket is developed. The lateral wound with the catheter is opened and the catheter is then tunneled to the pump.

27.2.2 Location of Catheter Tip

The location of the catheter tip at the time of implantation can vary depending on its desired effect. Vender et al[30] proposed placement at T6–T10 for patients with spastic diplegia and paraplegia, T1–T2 for spastic quadriplegia, and C5–T1 for dystonia and complex movement disorders. Grabb et al[31] found equal improvement of upper and lower extremity spasticity in children with catheter placement in the midthoracic spine. In this study, there is also good data demonstrating improved dystonia with higher catheter placement in the cervical spine.

27.3 Postoperative Management

27.3.1 Management of the Pump

Initial postoperative management of the intrathecal baclofen pump should consist of a multidisciplinary approach. Proper titration of the dose is important to optimize efficacy and minimize side effects. Many patients are well controlled on an initial low dose, but the magnitude of this effect dissipates over time, resulting in higher future dosing.[32] Dosing can be programmed various ways including continuous infusions or pulsatile bolus dosing.[7] Currently, no studies have compared the efficacy of simple continuous infusion to pulsatile bolus dosing. However, some centers have transitioned to bolus dosing as a result of finding a higher rate of satisfaction.[7]

After the initial titration during first few weeks after implantation, intensive physical therapy is recommended in particular to improve trunk control, as this can be problematic following implantation.[10] Patients can also be slowly weaned off some of their oral medications.[2] Comprehensive routine follow-up varies by institution, but it is recommended to have personnel involved in the patient care following implantation who have expertise and interest in the long-term management of dosing.

27.3.2 Complications after Intrathecal Pump Placement

While the safety and efficacy of intrathecal baclofen pumps has been evaluated,[13,15,27] there are still significant complications associated with their placement. Complications related to pump placement are well reported in the pediatric literature.[27,33,34,35,36,37,38] Medical, perioperative surgical, and postoperative surgical complications of intrathecal baclofen pumps are summarized in ▶ Table 27.1.

The incidences of catheter- and pump-related complications are variable in the literature. Complications include pump malfunction, pump hypermobility or malposition, catheter dislodgement, catheter breakage, and catheter malfunction. Armstrong et al[14] reported 10 catheter- or pump-related complications in 19 patients over 568 months. Rippe et al[39] reported a total of 264 catheter complications in 785 patients. In a review of 316 surgical procedures related to intrathecal baclofen pumps, Borowski et al[33] found that 39 of the 316 procedures (12.3%) were associated with device-related complications, including complications caused by catheter breakage (9), disconnection (7), and malfunction (16). Pump malfunction has been reported to be as high as 14% and can result from rotor malfunction, reservoir depletion, and programming malfunctions.[40,41] Complications related to catheters and pumps are a common reason for rehospitalization and reoperation.[23]

Wound complications and infections are also a common reason for rehospitalization and reoperation in patients after

Table 27.1 Complications of intrathecal baclofen pumps

Medical complications	Perioperative complications	Postoperative complications

• Vomiting
• Nausea
• Headaches
• Urinary retention
• Constipation
• Seizures
	• Bleeding
	• Cerebrospinal fluid leak
	• Baclofen overdose:
	  ○ Lethargy
	  ○ Seizures
	  ○ Respiratory depression
		• Cerebrospinal fluid leak
		• Infection: pump, cerebrospinal fluid
		• Wound dehiscence
		• Catheter-related complications:
		  ○ Breakage
		  ○ Dislodgement
		  ○ Malfunction
		• Pump failure
		• Seroma at pump site
		• Revision surgery

intrathecal baclofen pump placement. When infection does occur, there is a high reoperation and removal rate (44–59%) of the catheter and pump.[34,37] Overall, acute infection rates range from 4 to 10%.[33] Fjelstad et al[35] found the rate of infection after pump placement to be higher in children than in adults (10 vs. 0%). However, this may have been related to patient selection as more of the pediatric patients had a diagnosis of CP compared to the adult population. One study found a significant increase in infection rate with subcutaneous pump placement compared to subfascial placement (20.1 vs. 3.6%, $p < 0.001$) and thus recommend subfascial placement.[38] As discussed previously, the infection rate shows no difference whether pumps are implanted before, during, or after spinal fusion surgery.[25]

CSF leak can also occur. In a study by Motta et al[38], 4.9% of 430 consecutive patients developed a CSF leak. Another series reports a higher incidence of CSF leak of 17%.[36] Fifty-six percent of these patients recovered spontaneously, and 44% underwent revision surgery for treatment of the CSF leak or explantation.

Medical-related complications also occur at a frequent rate. Complications include vomiting (12%), headaches (12%), and meningitis (8%).[37] Urinary retention and constipation have also been reported. Borowski et al[33] found 46% of patients with new or increased constipation problems and 17% with acute urinary retention. New-onset seizures or worsening seizures have also been reported.[42]

27.3.3 Surgery after Intrathecal Pump Placement: Revision and Spinal Fusion

Revision

As stated previously, revision surgery occurs frequently secondary to infection and catheter/pump problems.[23,34,37] In one series, explantation was required in 44% of patients with wound complications.[37] Patients of smaller size, younger age, or with a gastrostomy tube were more likely to encounter complications necessitating explantation.[37] If cultures from around the pump and in the CSF are positive, then explantation is likely required followed by intravenous antibiotics.[28] If the pump and catheter are removed, baclofen withdrawal should be anticipated and patients should be managed with enteral baclofen. Hallucinations, confusion, agitation, seizures, hyperthermia, and severe

rebound spasticity can occur 12 to 72 hours after abrupt cessation.[43]

When pump or catheter failure occurs, this often needs to be addressed with revision of the malfunctioned component. For example, Borowski et al[33] had three pump revisions secondary to hypermobility or flipping of the pump, which has also been reported by other authors.[30] This issue can be resolved by directly addressing the pump problem with reoperation. Catheter fractures and disconnection are common and can easily be addressed operatively.[33]

Spinal Fusion after Intrathecal Pump Placement

Some surgeons have concerns when performing a spinal fusion when an intrathecal baclofen pump has been previously implanted. In these patients, there are options as to how to deal with the catheter. Surgeons can identify the catheter on their midline approach to the spine, keep it intact, and then work around the catheter. This requires significant care on the part of the surgeon to not injure/fracture/crimp the catheter upon placement of the spinal instrumentation.[24] This also puts the catheter at risk for inadvertent removal.

A second option for catheter management is to expose the catheter through the incision, cut, and remove it.[25] The dura can be sealed uneventfully and a new catheter placed after spinal fusion. A third option is to transect the catheter. Using a repair kit, a reanastomosis can be performed at the end of the case. No matter how the catheter is managed, it requires attention by the surgeon and preoperative planning to avoid complications of CSF leakage or postoperative catheter-related problems.

27.4 Conclusion

Intrathecal baclofen is an excellent treatment option for patients with spasticity or dystonia that is refractory to other medical management. Although concerns exist for progression of scoliosis after intrathecal baclofen pump placement, this progression is likely related to the natural history of the underlying disorder(s) rather than the pump placement. Timing of pump placement and spinal fusion do not appear to compromise the care of the patient. The complications of intrathecal baclofen are not insignificant, but the benefits appear to outweigh the complications. The decision to proceed with placement requires a conversation with caregivers regarding the benefits, treatment goals, complications, and potential for revision surgery.

References

[1] Vadivelu S, Stratton A, Pierce W. Pediatric tone management. Phys Med Rehabil Clin N Am. 2015; 26(1):69–78

[2] Khurana SR, Garg DS. Spasticity and the use of intrathecal baclofen in patients with spinal cord injury. Phys Med Rehabil Clin N Am. 2014; 25 (3):655–669, ix

[3] Sanger TD, Delgado MR, Gaebler-Spira D, Hallett M, Mink JW, Task Force on Childhood Motor Disorders. Classification and definition of disorders causing hypertonia in childhood. Pediatrics. 2003; 111(1):e89–e97

[4] Deon LL, Gaebler-Spira D. Assessment and treatment of movement disorders in children with cerebral palsy. Orthop Clin North Am. 2010; 41(4):507–517

[5] Lynn AK, Turner M, Chambers HG. Surgical management of spasticity in persons with cerebral palsy. PM R. 2009; 1(9):834–838

[6] Butler C, Campbell S, AACPDM Treatment Outcomes Committee Review Panel. Evidence of the effects of intrathecal baclofen for spastic and dystonic cerebral palsy. Dev Med Child Neurol. 2000; 42(9):634–645

[7] Skalsky AJ, Fournier CM. Intrathecal baclofen bolus dosing and catheter tip placement in pediatric tone management. Phys Med Rehabil Clin N Am. 2015; 26(1):89–93

[8] Coffey JR, Cahill D, Steers W, et al. Intrathecal baclofen for intractable spasticity of spinal origin: results of a long-term multicenter study. J Neurosurg. 1993; 78(2):226–232

[9] Scannell B, Yaszay B. Scoliosis, spinal fusion, and intrathecal baclofen pump implantation. Phys Med Rehabil Clin N Am. 2015; 26(1):79–88

[10] Dan B, Motta F, Vles JS, et al. Consensus on the appropriate use of intrathecal baclofen (ITB) therapy in paediatric spasticity. Eur J Paediatr Neurol. 2010; 14 (1):19–28

[11] Penn RD, Kroin JS. Continuous intrathecal baclofen for severe spasticity. Lancet. 1985; 2(8447):125–127

[12] Albright AL, Cervi A, Singletary J. Intrathecal baclofen for spasticity in cerebral palsy. JAMA. 1991; 265(11):1418–1422

[13] Gooch JL, Oberg WA, Grams B, Ward LA, Walker ML. Care provider assessment of intrathecal baclofen in children. Dev Med Child Neurol. 2004; 46 (8):548–552

[14] Armstrong RW, Steinbok P, Cochrane DD, Kube SD, Fife SE, Farrell K. Intrathecally administered baclofen for treatment of children with spasticity of cerebral origin. J Neurosurg. 1997; 87(3):409–414

[15] Gerszten PC, Albright AL, Johnstone GF. Intrathecal baclofen infusion and subsequent orthopedic surgery in patients with spastic cerebral palsy. J Neurosurg. 1998; 88(6):1009–1013

[16] Ginsburg GM, Lauder AJ. Progression of scoliosis in patients with spastic quadriplegia after the insertion of an intrathecal baclofen pump. Spine. 2007; 32(24):2745–2750

[17] Segal LS, Wallach DM, Kanev PM. Potential complications of posterior spine fusion and instrumentation in patients with cerebral palsy treated with intrathecal baclofen infusion. Spine. 2005; 30(8):E219–E224

[18] Sansone JM, Mann D, Noonan K, Mcleish D, Ward M, Iskandar BJ. Rapid progression of scoliosis following insertion of intrathecal baclofen pump. J Pediatr Orthop. 2006; 26(1):125–128

[19] Krach LE, Walker K, Rapp L. The effect of intrathecal baclofen treatment on the development of scoliosis in individuals with cerebral palsy: a retrospective case-matched review. Dev Med Child Neurol. 2005; 47 Suppl 102:14

[20] Burn SC, Zeller R, Drake JM. Do baclofen pumps influence the development of scoliosis in children? J Neurosurg Pediatr. 2010; 5(2):195–199

[21] Senaran H, Shah SA, Presedo A, Dabney KW, Glutting JW, Miller F. The risk of progression of scoliosis in cerebral palsy patients after intrathecal baclofen therapy. Spine. 2007; 32(21):2348–2354

[22] Shilt JS, Lai LP, Cabrera MN, Frino J, Smith BP. The impact of intrathecal baclofen on the natural history of scoliosis in cerebral palsy. J Pediatr Orthop. 2008; 28(6):684–687

[23] Caird MS, Palanca AA, Garton H, et al. Outcomes of posterior spinal fusion and instrumentation in patients with continuous intrathecal baclofen infusion pumps. Spine. 2008; 33(4):E94–E99

[24] Borowski A, Shah SA, Littleton AG, Dabney KW, Miller F. Baclofen pump implantation and spinal fusion in children: techniques and complications. Spine. 2008; 33(18):1995–2000

[25] Yaszay B, Scannell BP, Bomar JD, et al. Harms Study Group. Although inconvenient, baclofen pumps do not complicate scoliosis surgery in patients with cerebral palsy. Spine. 2015; 40(8):E504–E509

[26] Ford B, Greene P, Louis ED, et al. Use of intrathecal baclofen in the treatment of patients with dystonia. Arch Neurol. 1996; 53(12):1241–1246

[27] Albright AL, Ferson SS. Intrathecal baclofen therapy in children. Neurosurg Focus. 2006; 21(2):e3

[28] Albright AL, Turner M, Pattisapu JV. Best-practice surgical techniques for intrathecal baclofen therapy. J Neurosurg. 2006; 104(4) Suppl:233–239

[29] Ughratdar I, Muquit S, Ingale H, Moussa A, Ammar A, Vloeberghs M. Cervical implantation of intrathecal baclofen pump catheter in children with severe scoliosis. J Neurosurg Pediatr. 2012; 10(1):34–38

[30] Vender JR, Hester S, Waller JL, Rekito A, Lee MR. Identification and management of intrathecal baclofen pump complications: a comparison of pediatric and adult patients. J Neurosurg. 2006; 104(1) Suppl:9–15

[31] Grabb PA, Guin-Renfroe S, Meythaler JM. Midthoracic catheter tip placement for intrathecal baclofen administration in children with quadriparetic spasticity. Neurosurgery. 1999; 45(4):833–836

[32] Heetla HW, Staal MJ, Kliphuis C, van Laar T. The incidence and management of tolerance in intrathecal baclofen therapy. Spinal Cord. 2009; 47(10):751–756

[33] Borowski A, Littleton AG, Borkhuu B, et al. Complications of intrathecal baclofen pump therapy in pediatric patients. J Pediatr Orthop. 2010; 30(1):76–81

[34] Dickey MP, Rice M, Kinnett DG, et al. Infectious complications of intrathecal baclofen pump devices in a pediatric population. Pediatr Infect Dis J. 2013; 32 (7):715–722

[35] Fjelstad AB, Hommelstad J, Sorteberg A. Infections related to intrathecal baclofen therapy in children and adults: frequency and risk factors. J Neurosurg Pediatr. 2009; 4(5):487–493

[36] Motta F, Buonaguro V, Stignani C. The use of intrathecal baclofen pump implants in children and adolescents: safety and complications in 200 consecutive cases. J Neurosurg. 2007; 107(1) Suppl:32–35

[37] Murphy NA, Irwin MC, Hoff C. Intrathecal baclofen therapy in children with cerebral palsy: efficacy and complications. Arch Phys Med Rehabil. 2002; 83 (12):1721–1725

[38] Motta F, Antonello CE. Analysis of complications in 430 consecutive pediatric patients treated with intrathecal baclofen therapy: 14-year experience. J Neurosurg Pediatr. 2014; 13(3):301–306

[39] Rippe D, Tann B, Gaebler-Spira D, Krach LE, Gooch J, Dabrowski E. Complications of intrathecal baclofen pump therapy for severe hypertonia in children: a long-term follow-up review of 785 patients from four centers. Abstract. Dev Med Child Neurol. 2005; 47 Suppl 102:14

[40] Flückiger B, Knecht H, Grossmann S, Felleiter P. Device-related complications of long-term intrathecal drug therapy via implanted pumps. Spinal Cord. 2008; 46(9):639–643

[41] Penn RD. Intrathecal baclofen for spasticity of spinal origin: seven years of experience. J Neurosurg. 1992; 77(2):236–240

[42] Buonaguro V, Scelsa B, Curci D, Monforte S, Iuorno T, Motta F. Epilepsy and intrathecal baclofen therapy in children with cerebral palsy. Pediatr Neurol. 2005; 33(2):110–113

[43] Sampathkumar P, Scanlon PD, Plevak DJ. Baclofen withdrawal presenting as multiorgan system failure. Anesth Analg. 1998; 87(3):562–563

Index

Note: Page numbers set **bold** or *italic* indicate headings or figures, respectively.

A

Adults, spinal deformity associated with neurodegenerative disease in
- botox injections in **108**
- bracing in **108**
- case presentation **110**
- comorbidities in **104**
- deep brain stimulation in **109**
- disease-specific deformity characteristics in **104**
- disorder-specific techniques in **106**
- etiology of **104**
- in antecollis **104**
- in camptocormia *105*, **105**
- in lateral axial dystonia **105**
- lidocaine injection in **108**
- nonoperative treatment in **106**
- operative treatment of **106**
- outcomes in **108**, *110*
- pathogenesis of **104**
- perioperative considerations in **107**
- postoperative considerations in **107**
- rehabilitation in **108**
- scoliosis in **105**
- technical considerations with **107**
Airway
- difficult 3
- in cerebral palsy **40**
- in intensive care unit **161**
Ambulatory status **12**
Anemia of chronic disease 4, **4**
Anesthesia
- blood pressure management and 20
- cardiac arrest and 21
- in sagittal plane deformity **98**
- perioperative management and 21
- postoperative management and 21
- preoperative management and 20
- respiratory system and 20
- volatile agents in 21
Antecollis **104**
Anterior approaches
- mini-open **146**
- open **143**, *144–145*
- retroperitoneal lumbar *144*, **144**
- standard thoracotomy **143**, *144*
- thoracoabdominal **144**, *144*, *145*
- thoracoscopic **144**, *145*
Anterior diskectomy, indications for **146**
Anterior instrumentation, indications for *146*, **146**
Antifibrinolytics (AF) 23, **44**
Arthrogryposis **15**
Ataxia-telangiectasia (A-T) **17**

B

Baclofen pump
- as nonoperative management **8**
- catheter tip location with **181**
- complications and **151**
- complications with **181**, *182*
- in preoperative evaluation 3
- indications for **179**
- intraoperative management with **180**
- postoperative management with **181**
- preoperative management **179**
- revision surgery **182**
- spinal fusion after **182**
- surgical placement of **180**
- test dose with **180**
- timing of implantation of **179**
- tone management and **179**
- treatment goals with **179**
Baclofen withdrawal 3
Becker's muscular dystrophy, cardiomyopathy in 3
Biomechanical failure **168**
Biomechanics, in pelvic fixation **114**, *115*
Bladder, neurogenic 3
Blood loss 21, **22**, **44**, **125**, 151
Blood pressure management, in anesthesia 20
Bone density, in sagittal plane deformity **98**
Botox injections **8**, **108**
Bowel function 3, 21
Bracing 7
- *See also* Nonoperative management
- in adult spinal deformity associated with neurodegenerative disease **108**
- in cerebral palsy **42**
- in spinal cord injury **59**

C

Camptocormia *105*, **105**
Cardiac arrest, anesthesia and 21
Cardiac support **162**
Cardiomyopathy, in muscular dystrophies 3, **14**
Cardiopulmonary system, in preoperative evaluation **2**
Cardiovascular complications **34**
Cardiovascular health factors **11**
Cerebral palsy (CP)
- antifibrinolytics in **44**
- as heterogeneous disease 2
- bleeding and **44**, *125*
- bracing in **42**
- characteristics specific to **40**
- classification of scoliosis in **41**
- comorbidities with **173**
- complications in **46**
- functional effects of scoliosis in **40**
- fusion extent in **43**
- hip subluxation in *25*, **25**
- incidence of **40**
- instrumentation in **42**, *43*
- modular constructs in **122**, *123*
- natural history in **40**, *41*, **173**
- neuromonitoring in **22**, **44**
- nonoperative management in **8**, **42**
- outcomes in **47**
- pelvic fixation in **43**, *44–45*
- perioperative traction in **44**, *46*
- postoperative survival in **47**
- quality of life in **173**
- risk assessment in **31**
- seating modification in **42**
- seating position in **41**
- surgical indications *12*, **12**, **42**
- surgical management in **42**
- unit rods in **122**, *123*
- wound infections in **46**
Cervical extension *171*, **171**
Charcot-Marie-Tooth disease
- comorbidities in **81**
- deformity characteristics in **81**
- etiology of **81**
- neuromonitoring in **22**
- nonoperative management in 9
- outcomes in **83**
- pathogenesis of **81**
- surgical techniques in *82*, **82**
Chiari I malformation **88**, *89–90*
Child Health Index of Life with Disabilities (CPCHILD) **173**
Coagulopathy **165**
Cognitive status assessment 4
Comorbidities 2
- in adult spinal deformity associated with neurodegenerative disease **104**
- in cerebral palsy **173**
- in Charcot-Marie-Tooth disease **81**
- in Chiari I malformation **88**
- in Friedrich's ataxia **83**
- in Rett syndrome **78**
- in spinal muscular atrophy **73**
- in split cord malformation **92**
- in syringomyelia **88**
- in tethered cord syndrome **90**
Complication(s) **141**
- baclofen pumps and **151**
- blood loss as 21, **22**, **44**, *125*, 151
- cardiovascular **34**
- ethical considerations with **35**
- in baclofen pump **181**, *182*
- in cerebral palsy **31**, **46**
- in halo-gravity traction **128**
- in muscle diseases **31**
- in myelomeningocele **32**
- in osteotomies **135**
- in pelvic fixation **118**
- in spinal cord injury **62**
- incidence of *150*, **150**
- intraoperative **151**
- neurological **164**
- postoperative **152**
- prediction of *30*, **30**, *35*
- pulmonary **34**
- rates 2
- risk assessment and **30**
- surgical site **34**
Congenital muscular dystrophy, cardiomyopathy in 3
Continence 3

D

Deep brain stimulation (DBS) **109**
Diaphragm Intrusion Index (DII) **50**, *50*
Diskectomy, anterior, indications for **146**
Duchenne muscular dystrophy
- anesthesia and 21
- cardiomyopathy in 3, **14**
- Cobb angle in **67**
- glucocorticoid treatment in **66**, *67*
- natural history of scoliosis in **66**
- nonoperative management in **8**, *67*, *67*
- quality of life in **176**
- risk assessment in **31**
- surgical indications in **13**
- surgical management in **67**, *68*
Durotomy, incidental **151**

E

Early onset scoliosis (EOS)
- defined **136**
- growing rods in **136**, *137*
- magnetic growing rods in **137**, *138*
- Shilla procedure in **138**, *138*
Electrolytes **163**
Endocrine system, in preoperative evaluation 4
Epsilon aminocaproic (EACA) 23
Erythropoietin 4
Ethical considerations **35**
Evaluation, *see* Preoperative evaluation
Examination, physical 4
- *See also* Preoperative evaluation
Expectation management 7
Exposure **23**
Extubation **162**, *162*

F

Familial dysautonomia **16**
Family expectations 7
Fluid management **163**
Foot deformity, in Friedrich's ataxia **83**
Friedrich's ataxia
- comorbidities in **83**
- deformity characteristics in **83**
- etiology of **83**
- foot deformity in **83**
- nonoperative management in 9
- outcomes in **84**
- pathogenesis of **83**
- surgical indications in **16**
- surgical techniques in **83**, *84–85*

G

Galveston technique
- biomechanics of **114**
- in cerebral palsy **43**
Gastroenterological health factors **11**, **73**
Genetics, in spinal muscular atrophy **71**
Genitourinary health factors **12**
Glucocorticoid treatment, in Duchenne muscular dystrophy **66**, *67*
Gross Motor Function Classification System (GMFCS) 4, **40**, **173**
Growing rods *56*, **136**
- in cerebral palsy **12**
- in myelomeningocele *57*
- in spinal cord injury **61**
- in spinal muscular atrophy **15**
- magnetic **137**, *138*

H

Halo-gravity traction (HGT)

– apparatus *126*, **127**
– complications in **128**
– contraindications for **127**
– discomfort with **128**
– duration of **128**, *129*
– equipment for **127**
– halo application in **127**, *128*
– history of 126
– imaging with **128**
– in myelomeningocele *14*
– indications for **127**
– infection with **130**
– neurologic examination in **129**
– neurologic injury in **130**
– pin case with **129**
– preprocedure planning for **127**, *128*
– pulmonary disease and **128**
– setup **128**
– weight application in **128**
Head control 4
Health-related quality of life
– in cerebral palsy **173**
– in Duchenne muscular dystrophy **176**
– in myelomeningocele **176**
– in spinal cord injury **176**
– in spinal muscular atrophy **176**
Hematology
– in intensive care unit **165**
– in preoperative evaluation 4
Hip subluxation, in cerebral palsy *25*, **25**
History, in preoperative evaluation 2
Hydrocephalus, history of 3
Hypertonia **179**
Hypocalcemia **163**
Hypokalemia **163**
Hypomagnesemia **163**
Hypophosphatemia **163**

I

Iliac osteotomy, in myelomeningocele *54*, **55**
Iliac screws
– anatomic technique, biomechanics of **117**
– biomechanics of **116**
– double, biomechanics of **117**
– in cerebral palsy 43
– in myelomeningocele **55**
– in sagittal plane deformity **100**, **110**
– in spinal muscular atrophy **75**
– S2A1, biomechanics of **117**, *118–119*
Imaging
– in myelomeningocele **49**
– in preoperative evaluation **5**, **49**
– in spinal cord injury *60*, 61
– with halo-gravity traction **128**
Implant prominence **55**, *56*, **119**, **152**
Infections, surgical site **34**, **152**
– approach and **156**
– characteristics of *155*
– defined **155**
– in cerebral palsy **46**
– in halo-gravity traction **130**
– incidence of **155**
– intensive care unit and **163**
– microbiology of **155**
– nutrition and **156**
– outcomes and **158**, *159*
– prevention of **156**
– risk factors **155**, *156*

– treatment of early *157*, **157**
– treatment of late **157**, *158*
– vacuum-assisted closure and 157
Instrumentation failure **167**, *168*
Intensive care unit (ICU)
– assessment in *161*
– cardiac support in **162**
– electrolytes in **163**
– fluid management in **163**
– gastrointestinal system in **164**
– hematology in **165**
– infections and **163**
– information passed between, and anesthesiologist *161*
– mechanical ventilation in **161**, *162*
– neurological complications in **164**
– pulmonary support in **161**, *162*
– renal function in **163**
– skin in **165**

J

Junctional kyphosis 43, 96, **169**, *170*

K

Kugelberg-Welander disease 72
– *See also* Spinal muscular atrophy (SMA)

L

Lateral axial dystonia (LAD) **105**
Lidocaine injection **108**

M

Magnetic growing rods **137**, *138*
Malignant hyperthermia 21
Malnutrition 11, 21
– *See also* Nutrition
Marionette sign of Campbell 50
Mechanical ventilation **161**, *162*
Migration index (MI) 25, *25*
Mini-open approaches **146**
Modular constructs
– in cerebral palsy **122**, *123*
– in sagittal plane deformity **97**, *97*, **101**
Monitoring, *see* Neuromonitoring
Motor evoked potentials (MEP) 22, 162
Muscular dystrophy, *see* Duchenne muscular dystrophy
– Becker's, cardiomyopathy in 3
– cardiomyopathy in 3
– congenital, cardiomyopathy in 3
– risk assessment in **31**
Myelomeningocele
– confounding conditions with, fusion and 49
– Diaphragm Intrusion Index in 50, *50*
– functional assessment in **51**
– imaging in **49**
– medical management in *50*, **50**
– postoperative care in **56**
– preoperative evaluation in **49**, *50*
– quality of life in **176**
– risk assessment in **32**
– skin envelope in **51**, *51*
– spinal cord tethering in **52**, *53*
– surgical indications in *14*, **14**
– surgical planning in **51**

– surgical techniques with **52**, *54–57*
– treatment guidelines in *49*, **49**
– urologic protocol in **51**
– wound management in **56**
Myotonic contractures, anesthesia and 22
Myotonic dystrophy, cardiomyopathy in 3

N

Neurogenic bladder 3
Neurologic exam 4
Neurology, in preoperative evaluation 3
Neuromonitoring 22
– in cerebral palsy **44**
– in osteotomy **133**
– in spinal cord injury 61
Neuromuscular scoliosis
– as heterogeneous disease 2
– defined **136**
– nonoperative care for **136**
– operative care for **136**
– surgical indications in **11**
Nonoperative management, *see* Bracing
– and long-term risk of progression 7
– baclofen pumps in 8
– botox injections as 8
– bracing in 7
– diagnosis-specific considerations in 8
– in adult spinal deformity associated with neurodegenerative disease **106**
– in cerebral palsy **8**, **42**
– in Charcot-Marie-Tooth disease 9
– in Duchenne muscular dystrophy *67*, **67**
– in Friedrich's ataxia 9
– in Rett syndrome 9
– in sagittal plane deformity **96**, *96*
– in spinal cord injury **9**, **59**
– in spinal muscular atrophy 9
– wheelchair modifications in **8**, *8*
Nutrition 11, 21, 73, 156, **164**

O

Orthotics, in spinal cord injury **60**
Osteopenia 4, 97, 124, 151
Osteotomy
– iliac, in myelomeningocele *54*, **55**
– Ponte
–– complications **135**
–– in sagittal plane deformity **101**
–– preprocedure planning in **132**
–– setup for **132**
–– spinal cord monitoring in **133**
–– technique **133**
– vertebral column resection
–– complications **135**
–– in myelomeningocele 49, **52**
–– preprocedure planning for **132**
–– setup for **132**
–– spinal cord monitoring in **133**
–– technique **134**

P

Pain control **164**
Pancreatitis **164**
Parkinson's disease **105**

Patient expectations 7
Patient health factors **11**
Pediatric patients, as challenging 2
Pelvic fixation, *see* Spinal fusion
– biomechanics of **114**, *115*
– complications in **118**
– Galveston technique and **114**
– in cerebral palsy 43, *44–45*, **124**, *125*
– in sagittal plane deformity *99*, **99**, *100*
– unit rods in **114**
Pelvic obliquity **26**
Perioperative management, anesthesia and 21
Perioperative traction, in cerebral palsy 44, *46*
Physical examination 4
Pisa syndrome **105**
Pleural effusion 162
Ponte osteotomy
– complications **135**
– in sagittal plane deformity **101**
– preprocedure planning in **132**
– setup for **132**
– spinal cord monitoring in **133**
– technique **133**
Postoperative ileus 164
Postoperative management **141**
– anesthesia and 21
– in adult spinal deformity associated with neurodegenerative disease **107**
– in myelomeningocele **56**
– in spinal cord injury **62**
Postoperative planning 5
Preoperative evaluation
– cardiopulmonary system in 2
– endocrine system in 4
– hematology in 4
– history in 2
– imaging in **5**, **49**
– in myelomeningocele **49**, *50*
– in sagittal plane deformity **95**, **97**
– in spinal cord injury **61**
– neurology in 3
– physical examination in 4
– postoperative planning and 5
– review of systems in 2
Preoperative management
– anesthesia and **20**
– with baclofen pump **179**
Prior surgeries 3
Progression risk, nonoperative management and 7
Proximal junctional kyphosis (PJK) 43, 96, **169**, *170*
Pseudarthrosis 62, *64*, 152, **167**
Pulmonary complications **34**
Pulmonary function tests (PFTs) 3
Pulmonary health factors **11**
Pulmonary support **161**, *162*

Q

Quality of life, *see* Health-related quality of life

R

Rehabilitation, in adult spinal deformity associated with neurodegenerative disease **108**
Renal function **163**

Reoperation
– baclofen pump and **182**
– biomechanical failure in **168**
– cervical extension in *171*, **171**
– instrumentation failure in **167**, *168*
– junctional kyphosis in **169**, *170*
– pseudarthrosis in **167**
Respiratory disease
– anesthesia and 20
– halo-gravity traction and 128
– in preoperative evaluation 2
– in Rett syndrome 78
– in spinal muscular atrophy 73
Retroperitoneal lumbar approach *144*, **144**
Rett syndrome
– comorbidities in **78**
– deformity characteristics in **78**, *79*
– epilepsy in 78
– etiology of **78**
– nonoperative management in 9
– outcomes in **81**
– pathogenesis of **78**
– respiratory disease in 78
– surgical indications in **16**
– surgical techniques in **79**, *80*
Review of systems, in preoperative evaluation 2
Revision surgery, *see* Reoperation
Rhabdomyolysis 14, 21–22
Rib, prosthetic, *see* Vertical expandable prosthetic titanium rib (VEPTR)
Riley-Day syndrome **16**
Risk assessment **30**

S

Sacropelvic fixation, *see* Pelvic fixation
Sagittal plane deformity
– anesthesia in **98**
– bone density in 98
– etiology of **95**
– hyperlordosis in *101*, **101**
– infection and 98
– kyphosis in *100*, **100**, *101–102*
– medical considerations in **98**
– natural history in **95**
– nonoperative treatment of *96*, **96**
– outcomes in **102**
– pathogenesis of **95**
– patient assessment in **95**
– patient positioning in *97*, **97**
– pelvic fixation in *99*, **99**, *100*
– preoperative planning in **97**

– rigid hyperkyphotic and hyperlordotic deformity in **101**, *102*
– surgical treatment of **96**
Scoliosis, *see* Neuromuscular scoliosis
Seating modification, in cerebral palsy **42**
Seating position, in cerebral palsy 41
Seizures, history of 3
Shilla procedure *138*, **138**
Shunt, in preoperative evaluation 3
Sitting position 4
Skin, in intensive care unit **165**
Soft-tissue considerations, in spinal muscular atrophy **74**
Somatosensory evoked potentials (SSEPs) 22, 162
Spinal cord injury (SCI)
– bracing in **59**
– complications in **62**
– etiology of **59**
– hip stability in 62
– imaging in *60*, *61*
– intraoperative management in **61**, *63*
– lower extremity orthotics in **60**
– neuromonitoring in 61
– nonoperative management in 9, **59**
– outcomes in **62**
– postoperative care in **62**
– preoperative workup in **61**
– prevalence of **59**, *60*
– pseudarthrosis in **62**, *64*
– quality of life in **176**
– surgical indications in **15**, **60**
– T square in 62, *63*
– wheelchair modifications in **60**
Spinal cord monitoring 22
Spinal cord tethering, in myelomeningocele 52, *53*
Spinal dysraphism **89**
Spinal fusion, *see* Pelvic fixation
– after baclofen pump placement **182**
– blood loss in 22
– combined anterior and posterior **140**
– complication risk in **30**
– early posterior **140**
– ethical considerations with **35**
– in arthrogryposis 15
– in cerebral palsy *28*, *43*, **43**, *44–46*
– in Charcot-Marie-Tooth *82*
– in Duchenne muscular dystrophy 9, *13*, *68*, *68*
– in familial dysautonomia 16

– in Friedrich's ataxia 16, 83, *85*
– in myelomeningocele 51, *53*, *57*
– in Rett syndrome 16, *79*, **80**, *80*
– in sagittal plane deformity *99*, **99**, *100*
– in spinal cord injury **15**, *60*, *64*
– in spinal muscular atrophy **15**, **74**, *75*, *76*
– limited anterior with delayed posterior **140**
– neuromonitoring in 22
– pseudarthrosis in **62**, *64*
– surgical site infections in **34**
Spinal muscular atrophy (SMA)
– chest wall deformity in *73*, **73**
– classification of **71**
– comorbidities in **73**
– complications in **76**
– deformity patterns in **72**
– diagnosis of **71**
– disorder-specific techniques in **73**
– epidemiology of **71**
– etiology of **71**
– fusion techniques in **75**, *76*
– gastrointestinal issues in **73**
– genetic screening in **71**
– genetics in **71**
– growth-sparing techniques in **74**
– implant considerations in *74*, **74**, *75*
– nonoperative management of **9**
– nutritional issues in **73**
– orthopaedics and **72**
– outcomes in **76**
– pathogenesis of **71**
– perioperative considerations in **73**
– quality of life in **176**
– respiratory issues in **73**
– soft-tissue considerations in **74**
– spinal deformity in *72*, **72**
– surgical indications in **14**, **74**
– surgical management in **74**, *75–76*
– type II **72**
– type III **72**
– type IV **72**
Spirometry 3
Split cord malformation **91**, *92*
Stagnara wake-up test 22
Superior mesenteric artery syndrome **164**
Surgical approaches, anterior
– mini-open **146**
– open **143**, *144–145*
– retroperitoneal lumbar *144*, **144**
– standard thoracotomy **143**, *144*

– thoracoabdominal *144*, **144**, *145*
– thoracoscopic *145*
Syndrome of inappropriate antidiuretic hormone (SIADH) **163**
Syringomyelia **88**

T

T square 62, *63*
Temperature control 21
Tethered cord syndrome (TCS) **89**, *91*
Thoracoabdominal approach *144*, **144**, *145*
Thoracoscopic approach **144**, *145*
Thoracotomy, standard **143**, *144*
Tone management, with baclofen pump **179**
Tranexamic acid (TXA) 23

U

Unit rods
– biomechanics of **114**, *115*
– in cerebral palsy **122**, *123*
Urinary function 3
Urologic protocol, in myelomeningocele 51

V

Vacuum-assisted closure (VAC) **157**
Ventilation, mechanical **161**, *162*
Vertebral column resection (VCR)
– complications **135**
– in myelomeningocele 49, 52
– preprocedure planning for **132**
– setup for **132**
– spinal cord monitoring in **133**
– technique **134**
Vertical expandable prosthetic titanium rib (VEPTR) **138**
– in arthrogryposis 15
– in cerebral palsy 12
Volatile anesthesia 21

W

Wake-up test 22
Wheelchair modifications *8*, **8**, **60**
Windblown deformity *26*, **26**